Anthony M. Szema
Editor

Unusual Diseases with Common Symptoms

A Clinical Casebook

Second Edition

Springer

Editor
Anthony M. Szema
Global Psychiatric Epidemiology Group, Columbia University
New York, NY, USA

Donald and Barbara Zucker School of Medicine at Hofstra/Northwell
Hempstead, NY, USA

Divisions of Pulmonary/Critical Care and Allergy/Immunology
Department of Medicine, Northwell Health
New Hyde Park, NY, USA

Department of Occupational Medicine, Epidemiology and Prevention
International Center of Excellence in Deployment Health and Medical Geosciences, Northwell Health
New Hyde Park, NY, USA

Department of Technology and Society, College of Engineering and Applied Sciences, Stony Brook University
Stony Brook, NY, USA

Three Village Allergy & Asthma, PLLC
South Setauket, NY, USA

RDS2 Solutions, Inc.
Stony Brook, NY, USA

ISBN 978-3-031-40279-1 ISBN 978-3-031-40280-7 (eBook)
https://doi.org/10.1007/978-3-031-40280-7

This Springer imprint is published by the registered company Springer Nature Switzerland AG
The registered company address is: Gewerbestrasse 11, 6330 Cham, Switzerland

Unusual Diseases with Common Symptoms

Table of Contents

Abbreviations

AIDS	Acquired Immune Deficiency Syndrome
BDC	Bureau-De-Change
CAC	Corporate Affairs Commission
CAER	Centre for Australian Ethical Research
CAMA	Companies and Allied Matters Act
CBN	Central Bank of Nigeria
CEO	Chief Executive Officer
CGAP	Consultative Group to Assist the Poor
CIBN	Charted Institute of Bankers of Nigeria
CRIC	Corporate Responsibility Interface Centre
CRR	Corporate Responsibility Rating
CSR	Corporate Social Responsibility
CST	Catholic Social Teaching
DFI	Development Finance Institutions
EcoDes	Fundacion Ecologia y Desarrollo
EIRIS	Ethical Investments Research Service
EITI	Extractive Industries Transparency Initiative
FC	Finance Companies
FEAP	Family Economic Advancement Programme
FHG	Frankfurt-Hohenheimer Guidelines
GES	Global Ethical Standard
GDP	Gross Domestic Product
GNA	Good Neighbour Agreements
GSP	Global Sullivan Principles
HDI	Human Development Index
IMF	International Monetary Fund
Imug	Institut fur Markt-Umwelt-Gesellschaft
IPP	International Post-Graduate Programme
JSE	Johannesburg Securities Exchange
LDC	Least Development Countries
MDG	Millennium Development Goals
MDP	Modified Delphi Process
MFB	Microfinance Banks
MFI	Microfinance Institutions

MNC	Multi-National Corporations
MOU	Memorandum of Understanding
NAPEP	National Poverty Eradication Programme
NEEDS	Nigerian Economic Empower and Development Strategy
NGO	Non Governmental Organization
PBN	Peoples Bank of Nigeria
PLC	Public Limited Company
PMI	Primary Mortgage Institutions
PWYP	Publish What You Pay
ROSCA	Rotating Savings and Credit Associations
SEC	Securities and Exchange Commission
SEEP	Small Enterprise Education and Promotion
SHG	Self Help Groups
SME	Small Scale Enterprises
SRI	Socially Responsible Investments
TBL	Triple Botton Line
TRF	Tropical Rainforest
UAC	United African Company
UK	United Kingdom
UN	United Nations
UNEP	United Nations Environment Programme
VTA	Value Tree Analysis

Abstract

The Frankfurt-Hohenheim Guidelines (FHG) is an ethical-ecological criteriology designed not only to evaluate companies according to an ethical criteria, but also to help in mobilizing social and cultural pressures towards making businesses more ethical responsible to human society, human culture and human future. Built on a comprehensive and integral approach to the concept of sustainable development, this criteriology possesses an unparalleled potential to contribute to sustainable development and a new appreciation of social, cultural and ecological justice, as businesses and investments seek new ways of dialoguing with the concept and contexts for sustainable development.

This criteria originated from the German, hence western cultural ambient. And literature abound showing that western institutional, management, and cultural models exported or transplanted into other cultural environments or other regions of the world go with cultural baggage that are not always successful in those soils.

Added to that is the realisation that sustainability as a concept is social and culturally-specific. This is to say that its understanding vary from one context to another, and the issues around it vary as well and are framed, influenced and driven by whole gamut of social and cultural realities in any given environment.

The objective of this dissertation is to investigate the relevance of the social and cultural compatibility criteria of the Frankfurt-Hohenheim Guidelines in the Nigerian context. The purpose then is to examine how the microfinance banking industry in Nigeria view and appreciate the FHG and its implementation via the Corporate Responsibility Rating (CRR). The primary data was gathered through a field study done principally through questionnaires, and some telephone and online interviews conducted with a number of intimate participants in the Nigerian microfinance industry.

Studies show that the concept and practice of Corporate Social Responsibility (CSR) is relatively new in the Nigerian context and were ushered in through the activities of Multi-national oil concerns working in the Nigerian Niger Delta. And this has assumed a philanthropic character in the minds and policies of many companies across the country. But the concept of Ethical-ecological rating is non existent in the Nigerian context. Nigeria has never had a history of it, and there has been no framework for such in the Nigerian business environment, although the need for such a criteriology happens to be there.

The absence of such a criteriology does not mean that there is no basis for it, in the cultural and socio-ethical principles inherent in the local culture across Nigeria. There exist across the multitude of cultural traditions littering Nigeria, great traditional ethical-ecological understanding that has survived the ravages of time and history. But they have failed to find their way into the formal, mainstream theory and praxis of sustainability and corporate governance issues in the Nigerian public space and business environment. Ethical values such as as ***"onye egbukwala onye agbatobi ya"-'Let no one kill his neighbour'*** or what is validly framed as the ***"egbe belu ugo belu"*** philosophy, (live and let live) is a traditional value found in the Omenala principles of the Igbos of Southern Nigeria, which manifests itself in the way Igbos do their business and pursue their enterprise across the markets all over Nigeria and beyond. Another value "Ebe onye bi ka o na-awachi" mandate-(***One is bound to take care of wherever he lives or the environment in which he finds himself)*** principle is equally a core value and a sacred trust in Igbo omenala. This value which is more ecological in bent shows ontologically an unalloyed respect and reverence for "Ala"-The Mother Earth, which the Igbos in their cosmology believes is the mother of us all. These principles resonate with many of the principles resident in the bowels of the FHG, which is based on the Catholic Social Teaching. These Igbos principles are the reasons why Catholicism succeeded most in Igbo country than in almost all other parts of Nigeria. Both traditions; namely, Igbo Omenala and Catholic Social Teaching share intimate similarities that would always facilitate cooperation and dialogue between both traditions.

Although these traditional values have not been consciously evolved as to facilitate benchmarking them (Asa Helg, 2007), they still remotely influence the conceptual scheme of Nigerians as they make their decision about their lives, society, and economics. This is the basis upon which this project seeks dialogue between a foreign criteriology for evaluating companies, deeply rooted in the CST, and the Nigerian business environment, which is remotely influenced by traditional schemes like that found in the Omenala principles of the Igbos. This is to examine the relevance or otherwise of the FHG in the Nigerian business and socio-cultural environment. The results could be deployed not only be used in introducing Ethical-ecological rating and the FHG to the Nigerian audience, or used in constructing a culture-specific criteriology for evaluating Nigerian companies, investments and businesses; but also in facilitating dialogue between various stakeholders in the Nigeria business environment, with the aim of coming out with an evaluative and assessment framework that will satisfy the yearnings of all the stakeholders. Ours lay no claims to have comprehensively appropriated or examined the whole gamut of issues surrounding ethical-ecological rating or corporate responsibility in a complex environment like Nigeria; it is only a baseline study, which can be used as a basis for further research on the issue, with the aim of diffusing ethical-ecological consciousness in Nigeria.

Part I: Preliminaries

1. Introduction

1.1 Background

1.1.1 The Issues from a Global Perspective

In this age of globalization, the signs that the 'business as usual' mode is no longer a tenable position in the way we conduct human economic processes and systems are coming home for all to see.[1] News of upheavals engendered by the October, 2008 financial market crash, oil crisis, water conflicts, and declining food security daily deluge our media. The effects are globally felt, but most adversely at the global peripheries far from the epicentres of power.

As nations demand for their right to development and a share in the resources of the earth; and businesses transcend local boundaries seeking to carve niches of profitability for themselves and their shareholders in the global marketplace; our earth is exhibiting signs of acute environmental stress[2], and our relationships and values are increasingly experiencing radical displacements, leading to social imbalances and reduced quality of life across our communities. Nowhere are the consequences of this experienced as it is in sub-Saharan African, where Nigeria is located.

Over and above the socio-economic and ecological impacts, the cultural impacts are no less considerable. Granted that 'many of today's social systems, at the cultural level, have their own problems as levers of change, the fact remains that as small businesses rise in local contexts and as big ones cross boundaries in search of footholds in new markets, in an increasingly globalized marketplace, borne on the wings of deregulated capitalism and unfettered free markets, they like every other socioeconomic dynamic, are individually and collectively impacting on local synergies of social interaction, and straining cultural bonds of

1 The December, 2004 tsunami is South-east Asia; the greatest natural disaster in living memory, which wiped away hundreds of thousands of life, even far afield from the epicentre of the tragedy; and mostly recently the September 2008 World Market crash, which wiped away peoples savings and belched many workers once more into the unemployment quadrangle are cases in point here.

2 Sachs, W. & Santarius, T. (eds.) Fair Future: Resource Conflicts, Security and Global justice, London, ZED Books, 2007,p. ix

relationships, in their host localities across the world.[3] They attempt reorienting or reengineering the values of a community to tally in step with their visions and commercial projections; most times knocking them off their social tangents and trajectories.

This scenario is better pictured in the march of capital and its quest for profit maximization. Here recent occurrences have shown that the fears brilliantly articulated in the submissions of Robert Reich, to the effect that the march of rampaging and unrestrained capital is hijacking our governance structures and democratic ethos across the world is a fearful reality, which if left unchecked threatens to plunge what we know as civilization into an irreversible decline.[4] For Reich, the cause of this liberalisation of capital and the profit motive against every other consideration revolves around the fact that market competition, which in Adam Smithian economics, was supposed to engender a tide that ends up lifting all boats, has been so fierce in our times, that competitors are susceptible to being induced to cut socio-ethical and ecological corners, if that will assure their survival in the fiercely competitive market place. For him, the market is not designed to remedy this situation. The only institution, structure or system that can do is, is democracy. And democracy seems to be failing in this assignment at present.[5]

As new systems, structures, products, and vehicles with which to deploy capital in search of profit increased in their numbers and sophistication, they created or rather constructed and took along their own sociologies; introducing alien synergies and new networks of relationships into societies, with the kind of blitzkrieg effect that had decisive impacts on them.

These new entrants into local socioeconomies, most times trampled upon, or greatly eroded irreplaceable cultural heritages and values; consigning them to irrelevance as historical hangovers of human evolutionary infancy; and replacing them with values that serve the kind of knee-jerk consumerism that drives and worships the capitalist machine, as the absolute good. John Smart contended that after these capitalist surgeries, these reengineered orientations arising therefrom are then expected to aggressively perpetuate consumerist distractions in for instance, highly plutocratic societies. For him, today's United States, where the dominant youth heroes of today are athletes or entertainers bent on pushing you products; individuals who certainly play a valuable role in society but who have disproportionately displaced many of the great social welfare and justice role models of science, industry, medicine or politics that our 19th century youth idealized is a perfect example of this. To this end, our world at the instance of these

3 See: Barber, Jihad vs. McWorld.

4 Robert Reich, Supercapitalism: The Battle for Democracy in an age of Big Business, London, Icon Books, 2009, p.x

5 Ibid., p.9

dynamics enters an era of cultural poverty, where for instance dominant musical genres of the modern era celebrate sex, money, power, fame, and ego in simplistic terms rather than personal advancement, global awareness, empathy, and the more nuanced human needs.[6]

It has been recognized that unregulated and fundamentalist capitalism, the kind harshly criticized by Hoffmann[7], where market trumps morals, politics and ethics, in its bid to create and market new products, needs and utilities, has further watered down our down our values, weakened our relationships and compromised our ecological security on so many fronts-showing that capitalism is not a guarantee for social, cultural, ecological or political justice. Such fundamentalist constructs come with problems. These problems, which threaten not only the ecological stability and sustainability of our planet, but also the human society as we know it, arise because markets and the market system left on their own, do not always meet the ethical and aesthetic criteria of society.[8] This in our age has led to an increasing cognizance of the fact that the current form of economic growth is no longer of service to public welfare or to the preservation of the natural environment, but has become an end in itself-one that primarily serves the purpose of increasing monetary wealth, tending at the same time properly calculated-to reduce prosperity rather than raise it'.[9]

1.1.2 The Quest for Sustainable Development

Experts and authorities have been scrambling to proffer solutions to the threats, which this unbridled exploitation of our natural, cultural and human resources poses to mankind from a broad spectrum of fronts. Efforts in this regard have seen to a lot of initiatives at local and international levels; and have led to the publication of reports like the Club of Rome, Limits of Growth in 1972, and the convocation of the World Commission on Environment and Development, known as the Brundtland Commission, convened by the United Nations in 1983 to address growing concern about the accelerating deterioration of the human environment and natural resources, and the consequences of that deterioration for

6 John Smart, 'The Political-Economic Pendulum: The United States Example' in Didsbury H.F. & the staff of the World Future Society (eds.) Thinking Creatively in Turbulent Times, Bethesda Maryland, World Future Society, 2004, p.67

7 Johannes Hoffmann, Ethische Kritik des Wettbewerbsrechts, in Sustainability als Gestaltungsprinizip für die Rahmenordnungen von Finanz-und Gütermärkten: Symposium der Projektgruppe Ethisch-Ökologisches Rating, Frankfurt am Main, 2008, p. 19.

8 Heilbroner and Thurow, op. cit. p.30

9 Scherhon (1997) cited in Johannes Hoffmann/ Konrad Ott/Gerhard Scherhon (Hrsg.) Ethische Kriterien für die Bewertung von Unternehmen, Frankfurt am Main, IKO-Verlag, 1997, p.109

the economic and social development, and many others like the 1992 Rio Earth Summit and the World Social forum, all geared towards finding responses to the dangers posed by human onslaught on the various facets of our environment and socio-cultural institutions. Some others have equally been trying to mediate or find a midway between business and ecology and to subject businesses and corporations to the demands of social responsibility and ethical accountability. The forecasts and conclusions of most of these authorities converge on an increasingly portentous conclusion: If humanity does not retrace its steps in the direction in which it is presently headed-where the imperialism of unrestrained capitalism over every other consideration like ethics is absolute, and accepted or tolerated as such-we may be on the verge of paying a price for the greediest century in history.[10]

In the face of all these, the challenge then becomes clear. If humanity is to develop sustainably in the 21st century, the models and processes of development, which has led us virtually to the brink of socio-economic, ethico-cultural, and ecological collapse, must be reviewed. Urgent steps then becomes imperative towards reassessing and reforming the way we relate to our resources, ourselves and our environment, if we are not to plunge the earth into an irreversible process of destruction that would end in our annihilation.[11] Many authorities submit that the possibilities are looming that there would be a steep rise in the trend and incidence of environmental, resource and culture-inspired conflicts in the coming decades to come.[12] The extent to which this would lead to a clash of civilizations a la Huntington[13], or compromise the ability of our earth to sustain life, cannot yet be determined. But in whichever direction the sparks may fly, the facts as contended by Noreena Hertz are so very clear that a complex interplay of man-made factors at the economic, political and social levels has left our world in a precarious state; that the link between our economic processes and the major problems of the 21st century like AIDS, terrorism, war, poverty, and environmental devastation can no longer be denied.[14] These threats in the views

10 Stiglitz, J. The Roaring Nineties: Why we're paying the price for the greediest decade in history, London, Penguin Books, 2003. See also: Johannes Hoffmann, Ethische Kritik des Wettbewerbsrechts, in Sustainability als Gestaltungsprinizip für die Rahmenordnungen von Finanz- und Gütermärkten: Symposium der Projektgruppe Ethisch-Ökologisches Rating, Frankfurt am Main, 2008, p. 19. See also: Sachs, Wolgang & Santarius, Tilman (eds.) Fair Future: Resource conflicts, Security and Global Justice, London, ZED Books, 2005

11 Sachs, W. ibid.

12 See: Draman, Rasheed; Poverty and Conflict in Africa: Explaining a Complex Relationship, 2003. http://www.parlcent.ca/povertyreduction/seminarl_e.pdf accessed on the 1st of January, 2008

13 Huntington, S. The Clash of Civilizations, London, Simon & Schuster, 1996.

14 Hertz, Noreena, I.O.U. The Debt Threat and why we must Defuse it, London, Harper Perennial, 2005.

of James Garvey constitute some of the greatest moral challenges any generation has ever faced.[15]

These challenges as recognized by many, called for a multi-layered approach towards its resolution. There is this growing awareness that all powers in society will have to be mobilized in order to produce the cultural pressure necessary to enable the social market economy to mediate between liberalism and socialism, competition and solidarity, and between economy and ecology.[16] Reconstructing the bridge between ethics and economics has also been recognized as a veritable part of any set of solutions that would reverse this dangerous trend.[17] For this to happen, the gulf between markets and morality must be bridged. The imperialism of economics over ethics must be dethroned, if we are not to strip our ecological environment, cultural heritage, and social values and networks, of their ability to sustain our lives and scaffold our enterprise. In this purview therefore, Laissez faire as historically understood as 'leaving things alone' is no longer tenable or tolerable.[18] The idea of leaving the market alone to guide itself and create safeguards for its regulation, or laissez faire, which is the basic philosophy of capitalism, has since the dawn of that philosophy been perforated with concerns, which needs moderation, especially in our age. Markets alone have never been known to construct social justice. It has never been known to sustain ecological integrity or the sustenance of cultural values.[19] Wolfgang Sachs and his colleagues at the Wuppertal Institute for Climate, Environment and Energy, in Germany not only recognized this, they went a step further to lay the issues where they rightly belong. For them, it is not only an ethical issue that globalization and our socio-economic systems or processes must be sustainable. It concerns our self-interest as citizens of this one world. This is not only because of the fact that a long term transgression of the global limits of nature is only possible at the price of ecological crises and disasters, but that it can also set other processes in motion which

15 Garvey, James. The Ethics of Climate Change: Right and Wrong in a Warming World, London, Continuum Books, 2008.

16 Johannes Hoffmann/ Konrad Ott/Gerhard Scherhon (Hrsg.) Ethische Kriterien für die Bewertung von Unternehmen, Frankfurt am Main, IKO-Verlag, 1997, p.109

17 See the following: Karl Jaspers. The Future of Mankind, Chicago, University of Chicago Press, 1958, p.24. See also Sachs, Wolgang & Santarius, Tilman (eds.) Fair Future: Resource conflicts, Security and Global Justice, London, ZED Books, 2005, p. ix

18 It was said that a group of merchants called ion the great Colbert, French finance minster from 1661 to 1683, who congratulated them on their contribution to the French economy and asked what he could for them. The answer was "Laissez nous faire"-leave us alone. Since Colbert was a strong proponent of the complex regulation and red tape that tied up industry in France at his time, we can imagine how gladly he received this advice (Cf. Heilbroner and Thurow, Economics explained, New York, Simon & Schuster, 1994, p.24)

19 Heilbroner, R. and Thurow, L., Economics explained, New York, Simon & Schuster, 1994, p.30

could lead to conflicts and wars over resources and a breach of the peace.[20] This inheres in the fact that resource conflicts are fuel for minor and major confrontations, which may set villages or whole countries ablaze.[21]

1.1.3 Companies as Platforms of Ethical-ecological Sustainability

This scenario basically calls for a review of how companies relate to nature, culture and human future. Companies are the cells of the economic system. And since corporations have assumed a dominant role in modern economic society,[22] they retain the enviable position as the essential arena for any ethical-ecological revival of our economic system. The recognition has been gaining grounds that any attempt at making human enterprise responsive to ecological, social and ethical responsibility must commence at the doorsteps of this basic unit of the economic system. Consolidating this view, Sumantra, Bartlett and Moran writes:

> Modern economies are not market economies; they are organizational economies in which companies are the chief actors in creating value and advancing economic progress...(and) the foundation of a firm's activity is a new "moral contract" with employees and society, replacing paternalistic exploitation and value appropriations with employability and value creation in a relationship of shared destiny.[23]

In fact, to operationalize sustainability, companies, which are the centre pieces of the economic process holds a key. To this end, a new way of assessing and rating companies joined the fray as a part of this multi-pronged approach to restraining the onslaught of deregulated and unfettered free market on human future and destiny. It is believed in many quarters, that this would provide considerable impetus for the movement of entrepreneurial development in an ecologically oriented direction.[24] Companies need to be assessed for their performance not only based on their credit rating and financial performance, but also on other criteriologies, which takes cognizance of ethical, social, cultural and ecological impacts of their activities, products and operations on the human society. This is because since the business enterprise is the heart of the economic system, any factor, which can positively influence, motivate, or re-orient the behaviour of business enterprises to take a holistic view of what profit means for all stakeholders will be a great step in this direction.

20 Sachs, W. & Santarius, T. Op. Cit., p.ix

21 Loc. Cit.

22 Galbraith, John Kenneth. The Economics of Innocent Fraud, London, Penguin Books, 2004,p.10

23 Sumantra, G.; Bartlett, C.A & Moran, P. A New Manifesto for Management, in: Cusumano & Markides (eds.) Strategic Thinking for the Next Economy, San Francisco, Jossey Bass, 2001, p.10

24 Hoffmann, Ott & Scherhon, op. Cit. p.111

Prior to this advent, businesses were assessed according to the credit rating, which evaluates their financial status and profitability. And rating agencies have based their assessments of companies and company stocks on such criteria as 'financial standing', 'profitability', transaction stocks, validity periods, and tax considerations'.[25] As events and contemporary history proved this method to be notorious in its inadequacy[26], an ethical-ecological intervention, reorientation and criteria for assessing companies became imperative and absolutely necessary, if businesses were to be configured to contribute to the integrity of our cultural values, ecology and social processes, which confers meaning and significance on human life; and without which we would plunge ourselves into a cataclysmic collapse on so many levels of our existence.

The goal of business is to make profit. Abandoning this goal is ethically equally not sustainable. But the times demand a re-evaluation and expansion of the concept of profit to include and accommodate social good as well. To this end, innovations that are socially, environmentally and culturally compatible increasingly lent themselves to mediate between economic and ecology, in the drive to help curb the destructive potentials of our economic system. And these are the kinds of innovations native to ethical-ecological criteriologies of company assessment.

1.1.4 Nigeria in ethical-ecological perspectives

In the face of all this, the question comes down to concrete issues: where does Nigeria stand in all this? In spite of the global hullabaloo attending the discourse on the precarious nature of our environment ravaged by unconscionable exploitation, the unfortunate realisation remains that many developing economies are hell-bent on replicating the model of progress and developmental successes achieved by the developed ones, without taking considerable and accurate cognizance of the ethical and ecological mistakes that attended those journeys, which our world is collectively paying for today.[27] While movements are gaining global traction in

25 Johannes Hoffmann/ Konrad Ott/Gerhard Scherhon (Hrsg.) Ethische Kriterien für die Bewertung von Unternehmen, Frankfurt am Main, IKO-Verlag, 1997, p.110

26 See: O'Brien, Justin. A Corrupted State?: Wall Street on Trial, West Sussex, John Wiley & Sons, 2003.

27 Suffice it to note that since the dawn of the civilization, economic and production processes have raised ethical and ecological questions. These questions have received various treatments and attempts at answers in various epochs and societies. Not until the Brundtland Commission did we have a comprehensive accent placed on sustainable development as the way to go if we entertain any hope of saving our environment and ensuring that future generations are able to meet their developmental needs as well. But many countries like China are not been deterred by the ecological argument in their bid to develop.

the developed economies, to question the ethical and ecological damage perpetrated on the human person, society and environment in the name of development and business, with the aim of creating enough cultural pressures to bring ethical-ecological issues to the table of social discourse and behaviour; most of the developing ones are still dreaming of attaining the kind of resource intensive development, quite oblivious of its social and ecological costs.

A perfect example of this could be seen in the Nigerian context. There are no known ethical-ecological criteria for rating companies in Nigeria, although the assessment of companies on social, environmental, cultural and economic issues has evolved into an established information services market with many facets, agents and technologies-all in a 'lively biotope', on the global scale.[28] Outside a scattered and isolated pocket of legislations gracing statute books, there is nothing equalling a comprehensive procedure or criteria tasking companies to be ethical and ecologically efficient in their business practices. In fact, this country which happens to be the most populous Black nation in the world, and the largest market in Africa, lacks a coherent and socially-pervasive ethical-ecological awareness in the economic and business practices and products of companies operating in the local economy.

Many companies operating in the country have the principles of corporate social responsibility inscribed in their mission statements. But in most cases, there are no corporate structures or activities to support most of those loftily and brilliantly articulated visions.[29] Some studies have questioned whether these inscriptions evolved out of indigenous practices or whether it is simply an attempt to mimic western conceptual schemes.[30] This may not be totally unrelated to the fact that crises in the Niger-Delta, which happens to be one of the major ecological issues in the country, gained traction at the instance of international pressures exerted on the oil multi-nationals working and polluting the Niger-Delta. To that end, many companies joined the bandwagon to showcase their subscription to Corporate Social Responsibility in their mission statements, although no concrete proofs of their actions in this regard are there to be seen. Even in the face of these international concerns, there has not be a major move on the part of the Nigerian authorities to lay down specific guidelines that will affect every other aspect of social justice, ecological integrity and ethical guidelines for business and investment in Nigeria, outside dormant and watered down regulations in our statute books. The companies themselves are not doing better. The motivations to cheat

28 Schäfer, H., Jana Beer, Jan Zenker, & Fernandes, P., Who is who in Corporate Social Responsibility Rating: A survey of internationally established rating systems that measure Corporate Responsibility, Bertelsmann Foundation, 2006, p.1

29 See: Amaeshi, et al. Op. cit.

30 Schäfer, H., Ibid.

in this regard are seductive and many. This is what led many to conclude that ethical-ecological concerns seem to be the exclusive province of underfunded and understaffed NGOs struggling for relevance.[31]

This meagre and most times empty attention paid to CSR is most times advertised ad nauseam, even when no actions support them on the ground. And as it were, this pretence runs the risk of showing a pervasive concern for ecology and ethics in business in Nigeria. But our research has shown that this concern has neither been pervasive nor significant. A proof of this is the non-existence of coherent, culture-specific ethical-ecological criteria in Nigeria, for the assessment of the performance of companies or business institutions, and/or their products, services, and practices. And this situation is really worrying because the 'capacity of a society for solving the social and economic problems that emerge in it depends to a decisive degree on the moral understanding at its disposal; i.e. on the basic stock of its tradition and conscience, as it were, which can be mobilised for problem solving.[32]

This lack has not augured well for the Nigerian economy, which plays host to a lot of businesses with some extraordinary baggage of ethical-ecological, social and cultural issues and questions. Most of these concerns have been known to most times spin violently out of control into the social arena and public discourse; sometimes attracting local and international concern and outrage, like the Niger Delta ecological disaster playing out before our very eyes; consequent on the ecological irresponsibility of oil companies like Shell BP, ExxonMobil, ChevronTexaco, and the rest. In lieu of this absence, indigenous firms, businesses and companies perceive and practice pedestals like Corporate Social Responsibility as corporate philanthropy aimed at addressing socio-economic development challenges,[33] not as a socially relevant strategy or rationality aimed at subordinating economics to the service of integral human development and welfare in the Nigerian context.

In the Nigerian context, the oil industry happens to be the major culprit and target of international and local concern and outrage as it relates to corporate irresponsibility. This is not only because of the immediate impact of its activities on the environment and on the people of the Niger Delta; but also due to the fact

31 See: Amaeshi, et al. op. cit.

32 Project group Ethical-Ecological Rating/oekom research AG (eds.) Ethical-Ecological Rating: The Frankfurt-Hohenheim Guidelines and their Implementation via the Corporate Responsibility Rating. Munchen, oekom Verlag, 2003, p.21

33 Kenneth M Amaeshi, Bongo C Adi, Chris Ogbechie & Olufemi O Amao, Corporate Social Responsibility (CSR) in Nigeria: western mimicry or indigenous practices? International Centre for Corporate Social Responsibility, Research Paper Series, ISSN 1479-5124, http://www.nottingham.ac.uk/business/ICCSR/pdf/ResearchPdfs/39-2006.pdf accessed on 12th of November, 2008

it attracts instant international attention due to the economic and geopolitical importance of oil. But the fact remains that it is not the only sector, where corporate irresponsibility festers below the radar. Other sectors of the Nigerian economy are not spared this invasion of corporate unconcern on the activities of companies and their impact on the Nigerian people and on the Nigerian environment.

Corporate irresponsibility of big and small companies in Nigeria has taken a life of its own, and is simply a symptom of an environment where corruption and corporate dysfunctionality of Nigerian regulatory institutions merged to create a monstrous hybrid of corporate irresponsibility.[34] The failure of the firms to conduct themselves according to the best practices in the field is rife, and regulatory bodies have been unable or unwilling to do their job in this regard.

In the Nigerian financial services and banking sector, a spate of frauds, ethical misconduct, falsification of returns by the banks to the Central Bank, unprofessional use of female staff in some banks in the name of 'marketing' have all been witnessed.[35] The case has been strongly making the rounds that women in the Nigerian banking industry are forced by the unwritten but morally questionable conditions of service prescribed by their employers, into 'corporate prostitution'; in order to bring in customers to invest in their banks.[36] According to Uche Nworah:

> The code is red for the young women to do whatever is required to meet their targets, if they wriggle out this month with some excuse for not meeting the target, there is the next month to think of as well, it is a heart wrenching job. The working hours are nightmarish, in an unsafe country like Nigeria with epileptic transport situation, some of the women are known to come back home as late as 11PM or even later, these women are loosing out on the home front as well, they no longer have the time to care for their children nor for their husbands. Relationships and marriages are down and the banks are smiling, and declaring Billion Naira profits. The women do not have too many appealing option; it is only the banking sector that offers any real employment hopes… It does not matter in what culture it is practiced, soliciting is morally wrong, the banks can not claim that they do not know that their female employees get into all sorts in other to bring home the goods.[37]

34 Kingsley Dike, Halliburton and Corporate Malfeasance in Nigeria, http://www.nigerdeltacongress.com/harticles/halliburton_and_corporate_malfea.htm accessed on the 4th of January, 2009

35 Soludo, Charles Chukwuma: Consolidating the Nigerian banking industry to meet the development challenges of the 21st century: An address presented of the Central Bank of Nigeria Governor, at the special Meeting of the Bankers' Committee, Abuja, 6th July 2004.

36 Nwankpele, Chidi. The Bizarre World of Marketing in the Nigerian Banking Industry, http://www.incorporatenigeria.com/magazine/corporate-lifestyle/76-the-bizarre-world-of-marketing-in-the-nigerian-banking-industry accessed on the 12th of January, 2009

37 Uche Nworah, ‚Banks, Women and Corporate Irresponsibility' http://www.nigeriavillagesquare.com/articles/uche-nworah/banks-women-and-corporate-irresponsib.html accessed on the 3rd of January, 2009

It is alleged that these banks give these employees, a target of hundreds of millions of Naira to bring in, and if they fail, their job goes; thereby subjecting them to a moral obligation/hazard beyond their ability to fulfil, which is goes against the ethical principles, which counsels that no one should be subjected to moral obligations beyond their ability to fulfil them. Although the Nigerian banking industry experienced a cleaning and consolidation exercise, in 2006, which weeded out the weak institutions and merged the weaker ones that could be salvaged, it does seem that this exercise did not touch on fund soliciting from customers, or the conditions under which workers, especially women are compelled to work, to bring profits to the banks at the expense of their dignity.[38]

Further proofs and effects of corporate irresponsibility in the Nigerian context could equally be seen in the way companies and individuals dispose their refuse in Nigeria.[39] According to Ogbonna, Ekweozor & Igwe:

> Indiscriminate disposal and dumping of waste has become a common practice in Nigerian cities. Most of the waste dumps are located close to residential areas, markets, farms, roadsides, and creeks. The composition of waste dumps; varies widely, with many human activities located close to dump sites. Familiar examples include domestic and industrial wastes. Industrial wastes are generated from industrial activities such as chemicals, pesticides, paints, grease, inorganic materials, oil sludge, and so on. Domestic wastes are those generated from commercial establishments and household activities. They occur in different forms, water-borne waste from households, including sewage and sullage water, rubbish, human and animal remains as well as chemical and laboratory wastes…As is common in most developing economies, Nigerians seem to see pollution by domestic and industrial wastes as a necessary outcome of development…Domestic waste production is increasing and is compounded by a cycle of poverty, population explosion, decreasing standards of living, bad governance, and the low level of environmental awareness.[40]

The fact must be emphasized that although that there is no ethical criteria for the assessment or rating of companies in Nigeria, that does not does not mean that Nigerians or the various peoples existing across the country existed or are existing in an ethical vacuum. The customs and traditions of various culture groups across Nigeria show a very developed sense of respect for the human person, his society and his environment. This could be said of so many other African cultures.[41] And these values were configured to bear on the socio-economic and cultural life and processes of these traditional societies. Most of them have quasi-religious

38 Nwankpele Chidi, loc. Cit

39 Ajiwe V.I.E., Nnabuike B.O., Onochie C.C., and Ajobola V.O. 2000. Surface water pollution by effluents from some industries in Nnewi area, Nigeria. J. Appl. Sci. 3,1265–1280

40 D.N Ogbonna, I.K.E. Ekweozor, and F.U. Igwe, 'Waste Management: A Tool for Environmental Protection in Nigeria', AMBIO: A Journal of the Human Environment, Vol. 31, Issue 1, February, 2002, pp.55-57

41 See: Mbiti, J.,African Religions and Philosophy, (1969) Onwubiko Oliver, African Thought and Culture, Enugu, Snaap Press, 1994.

character, as taboos were used to enforce adherence and general application. For instance, in Igbo traditional society, 'Omenala'-meaning ***'the law of the land'*** ...offers an important principle and philosophy in understanding the interplay between community and individual; forces of nature and forces of nurture; religion and business; the environment and humanity; and generally helps us better understand various factors and values that ensured sustainability and stakeholder participation among the traditional Igbo people.[42] Laced with taboos and millennia of praxis, these pedestals were rational mixture of experience and the need to sustain the environment which sustains them; and were hard thought-out modes of allowing the earth replenish itself, recover its elasticity from excessive human use in order to sustain the people and their posterity. Under this corpus of laws, it is elevated to the level of an ***'aru'***-abomination or violation of the land,[43] for one to cut a tree in the communal forest, or fish in the river during the season, when it was forbidden to do so. It is equally an 'aru' for one to produce, package, and sell poisonous, damaged, or rotten goods or food in the market, no matter how it is packaged.[44]

Cultural pedestals as these were basis upon which ethical-ecological consciousness could comfortably be created from within. But most of these cultural values failed to cross the threshold of their traditional ambience to stamp their impress on the post-colonial, urban Nigeria business life and environment. In fact, they failed to transcend the socio-cultural flux provoked by the colonial and post-colonial dynamic, into the modern/urban business culture in many sectors of the Nigerian economy. To this end, there was no broad, comprehensive or coherent transplantation of these cultural values into the policy environment of modern Nigerian economy.

---

42 Nnoli-Edozien, N., Ownership and Management Structures in the Economy: African Traditonal Values Applied to Modern Issues of Sustainability, Enugu, CIDJAP Publications, 2007, p.20

43 Ala-the Land in Igbo cosmology is the mother goddess that owns us all. A violation of Ala or her ordinances is a great crime that requires not only cosmic restitution, but also a social restitution that is costly in the extreme the offender. Offences that constitute this violation include incest, stealing yams, killing someone at a funeral, swearing falsely while calling 'Ala' as your witness, and so on. 'Aru' is any act that violates the ordinance or the sanctity of 'Ala'. And punishment for this violation include banishment, ostracism, exile and in extreme cases death. 'Ikpu aru'-Placating 'ala' is the restitution imposed by ala for such violations.

44 Most of these prohibitions were time-tested methods with which these societies sought to protect their environment by giving it time to recover from the yields it gave the community in the previous season. In these practices, one can see a highly developed sense of respect for the environment, for nature and nature's gifts. For the traditional Igbo, nature is so holy that to violate her is a crime attracting the highest repulsion from the community. (See: V.C Uchendu: The Igbos of Southeast Nigeria. See also: Nnoli-Edozien, Ndidi; Ownership and Management Structures in the Economy, Enugu, Cidjap Publications, 2007, p.228)

Consequent on this realization that there are no ethical-ecological criteria or criteriology in existence to assess companies and enterprises in Nigeria; and aware of the fact that the 'factual power of the normative wisdom possessed by the various cultures can be put to conscious use for the regulation of the normative power in existing processes in science, economic life and technology;[45] our research then assigned itself the task of attempting to suggest a direction, and offer an ethical criteriology for the assessment of companies in Nigeria. For us to achieve that, it became imperative to find out what Nigerians, against the backdrop of their context, would like to have in any ethical-ecological criteriology, channelled towards the assessment of companies, investments, or businesses in their environment. We are aware based on inferences from other lands,[46] that for any such projects to have any chance of success, it must consult the people, in whose environment it is designed or intended to operate in. And since there were no local frameworks in that direction to guide us, we undertook a search and examination of foreign criteriologies with the aim of settling on the one, which have a preponderance of similarities with the ethical pedestals of some of our cultural traditions; and then subjecting it to a relevance test in the Nigerian context. The relevant test we deployed consisted of asking Nigerians through the instrumentality of a questionnaire whether they think that the criteria we have chosen are of any relevance to their context, and conducting a systematic analysis of the responses.

The criteriology that we intended to use must be to an extent, compatible to the Nigerian cultural context. This is because Culture is the foundation of every ethics. To this end, no ethical criteria for assessing companies would survive the transplantation rigours, if it fails to take cognizance of the culture, where it is expected to operate or take a life. Amartya Sen in *Development as Freedom* contended that social values and prevailing mores influence the freedoms that people enjoy and have reason to treasure. This is as a result of the fact that shared norms can influence social features such as gender equity, the nature of child care, family size and fertility patterns, the treatment of the environment and many other arrangements and outcomes. It also affects the presence of absence of corruption, and the role of trust in economic or social or political relationships.[47] As reiterated earlier, studies in India have shown that foreign criteriologies for assessing companies, which are arbitrarily and uncritically implanted into other cultural contexts to ethically assess companies, have been shown to fail more often, than attempts to create synergies between a comprehensive criteriology and local realities.[48]

45 Project group Ethical-Ecological Rating/oekom research (eds.) Op. cit. p.21

46 See: Agi, Makil's work in the Indian context.

47 Amartya Sen, Development as Freedom, Oxford, Oxford University Press, 1999, p.9

48 Makil, Agi, James. Ethisch-okologische Bewertung von Unternehmen in Indien auf Basis des Frankfurt-Hohenheimer-Leitfadens und des Corporate Responsibility Ratings-Prufung der

From a very rich list of assessment criteriologies,[49] we chose one which would to an extent capture the local realities relevant to the Nigerian cultural context as well as the environmental concerns which are of importance to Nigerians in their day to day lives and businesses. The Frankfurt-Hohenheim Guidelines won our attention as a comprehensive criteria, with far reaching tentacles that could be configured to fit various cultural environments, in the battle to make our business processes and products more ethically sensitive, socially just, eco-friendly, and able to contribute its quota towards stabilizing our precarious environment and socioeconomic system. The Guidelines,-a product of a project group in the German-cultural environment passed our preliminary tests for further evaluation in the Nigerian context. This is not only because of its general realisation to the effect that more justice in the world cannot be achieved by simply globalizing the Western model of prosperity[50] but because it advocates and contains in itself, the seeds for the development of a culture-specific assessment of companies.

Culture happens to be the raw material of development and progress. The core values of a culture and its dynamism determines to a very great extent the depth and level of development it can engineer, accommodate, or support. A culture-specific response commanded our attention as the way to go because various environments are made up of various contexts on the social and cultural levels. And for development to be really sustainable, it must have roots in the culture. And any criteriology that lacks this facility cannot bear the Nigerian context any good.

In lieu of this, the FHG passed the similarity test in the sense that it was built on the basis of Catholic Social Teaching, which has deep similarities both at the ontological and practical level, with Igbo cultural ethics represented by the 'Omenala' principle as has been brilliantly shown by Nnoli-Edozien.[51] The preliminary research we did at the commencement of the study, which was confirmed by the responses we got to the questionnaires, show that there is a need for such a criteriology in Nigeria. Companies, investors, workers and the Nigerian public need such a guide. This inheres in the fact that sustainable investments contribute to a sustainable development[52], which ends up impacting on all and sundry. And

---

interkulturellen Brauchbarkeit vom Frankfurt-Hohenheimer-Leitfaden und des Corporate Responsibility Ratings fur die Messung und Forderung von Nachhaltigkeit im Indischen Kontext: Doctoral dissertation submitted to the Faculty of Catholic Theology of the Johann Wolfgang Goethe University, Frankfurt am Main, 2008

49 See: Henry Schafer, Jan Beer & Pedro Fernandes, Who is Who in Corporate Social Responsibility Rating? Guterslohn, BertselsmannStiftung, 2006

50 Sachs, W., loc. Cit.

51 Ndidi-Nnoli Edozien, Ownership and Management Structures in the Economy: African Traditional Values Applied to Modern Issues of Sustainability and the Corporate Governance Function, Enugu, CIDJAP Publications, 2007

52 Hoffmann, J.; Scherhorn, G. & Busch, T. (eds.) Darmstadt Definition of Sustainable Investments, Frankfurt am Main, CRIC e.V, 2004, p.8

to that end, economic concerns, business processes or investments in Nigeria cannot afford to focus on profit maximization alone in both the short and the long term. They also have to contribute to the sustainability of our ability to attend to our needs at the social, cultural and environmental level, and not endanger or compromise the ability and right of future generation of Nigerians to meet their own needs. This is where the Frankfurt-Hohenheim Guidelines (FHG) made its entrance as a part of this drive to restrain/minimize the negative impact of businesses on human socio-economic and cultural environments, and swing businesses to recognize and honestly aspire to the demands of the ethical responsibility it owes all the stakeholders to its operations, products and activities.

The FHG is an ethical criteriology for the assessment of companies and investments developed in Frankfurt am Main by an interdisciplinary project group Ethical-ecological Rating, led by Professor Dr. Johannes Hoffmann of the Faculty Catholic Theology of the Johann Wolfgang Goethe University, Professor Dr. Gerhard Scherhon, a consumer-affairs economist at the Hohenheim University in Stuttgart, as well as the Wuppertal Institute for Climate Change, Environment and Energy; Prof. Konrad Ott of the Centre for Ethics in Sciences at the University of Tübingen. This criteriology is one of the most comprehensive guidelines for the ethical assessment of companies. The guidelines assess companies based on the company's responsibility towards the natural environment (ecological compatibility), the internal and external stakeholders of a company (social dimension) as well as toward the society and culture in a more general sense (cultural dimension).[53] The FHG is a set of criteria for the ethical assessment of companies and enterprises, and the FHG is designed to analyse dimensions of environmental, social and cultural sustainability of companies. But sustainability, its definition, and application is and would remain culture and environment specific. To this end, the set of factors that are valid and relevant in one cultural context may need some re-evaluation in another. To this end, our research essays to examine the contextual relevance of the FHG when it confronts the Nigerian situation; the implications, challenges and possibilities awaiting it. This is the basis upon which we undertook to investigate if the Frankfurt-Hohenheim Guidelines for the assessment of companies could be relevant in the Nigerian context, and measure the extent of this relevance.

53 Reisch A. L, and Konrad Ott, Ethical-ecological Investment: A Strategy for sustainable Consumption, in Reisch (ed.) Ethical-ecological Investment: Towards Global Sustainable Development. Frankfurt am Main. IKO Verlag, 2001, p.13

1.2 Statement of Problem and Research Objectives

Nigeria has no history of ethical investments or ethical-ecological criteria for assessing companies or investments. This absence could be attributed to a mixture of factors like Nigeria's history, the corporate governance framework which evolved on the basis of this history as well as the geopolitical and socio-economic trajectory taken by the country which all came together to make the Nigerian business context and public life what it is today. The country for instance never generated the climate or manufacturing base, which created the kind of evolutionary conflict, which would have refocused the accent of the economic process equally on the ethical behaviour of companies, like was the case in industrial societies.

Contemporary motivations for the germination or emergence of an ethical-ecological consciousness in the public and business life are equally lacking in Nigeria. In a country where unemployment rate is 40% and 70% of the 150 million citizens are living on 1$ dollar a day, and bad government and corruption reigns supreme, with the government as the greatest employer; many companies haven't got a lot of motivation to be ethical in their relationship with their broad stakeholder base. Add this to the fact that no Nigerian company is a global player in the real sense of the word; and to this end, international conventions and sanctions are not directly of consequence to their operations and profits. Throw a company law that supports a contractarian viewpoint, which sets its accent on the profit for shareholders as narrowly defined by the company, then ethical criteria in business stands no chance of survival.

This absence of criteria for ethically evaluating companies in Nigeria does not augur well for the country. This could be seen in ecological damage engendered by oil companies in the Niger Delta and the impoverishment and hazards that engenders. It could equally be seen in the failure of many banks and financial institutions, predicated on fraud and other sharp practices by the bank officials. It could equally be seen in the unethical practices of some companies in almost all sectors of the Nigerian economy, whose investments, activities and operations destroy the Nigeria environment, degrade the dignity of their employees and endanger the life and wellbeing of the consumers across the country. In Nigeria, for instance, the relationship between employers and their employees are in certain cases akin to that between a house slave and his master. In some companies, strikes are construed as the exclusive province of those in public service or government employ, never for those who work for companies. This is a terrible situation and could be explained that since companies hold the lifeline over the livelihood of these people against the backdrop of the fact that unemployment rate is 40% and graduates are coming out of the university daily; joining the already swollen and bursting unemployment market, companies most times feel that if a worker joins a strike, he risks losing his job, which a million others are ready and waiting to snap for half the salary.

The fact that there are no ethical-ecological criteria for evaluating companies in Nigeria does not mean that the basis for such does not exist. Research[54] has shown that some local cultures across Nigeria, like the Omenala principle; a very ancient body of laws of the Igbos of Southern Nigeria, dating back to much more than 450BC, are in agreement with the basic tenets of the FHG which is the Catholic Social Teaching. This is a cultural soil upon which such criteriologies could be engrafted into the Nigeria business consciousness. For instance, due to the fact ethics has forever been a living, breathing part of the traditional cultural fabric, there were pre-colonial agitations in relation to the behaviour of government parastatals. The 1929 Aba women riots, which was embarked upon to protest the injustice of arbitrary taxation is construed by many historians, more as a political agitation, than as the action of workers protesting better conditions of service. But the 1949 coal miners strike in Enugu and the consequent massacre of the coal miners by the colonial authorities was more of the search for better conditions of service by the workers. It directed the searchlight on the colonial machine's treatment of its workers. The colonial administration reacted with the kind of brutality that we still witness sometimes in subdued tones in the relationship between the Nigerian government, which is the largest employer of labour, and workers. Many labour leaders have done time in government jails, because they protested the bad conditions of service or the hunger wage they have been paid in the course of Nigerian history.

Nigeria is a new, expanding and important investment market in Africa. After years of political instability and military tyranny, this country of over 150 million people, was welcomed into the committee of democratic nations in 1999. To this end, many foreign companies are already locked and struggling for the market share in the oil sector. The banking industry is stabilizing after the consolidation exercise of the CBN in 2005. Many foreign investors especially Chinese are showing greater interest in Nigeria. It is against the different backdrops listed above that an ethical-ecological criteria for evaluating companies and institutions becomes imperative.

In the face of all these, the question which faced us then became: how does one go about trying to redress this scandalous lacuna? There exists no local framework in this direction upon which to build. The choice was either to abandon the enterprise and mourn its absence in Nigeria, or to extend the search for a framework to other business environments, where that exists to see what could be taken. Importing an alien framework to lead this paradigm shift is not without

54 See: Nnoli-Edozien, Ndidi; op. Cit.

its cultural, hermeneutic and epistemic implications. Ethical criteriologies in this regard in other to be functional are essentially culture-specific. What obtains across Nigeria are cultural and epistemological basis that could act as authentic scaffolds for the introduction of an ethical criteriology from another cultural environment into the local Nigerian context, but not a criteriology. That is screaming to be developed. Our search for a framework concentrated on one that could align with Nigerian cultural pedestals with as little risk of rejection as possible. Such pedestals are the ones provided by for instance. That was what led us to the FHG. We hypothesized and argued that the FHG could be a basis for the development of an ethical criteriology for the assessment and evaluation of companies in the Nigerian context.

The FHG is a comprehensive criteria for evaluating companies according to criteria that conduce to sustainability on the environmental, cultural and social levels. But since sustainability is culture specific, it is impossible to import and transplant an alien set of criteria into Nigeria, without taking cognizance of its relevance on the social and cultural level, how does one go about suggesting a culture-specific ethical criteria for the assessment of companies that will be relevant in the Nigerian context

In lieu of this, since the development of this criteriology took place in and was informed by the German cultural ambient, any deployment of it in other cultures must be reassessed in the light of the recipient culture and readapted to suit the demands and peculiar exigencies of that culture. This is more important in the areas of cultural and social sustainability more than it is for ecological dimension, which as it were is less culture sensitive.[55] This informed our conclusion that since there is no ethical-ecological criteria for assessing companies in Nigeria, that we could readapt the FHG and examine whether it can be of relevance in the Nigerian context for the assessment of companies, especially as it regards their social and cultural compatibility to sustainable development.

Since Nigeria is a very broad entity with so many sectors in its economy, we selected the microfinance sector as the case study for our research. This selection was informed by the fact that poverty is the central problem facing Nigeria at the moment, and that microfinance is an instrument deployed in poverty alleviation. To that end, our decision to use the microfinance sector inheres in our belief that poverty alleviation must equally take cognizance of some ethical principles which conduce to sustainable development and corporate social responsibility values. Microfinance is recognized as an anti-poverty instrument that gives voice to the concerns of the poor. Our thesis sought to find out whether a coherent ethi-

55 Reisch, Lucia, Steps towards a Worldwide Ethics of sustainable Development: An Introduction, in Reisch (ed.) Ethical-ecological Investment: Towards a Global Sustainable Development, Frankfurt am Main, IKO Verlag, 2001, p.1

cal criteriology and sustainability issues like the ones contained in the Frankfurt-Hohenheim Guidelines are relevant to the Nigerian context, with the aim of advocating or recommending their being consulted in the ratings of the viability of companies in the Nigerian Microfinance Banking sector.

To do this, the research looked at the Nigerian business environment to ascertain what exists there in the form of corporate social responsibility principles, its level of operation in the policy and products offered by the microfinance industry, and how the Frankfurt-Hohenheim Guidelines could be applied in bettering the appreciation and application of ethical-ecological concerns in the banking policies of these institutions geared towards poverty alleviation. Our research hopes to introduce, refocus attention on, and reposition the FHG into a facility that would augment accounting standards to improve not only MFI reporting in Nigeria and the African context, but equally bring or consolidate an ethical-ecological awareness and orientation, which would take long-term looks at its approach to poverty alleviation and sustainability issues.

Suffice it to note that the Consultative Group to Assist the Poor (CGAP) have developed disclosure guidelines to specify information that should be included in MFI financial reporting. But these are not necessarily ethical-ecologically oriented. To this end we worked with the ethical-ecological rating derived from the Frankfurt-Hohenheim Guidelines to assess what the Management of Microfinance banks in Nigeria think about social sustainability and the clientele about cultural sustainability.

The Frankfurt-Hohenheim guidelines are not accounting standards per se. The criteria canvassed here revolved around the social and cultural compatibility of the operations, products and policies of the microfinance industry. The stand adopted here cannot agree more with the views canvassed by Ike and Edozien (2003) that business should not be about profit alone. Ethics and the impact on the people are equally valid considerations, which businesses must be configured to owe and show responsibility to, in their operations and products.

To this end, the over all aims of the research presented here could be articulated as follows:

1. Since there are no ethical criteria for assessing companies and investments in Nigeria, or any rating agency that deploys an ethical criteriology in the assessment of companies and investments in Nigeria; this project assigns to itself the task to find out the relevance or otherwise of the Frankfurt Hohenheim Guidelines for the ethical assessment of companies and investments (FHG) in the Nigeria context, and the extent of that relevance in the Nigerian socio-economic environment. At this determination, the results would then be recommended as a basis for further research in this direction and its possible operationalization by rating agencies, who would desire to work in the Nigerian environment.

2. We want to offer a potential criteria based on the empirical work undertaken here to evaluate Microfinance Institutions in Nigeria.
3. Ethical assessment of companies, although alien in the Nigerian business space is a very wide and extensive area, which a dissertation of this nature cannot claim to exhaust. For purposes of precision, the work concerns itself with the Social Compatibility and Cultural Compatibility of the FHG and its implementation via the CRR. To do this, we would be readapting to the Nigerian context, the questionnaires developed by the project EOR in concert with oekom Research AG and adapted for a similar study in the Indian context by Agi James Makil.
4. Since the main purpose of our work is to test the relevance of the FHG in the Nigerian context, in the process of doing this, we equally intend to create an essential arena for dialogue between the ethical pedestals of the FHG and that of the Nigerian cultural and business environment.

1.3 Hypothesis

The hypothesis we are out to test is the proposition that that the Frankfurt-Hohenheim Guidelines (FHG) criteria of Social and Cultural Compatibility/Sustainability are relevant in the Nigerian context. This hypothesis took its life from the results that this guideline is already gaining broad interest as being of relevance in the German context. Studies of its relevance is alongside ours here being conducted in the Indian context to seek the validation or otherwise of proposals or hypothesis such as we have assigned ourselves here.

1.4 Methodology

The methodology employed for our research was a mixture of three approaches. On the ethical criteria for the appraisal of companies, we effected a review of existing literature in this regard as well as in the role of ethics in business. This was done through literature review and library research. We carried out further literary research on ethical investments and the ecological implication of business decisions by companies. Here we employed library research using the historical-analytical style of reviewing and analysing relevant literature in relation to other areas like the Nigerian corporate governance framework and the socio-economic context in which businesses operate there; the microfinance industry, the case for ethics in business, sustainability, and the Frankfurt-Hohenheim Guidelines.

The second methodology entails the empirical work, where we attempted to test the hypothesis we formulated at the beginning as the framework upon which the work revolves. On the third methodology, we employed the participant-observer methodology in our contextual discourse on Nigeria. Due to our acquaintance and intimate participation in the Nigerian project as informed citizens, social activist, and researcher, and our contact with Nigerians of all walks of life, we were able to synthesize the myriads of opinion on the direction of the Nigerian state.

The methodology for testing this hypothesis is principally the appraisal and analysis of the opinions and views of a select target audience, drawn from the Nigerian financial industry on what they think should be of relevance to the Nigerian context in relation to pedestals or criteria of assessing companies and businesses to determine their ethical-ecological strengths and weaknesses. This work researched what would be the possible contents of any ethical-ecological criteriology for rating firms in the microfinance industry in Nigeria. This research was conducted using the Frankfurt-Hohenheim Guidelines (FHG) as the theoretical and practical framework. Our choice of the FHG was informed by the comprehensive nature of this criteriology.

On the questionnaire design, we employed a readapted version of the Frankfurt-Hohenheim Guidelines questionnaire developed by CRIC, eV. and Oekom Research A.G; and first deployed in such a fashion by Dr. Agi, James Makil in the Indian context, as our criterion of measuring and testing the relevance of the FHG in Nigerian context using the Microfinance Banking industry as our case study. We redacted the questionnaires to reflect the Nigerian reality and cultural context before administering it to our target respondents.

For our empirical research, a total of 600 questionnaires were distributed in two batches. 300 questionnaires were for measuring Cultural sustainability and were distributed to clients of microfinance banks, or anyone who has ever borrowed money from microfinance banks across Nigeria. We distributed 100 questionnaires each in the three major cities, where the three major tribes in Nigeria live and do business: namely Kano, Lagos and Enugu. The Hausas that are a Muslim majority live in Kano, the Yorubas that are a mixture of Christians and Muslims live predominantly in Lagos, and the Igbos that are predominantly Christian live predominantly in Enugu. This is to make sure that the work covers at least the major parts of the country. We could not distribute to other states or regions due to the logistics and financial implications of such a wide study, which is beyond the immediate scope of this dissertation. We wanted a representative sample that shows the major socio-cultural currents in Nigeria. And it is our opinion that these major cities can provide us with the trends that one can see across the Nigerian nation. The three major cities we selected happen to be the business hubs of the nation in those regions.

Out of the 300 Cultural Sustainability/compatibility questionnaire distributed, a total of 275 came back to us. 25 of these were mangled by illegibility and non-observance of the instructions and where hence declared null and void. We worked with 250 questionnaires representing 83.3% of the total questionnaires distributed for Cultural Compatibility test.

For Social Sustainability, we distributed 300 questionnaires to CEO and Manager-level officials of 300 microfinance banks out of the 774 microfinance banks registered by the CBN so far. We chose people at this level because of the fact that by virtue of their positions, they should have sufficient knowledge of their companies and the industry in general. Out of this number, 250 questionnaires were returned representing 83.3% of the total. 20 representing 6.6% of the total were declared invalid due to problems ranging from illegibility in filling out the questionnaires to non-filling out of the questionnaires. The number which we worked with was 230 questionnaire representing 76.6% of the total. That for us is a good number as it represents over 50% of the total questionnaires distributed for the study. Our analysis and conclusions on Social Sustainability/compatibility were based on this number.

Questionnaire Type	**Total Distributed**	**Number Returned**	**Number not valid**	**Number Valid**
Social Compatibility	300 (100%)	250 (83.3%)	20 (6.6%)	230 (76.6%)
Cultural Compatibility	300 (100%)	275 (91.6%)	25 (8.3%)	250 (83.3%)

For our test, we randomly chose the Microfinance banks, which the CEOs or Managers are to take part in the study. This is as a result of the fact that microfinance Banking formally took off in Nigeria in 2005 at the introduction and promulgation into law of the Microfinance Supervisory and Regulatory Framework. To this end, many of the banks share contemporary experience in microfinance banking except those which transmuted from Community Banks to Microfinance banks. But those were not our primary concern.

For our cultural compatibility test, we randomly chose men and women, who were 18years and above for the study. But the factor that runs through in all of them is that all of them either have borrowed money from, or have done one business or the other with a microfinance bank. This is a difficult thing to come by in a country where over 65% of all business activities are done in the informal sector and most of the poor people who constituted a bulk of those who took part in the cultural sustainability study patronize other financial intermediaries other than banks.

We transcended the geopolitical divisions in Nigeria, which divided Nigeria along political areas of influence. For the selection of our respondents, we divided Nigeria broadly into North and East and West. This was done to elicit responses from the culture centres of the three major tribes in Nigeria and the three major business hubs occupied by these people. This helped us to determine whether a trend existed or whether there existed fundamental differences in the ethical dispositions of the groups to issues of ethics in business and ecological governance. Our results yielded no particular distinctions that suggested broad religious differences in the way the groups approach ethical-ecological issues. Whether their religious persuasions played a role in their decisions or answers, could not be determined from our work consequent on the fact that no pattern for that established itself in the responses to our questionnaires, and the reasons that informed their answers.

We have two questionnaires as reiterated earlier, one was for cultural sustainability and the other was for Social sustainability.[56] Both questionnaires have 35 questions apiece. In both questionnaires, every criterion represents one question and potential answers to the questions were as follows:

1. Relevant as it is (+2)
2. Relevant but with modifications (+1)
3. Undecided (0)
4. Not Relevant (-1)
5. Totally not relevant (-2)

And if a criterion garners relevant affirmation greater than 50%, then it is positive and relevant to the Nigerian context; if not, then the obverse obtains. At a > 50% affirmation, then our hypothesis is positive. At the end, we gathered the positives and the negatives together and did a comparative analysis of them for each of the questionnaires. And the trend that garners more than 50% becomes the answer to our hypothesis.

1.5 Delimitation of Scope

To find out whether the Frankfurt-Hohenheim Guidelines is relevant in the Nigerian context is the object of this dissertation. Our work does not tout the FHG as the solution to the corporate governance problematic and challenges which confront one in the Nigerian business environment, it only examines the roles such a criteriology could play in a set up in need of such a criteriology, like Nigeria

56 Cf. Annexes 1 & 2

is. It does not equally posit microfinance as the solution to poverty. Its wide currency directed our attention to a central problematic in Nigeria, which is poverty. And we used the microfinance banking industry as a pedestal to examine the relevance of the FHG. It is not a judgement on the efficacy of microfinance.

Our work did not examine the whole broad spectrum of the Nigerian economy. That is a logistic impossibility for a dissertation such as this. We concentrated attention on the microfinance sector, choosing 300 microfinance banks out of over 700 of such banks that are presently in operation in Nigeria. We tried to be equitable by choosing equal number of banks from the three regions that occupied our attention. We could not find 100 microfinance banks in a State, so we extended our span to include a whole region. For instance, Enugu is the Southeast region. Since we could not find 100 microfinance banks in Enugu, we extended our span to Imo, Abia, and Anambra States, within the same cultural or tribal group. The same applied to Kano and Lagos.

The work showed itself capable of reviewing the concepts which it employed, but it could not go into details in relation in so many instances due to the peripheral role they play in the whole work. It chose the points that are of relevance to the work and the over all presentation of our findings.

The research focuses on the responses of a randomly selected assemblage of microfinance bank management and their clients to a readapted questionnaire, asking if they find the concepts and pedestals of the FHG relevant for the Nigerian context. The study one must reiterate did not cover the whole Nigeria. It considered only about 3 States, one from each of the three selected regions; namely the North (Kano) The West (Lagos) and The East (Enugu) in order to infer if a trend and paradigm for what is potentially possible in Nigeria if resources are directed to the full development of such a criteriology could be seen. In other words, Nigeria is our contextual problematic, and we are investigating responses, which could show trends that could have wider implications in the appreciation of the FHG across Nigeria.

1.6 Structure of Work

The work is structured and principally divided into eight chapters. In the beginning was an abstract. It tried to summarize the whole thesis. Chapter 1, dealt with the preliminary considerations comprising a general introduction into our theme, the statement of problem and objectives of the research, the hypothesis we were out to examine, the methodology employed the scope and limitation of the thesis, and the structure of the work. Suffice it to note that the justification of the study, which is built into principal parts of the work portrays and emphasised the interdisciplinary nature of the work.

The Second chapter introduced the context of our investigations. It looked at Nigeria, which is our geographical context and at microfinance, which in the Nigerian context is the sector of the economy we used in the verification of our hypothesis.

The third chapter was the commencement of our consideration of the theoretical framework upon which the whole thesis revolved. It overviewed the concept and traced the historical evolution and development of the ethical assessment of companies. It traced the history and present stand of the discourse and praxis of ethical assessment of companies. It dwelt extensively on this, building a basis for the consideration of the FHG as the most plausible and comprehensive criteriology that could be applied in the Nigerian situation.

Chapter 4 introduced and x-rayed the Frankfurt-Hohenheimer Guidelines, its major pedestals and its implementation through the Corporate Responsibility Rating (CRR) as the core framework which we employed in examining the relevance or otherwise of the FHG in the Nigerian context.

Chapter 5 led us through the empirical work and analysis of our questionnaire results in relation to the Cultural Compatibility criteria. The questionnaires took the centre stage for extensive dissection and appraisal. It drew the curtains on the analysis of the relevance test Cultural compatibility in the Nigerian context. Chapter 6 took up the same analysis for the Social Compatibility. Both together comprise the centre of the whole work.

The entire work was subjected to a synoptic recapitulation and systematic appraisal in chapter Seven. Here, an appraisal of the advantages of our findings was extrapolated from the insights gained from the facts examined during the research. The appraisal equally reviewed the strengths and weaknesses of FHG in relation to the Nigerian context. This is where we analysed our findings and took our stand on what we believe is the importance of the work and what it portends for future research and what it could be applied to achieve in the Nigerian context. Chapter eight was designed to shoulder our closing reflections and conclusions.

2. The Context of our Study

2.1 Nigeria

2.1.1 A Brief Introduction of the Country

Nigeria came into existence in 1914 when the British colonial government amalgamated the Lagos colony and the Northern and Southern Protectorates for administrative purposes. Previously, for outsiders, Nigeria consisted of four different empires: The Northern Empire, the Calabar Kingdom, the Oduduwa Empire and the Benin Empire. This is a far outcry of the reality on the ground, which demonstrated that Nigeria consisted of different ethnic nationalities beyond the pale of what was known to outsiders. The Igbos of Southern Nigeria for example lived in a republican nation devoid of centralized leadership as was the case in most other kingdoms in Nigeria.

Nigeria is a country of nations. It is an amalgam of over 250 different ethnic nationalities, tribes and tongues, brought together many contend to serve British colonial interests. It is and remains a huge boiling pot of divergences. The major tribes are the Igbos in the Southeast, the Hausa-Fulani in the North and the Yoruba in the West. And the three largest religious persuasions in the country are African Traditional religion, Christianity and Islam.[57]

The country got her independence from Britain on the 1st of October 1960. This saw to the formation of a federal government. The country is at present made up of 36 states, with the Federal capital located in Abuja. The country for much of her post-independence history was under military dictatorship. In 1999, a new democratic dispensation was ushered in which in spite of its teething problems still paddles on in search of answers to the development challenges facing the country.

57 John Nwafor, Church and State: The Nigerian Experience: The relationship between the Church and the State in Nigeria in the areas of Human Rights, Education, Religious Freedom and Religious Tolerance. Frankfurt am Main, IKO Verlag, 2002, p.25

2.1.2 Geopolitical and Socio-economic Context

2.1.2.1 Introduction

By geopolitical and socio-economic contexts, we mean the actual situations in which companies found themselves in a given locality, this time in Nigeria. We are aware that the nobility of ideals which a firm aspires to is to a great extent tempered by the geopolitical and socio-economic reality environing it. Most of these conditions compel firms to water down their corporate ideals and visions, some of them frustrate their efforts, while some others are supportive of it. All these as variously emphasized in this work, are thanks to the admixture of Nigeria's history; the trajectory of its geopolitical development, and its social and legal framework.

It is necessary to x-ray the Nigeria through the prisms of its social and economic situation, in order to show why we chose microfinance as the economic sector to test the relevance of the FHG ethical criteria in the evaluation of businesses in Nigeria. The aim is to show the actual situation and to situate poverty as the central and most important development challenge confronting Nigeria at the moment. And that poverty of the majority colours every other relationship in Nigeria, like the one between government and citizens, between businesses and citizens, etc. This makes the context in which firms and businesses operate in Nigeria a very difficult and complex one. This is well articulated in to the Nigerian Economic Empowerment and Development Strategy (NEEDS) documents as follows:

> Businesses wishing to operate in Nigeria face many constraints, including poor infrastructure, particularly road networks and electricity supply; inadequate physical security; corruption; weak enforcement of contracts, and the high cost of finance. These factors have deterred foreign entrepreneurs from investing in Nigerian and induced many Nigerians to take their money and skills abroad.[58]

Situating this is equally vital to our argument that poverty alleviation must take cognizance of some ethical principles which conduce to sustainable development and corporate social responsibility values. Microfinance is increasingly being recognized as an anti-poverty instrument that gives voice to the concerns of the poor, as well as a new sustainable investment vehicle. The Consultative Group to Assist the Poor (CGAP) have developed disclosure guidelines to specify information that should be included in MFI financial reporting. But these are not necessarily ethical-ecologically oriented. Our thesis seeks a way to introduce and engraft the ethical values and sustainability issues like the ones contained in the Frankfurt-Hohenheim Guidelines on ethical and sustainability structures present

58 NEEDS documents, xv.

in some Nigerian cultural principles, and test whether it would be relevant in hoisting and contributing to a comprehensive ethical-ecological criteriology for rating companies in Nigeria.

2.1.2.2 Brief But Salient Facts About Nigeria

Nigeria with a GDP of $ 294.8 billion ranks 40 on the global scale of largest economies in the World. She is the 3rd largest economy in Africa after South Africa and Egypt.[59] The nation is oil-rich and virtually a mono-economy due to its over-dependence on the capital intensive oil sector, which is responsible for 20% of the GDP and 95% of the foreign exchange earnings, and as much as 80% of budgetary revenues. The agricultural sector which is largely subsistence, has failed to keep up with the booming population growth so much so that the country which was a net exporter of food now depends on food imports to feed her population. The country's GDP rose strongly in 2007 due to high global crude oil prices.

In spite of this, two thirds of the population live below the poverty line and one third survive on less than a dollar a day. Over 40% of the adult population is illiterate and less than half of the population have access to safe water and adequate sanitation.[60] The country lacks basic infrastructures like good roads network or efficient transportation system. Corruption is rife in public life, and crippling sectarian political disputes dominants the political discourse.[61] To this end, the majority of the Nigerian population survives in a state of destitution; while an insignificant minority basks in obscene affluence is a skewed economic relation, which does not reflect the geographical spread of resource endowment, but rather a product of classical greed, injustice and selfishness which transcends every rational economic principle.[62]

There is a highly unequal distribution of wealth in Nigeria. This places the country among the 20 poorest countries in the world. This is against the backdrop the fact that the country has earned more than $320billion from her oil wealth since 1970. But this sum has been squandered, mismanaged and stolen by a cor-

59 ClickAfrique.com Magazine, November, 11, 2008, 'Africa's Ten Largest Economies' http://www.clickafrique.com/Magazine/ST014/CP0000002788.aspx accessed on the 12th of January, 2009

60 Tunde Obadina, Nigeria's economy at the crossroad: New government faces a legacy of mismanagement and decay, Africa Recovery Online, http://www.un.org/ecosocdev/geninfo/afrec/vol13no1/nigeria1.htm accessed on the 8th of March, 2008

61 Loc. cit

62 Osinubi, T.S, Macroeconomic Policies and Pro-Poor Growth in Nigeria, a paper submitted for presentation at the World Institute for Development Economics Research (WIDER) Conference on Inequality, Poverty and Human-Well Being, Helsinki, Finland 30-31 May 2003., http://www.wider.unu.edu/conference/conference-2003-2/conference%202003-2-papers/papers-pdf/Osinubi%20060403.pdf accessed on the 20th of March, 2007

rupt few who have infected the moral fabric of society, contributing to group rivalries and a loss of national direction. In the wake of this, Nigeria's agricultural potential has been sadly neglected over the years, which obliged the country to import foods that it used to export.

Manufacturing industry has also suffered from serious lack of investment. And the economic indicators have been fluctuating southwards since then, with minor improvements in growth rates.[63] The exploitation of the nation's oil resources, and the management of oil windfalls, have dominated the progress and decline of Nigeria's economy over the past two decades, and have significantly influenced evolution and perception of poverty. The economy is currently characterized by a large rural, mostly agricultural based, traditional sector, which comprises about two-thirds of the poor, and a smaller urban capital intensive sector, which has benefited most from the exploitation of the country's resources and from the provision of services that successive governments have provided[64].

All these are not without serious impacts on the social life of the people. For instance, socially, the lives of many Nigerian women are plagued by ignorance, illiteracy, high fertility and a lack of recognition. They are generally poor, underemployed, and unfairly rewarded. They are politically they are ignored, as attested to by the insignificant number of women in positions of power in Nigeria, which would have enabled the voices of poor to be heard.[65]

The case of Nigeria's political state, since independence in 1960, has been one of rivalry and suspicion between the traditional, Muslim, Hausa and Fulani groups of the north and the more modern, Westernized Yoruba and Ibo of the south. Initially composed of a number of ethnically based kingdoms and states, the area of modern Nigeria was brought under British rule in 1906. It became an independent state on October 1, 1960[66]. The country has survived a civil war and has been on the brink of implosion on so many occasions. These vacillations have no doubt had some serious implication on the social and economic development of the country.

63 Pyke & Akajiak, Measuring Poverty in Nigeria, Oxfam Report, 2003, p.2 (cite properly)

64 IMF. Poverty in the Midst of Plenty: The Challenge of Growth with Inclusion. See http://wbln0018.worldbank.org/dg/povertys.nsf/0/e4b16f6afdb8133685256b22005c3e38?OpenDocument (accessed August 24, 2006)

65 Oxfam, Measuring Poverty in Nigeria, p.8

66 UNDP, http://www.uncdf.org/english/microfinance/documents_and_reports/country_feasibility/nigeriadb.doc accessed February 13 February, 2007

2.1.2.3 Poverty in Nigeria

Although ranking as one of the most ancient and universal problems native to human social history[67], poverty's onslaught has continued in our time in spite of the stupendous heritage of progress accumulated by humankind across the ages. In our time and age, incredible wealth exists side by side with incomprehensible squalor. This is to the extent that poverty and inequality has come to assume the role of the central developmental challenge facing many countries today, especially those in the global south.[68] In Nigeria, it has assumed a very intimidating proportion.

Poverty in the Nigerian context transcends ethnic, geographical and regional boundaries. Its incidence and effects could be seen across the country, both in rural and urban centres. In spite of the fact that the incidence of poverty is higher in the rural areas than in the urban centres, the urban slum dwellers form one of the most deprived groups in Nigeria.[69] The fact that Nigeria substantial revenue gains generated over the years from her oil resources, has not translated to better life for her population lies in the fact that the country has been in the thraldom of a corrupt political and management system, which succeeded only in frittering these revenues, and locking the country in a debilitating poverty situation. Nigeria's oil resource and the rent-economy, which it created, helped to create and nourish an overdependence on an undiversified economic base, represented by oil. This has neither brought some benefit to the economy nor to the masses. It has only essayed to concentrate massive wealth in the hands of a few elites.[70] This is the situation, which informed Achebe's observation that the trouble with Nigeria remains squarely, a failure of leadership.[71]

Nigeria is the most populous nation in Africa with over 150 million citizens. She is one of the wealthiest countries on the African continent in terms of resources and manpower, as well as the 6th largest exporter of crude oil in the world. The country has earned over 400 Billion dollars from her oil resources since 1956, but that has not translated to a better quality of life for her teeming population. Statistics show that over 70% of her citizens are living below the poverty

67 See: CEDS-Paris & Scientific Committee of The World Political Forum, 2004: Poverty, a Challenge to Globalization, http://www.theworldpoliticalfum.org/files/ricerca/stresaReportl-EN-dh3.doc accessed on the 9th of March, 2007.

68 Hilderbrand, M.E: Capacity Building for Poverty Reduction: Reflection on Evaluation of UN System Efforts, Cambridge, Harvard University, 2002, p.1

69 Loc. Cit.

70 Schubert, Samuel. R., Revisiting the Oil Curse: Are Oil Rich Nations Really Doomed to Autocracy and Inequality? Vienna (National Defense Academy in Austria: Institute for Human and Social Studies) http://www.ogbus.ru/eng/authors/Schubert/Schubert_1.pdf

71 Achebe, Chinua. The Trouble with Nigeria, Enugu, Fourth Dimension Publishers, 1983, p.1

line.[72] This means that more than 105 million people are living in poverty. 35% of these are living on less than 1$ dollar a day. Life expectancy in Nigeria is 47-49 years, indicative of underdevelopment. Inequality is scandalous to the point of obscenity. The World Bank contends that about 1% of the Nigerian population own over 80% of the wealth in the country. Unemployment rate here is 40% in a country where over 60% of her total population are young people. 60 million Nigerians are illiterate and can neither read nor write. These are the indices which qualified Nigeria to be classified among the 20 poorest countries in the world.

Poverty in Nigeria is especially severe in rural areas, where social services and infrastructure are limited or non-existent. The great majority of those who live in rural areas are poor and depend on agriculture for food and income. About 90 per cent of the country's food is produced by small-scale farmers cultivating tiny plots of land who depend on rainfall rather than irrigation systems. Surveys show that across the country 44 per cent of male farmers and 72 per cent of female farmers cultivate less than 1 ha per household. Women play a major role in the production, processing and marketing of food crops. The poorest groups eke out a subsistence living but often go short of food, particularly during the pre-harvest period. A high proportion of rural people suffer from malnutrition and other diseases related to poor nutrition. The HIV/AIDS pandemic has also taken a heavy toll among the rural population.[73]

In the search for answers to the poverty of majority of her citizens, the Nigeria government had on various occasions, designed and implemented five National Development Plans since independence. It has financed a Green Revolution; an Austerity Measure; a Structural Adjustment Programme-a mandated prescription of the IMF, all in search of ways of repositioning its economy to attend to the needs of its population for development. But all these have failed to yield considerable fruits. In the 2006 United Nations Human Development Report, Nigeria's Human Development Index (HDI) was ranked at 0.448 which ranks the nation 159th out of 177 countries. This ranking summarizes other indicators like life expectancy at birth, literacy level measured by the percentage enrolment in the primary, secondary and tertiary levels of education. These show that Nigeria is seriously losing it. The poverty situation creates and sustains unhealthy impacts on various dimensions of social life. Education, health, politics, economics, security are sectors where poverty illustrates its impact with serious deficiencies. In the economic sector, low productivity, low investments, mass unemployment, price fluctuations and perennial inflationary trends are the daily issues which Nigerians grapple with. In the health sector, primary health care for majority of

72 See: http://www.ruralpovertyportal.org/english/regions/africa/nga/index.htm accessed on the 9th of March, 2007

73 Ibid.

the population is a luxury superlatively unaffordable. To wit, poor Nigerians are compelled to patronize unorthodox healers, which such situations call into existence. Poor infrastructural provisions and the absence of basic social amenities characterize the social sector and have led to the deaths of thousands of Nigerians annually, who lose their lives to things like road accidents across the country, consequent on bad roads.

2.1.3 The Context in which Businesses Operate in Nigeria

The Nigerian economy is medium sized, when one goes by the World Bank classifications.[74] Nigeria is one of the largest economies in Sub-Saharan Africa. She has ranked second after South Africa for long but took a notch deeper to the third place after Egypt.

The country prior to independence till the early 1970s was an agrarian economy. During this era, agriculture and commercial activities constituted the country's economic based. This was displaced by the explosion in global oil prices, which saw Nigeria's earning skyrocketing from revenues accruing from oil. This oil boom degraded attention to other sectors of the economy; to the extent that today over 86% of Nigeria's GDP comes from oil and over 95% of her foreign exchange earnings.

The structure of the economy tilts towards primary production and services, with primary production in the oil, mining and agricultural sectors taking up to 60%, manufacturing with 6.5%, services with 33.1% and financial services with 9.6%.[75]They key segments of the Nigerian economy are as follows; the petroleum/oil industry, the organized private sector, the public sector-where the government constitutes the largest employer of labour; and the informal sector where over 65% of all business activities in the Nigerian economy takes place. Growth has been considerable in the telecommunications sector although Nigerians are still paying comparatively higher tariffs to make phone calls. Many other sectors of the economy have not seen such growth.

The banking in spite of the 2005 consolidation exercise has shown relative stability. The sector has been described as a high risk one in a global context.[76] The high operational risks identified here include unstable politics, a weak judiciary, poor corporate governance, internal security problems, and infrastructural defi-

74 Cyril Chukwuma, Entry Strategies in the Nigerian Banking Industry: Key Factors for Foreign entrants.

75 Loc. Cit.

76 Obajenu, Moses, Nigerian Banking Sector, High Rist-S&P, http://www.stockmarketnigeria.com accessed on the 21st of December, 2008

ciencies. These risks are a legacy from the old military dictatorships, which by means of chronic underinvestment and economic mismanagement have caused poor infrastructure, low wealth, and poor development levels.[77] But the consolidation in the banking sector has opened this sector to marked increases in transparency, innovation, and competition. But generally in Nigeria, low individual wealth levels, an underdeveloped private sector, and a highly liquid public sector have kept financial intermediation levels low in Nigeria

The manufacturing sector of the economy accounts for a negligible proportion of the GDP. Many companies in this sector have virtually disappeared due to the inclement business environment,-which is a mixture of poor government policies in this regard, high cost of raw materials, and inability to stand to cheap competition from abroad. Those that survived were swallowed up by multinationals

The economy is highly import-dependent. Manufacturing depends on import for between 40 and 70% of its raw materials, machine spares and industrial good. As reiterated earlier, incentives in the economy are largely unfavourable to manufacturing. Factors like poor physical, legal and social infrastructure, epileptic power supply and other utilities from inefficient government monopolies, highly unstable and volatile exchange rates, highly unstable and volatile exchange rates, low purchasing power, persistent budget deficits financed by domestic borrowing, large non-taxable informal sector, high production costs, and high cost of maintain world standards in any sector of the economy, are all there militating not only against manufacturing, but also against other sectors of the economy.

In the Nigerian economy, the government remains the biggest player as well as the largest employer of labour, while the private sector is still small and unsophisticated, even in the presence of pockets of highly skilled world class technocrats. The government is involved in key sectors of the economy like oil and gas and utilities.

Today, the business environment is not all that stable due to the weakness and instability of democratic mores at this time. Many have forecast that the country's young democracy may not be up to the challenges ahead, and there is the fear that the underlying currents of conflict may constitute threats to stability. The major dilemmas that the country faces at this time include corruption, violence in the Niger Delta, a weak business environment. Inflation poses a risk to the economy, as does oil production shortfalls brought on by conflict in the Niger Delta.

In summary, most of the businesses operating in Nigeria face huge and unpredictable transaction costs, which are often passed to the consumers. The lack of basic infrastructure, an inclement business environment and unstable political situation are a contributory factor to this. Åsa Helg articulated this problematic well in relation to its implications for Corporate Social Responsibility thus:

77 Standard & Poor, cited in ibid.

For most businesses operating in Nigeria whether small or large, local or national, the transaction cost of operating is often unpredictable. At the heart of this difficulty is the obvious problem of lack of infrastructure as well as the not so obvious problem of operating in a low trust economy. For many businesses the cost of paying upfront on cash flow or delayed payment; the difficulty of investing in people development; the challenge of high volume cash transactions are all part of a severely eroded social capital. At the core of this issue is the role of business partnership with government and others to exemplify and model behaviours that restore optimism and improves trust. The challenges that face a business in Nigeria are unique because Corporate Social Responsibility can probably not be optional in such a climate. In a country where the social, health, education and environmental needs are so prevalent, where government resources are so stretched, where everyday people live on the breadline, business any other way is not only unethical, it is most probably not sustainable. [78]

2.1.4 A Brief History of Evolution and Development of Companies in Nigeria

In Nigeria, companies as institutions of socio economic production and exchange came into being, like the country itself, in the context of colonialism.[79] Nigeria as a nation was a colonial invention.[80] [81] This being the case, the early development of companies towed the same trajectory directed by the colonial project.

Prior to the contact with the Europe, the mode of production across the conglomeration of ethnic nationalities constituting what is Nigeria today was primarily agrarian and subsistent in nature. The people inhabiting this stretch of territory from the Sahel Savannah in the North to the tropical rainforest basin and mangrove swamp regions due south, were mainly involved in agriculture, hunting, fishing, cattle rearing and trading. They had trade contacts with their internal neighbours and with the north of Africa in what is termed the trans-Saharan trade. This was the situation till the contact with the Europe, when trading in slaves, palm oil, ivory and so many other articles took off at magnitude greater than was earlier known.[82] The slave trade saw to the rise of many trading houses around and about the Niger Delta creeks bordering the Atlantic Ocean. These were firms in their own right at that point in history and they subsisted till

78 Äsa Helg. Corporate Social Responsibility from a Nigerian Perspective. Masters thesis submitted to the Göterborg University Sweden 2007, p. 12

79 Amaeshi, et al, loc cit.

80 See: Ogbunwezeh, Emmanuel Franklyne, The Evolution of a Hoax, http://nigeriaworld.com/articles/2004/feb/271.html accessed on January 23rd 2008. See also: Ogbunwezeh, E.F., Africa: The Ontology of Failed States, http://www.dawodu.com/ogbunwezeh1.htm accessed on ditto

81 See: Richard Akinjide, 100 years after the Invasion of Benin, Institute for Benin Studies, http://www.greatbenin.org/Akinjide.html accessed on the 28th of December, 2008

82 See: Kenneth Onwuka Dike & Felicia Ekejiuba, The Aro of South Eastern Nigeria 1650-1980, Ibadan, University Press Limited, 1990

the end of the slave trade made it imperative for a new economy and new forms of trade.

The first generation of Nigerian companies came into being in this immediate post-slave trade era.[83] The United African Company (UAC) was one of the first companies in Nigeria. This company was founded by George Tubman Goldie in 1879, exactly a hundred years after the French revolution, and four years before joining the British delegation to the 1885 Berlin conference chaired by Otto von Bismarck, to stake claims to the area around the lower Niger for the British crown.

History records that it was this firm that was in custody of the British concession for control of areas around the River Niger under the charter of the Royal Niger Company as of 1886. The possession of this concession never nullified the fact that competition was fierce; coming from some other British merchants; who as retired slave traders had no option of survival save in scrambling out firms to compete for the booming commerce in palm oil from the oil Rivers. These companies fought and competed for every inch of the market. It was a ruthless market with cutthroat competition. Force was sometimes employed to stake claims to market shares, and to compel local trading partners to succumb to the terms of exchange fixed by these companies. This lends credence to the contention of some authorities that the abolition of slavery did not eliminate the room for sharp practices by these traders. It coloured the trade in other articles of commerce in Nigeria. In the relationship of these companies with indigenous population, even after the abolition of slave trade, the slave raiding instinct was most times allowed leeway and the merchants in many cases resorted to outright banditry. Amaeshi et al, articulated this situation well. They wrote:

> …banditry characterized the initial strategy of colonial firms in their dealings with the indigenous people of Nigeria. The case of the Niger Delta versus the Nigerian State and Oil corporations therefore, has a rich historical antecedent.[84]

With the abolition of slave trade, followed by the 1885 Berlin conference scramble for Africa, the British stamped their authority over the areas of the lower Niger and settled to administer the country. This time saw a rapid growth in both internal and external trade. The early companies in this environment were British firms. And the laws applicable to companies at this time were the English Common law, the Doctrines of Equity and the Statutes of General Application in England on the first day of January, 1900, subject to any later relevant statute. This was by the virtue of colonial statutes enacted between 1876 and 1922.

The significance of this is that the common law concepts such as the concept of the separate and independent legal personality of companies as explicated in

83 Amaeshi, ibid.

84 Amaeshi, et al. Op. cit. p.9

Salomon v. Salomon was received into the Nigerian company law and has since then remained a part of the law.[85] Be that as it may, as volume and extent of trade grew, the need to create laws facilitating business activities arose. In response to this, the colonial government enacted the first company law in Nigeria; which was the Companies Ordinance of 1912. This law was a local adaptation or re-enactment of the English Companies (Consolidation) Act of 1908. The colonial inspiration for Nigerian company laws did not cease or end with this ordinance. In fact the present Nigerian Company law known as The Companies and Allied Matters Act 1990 (CAMA), was basically modelled on the U.K Company Act of 1948.

Although modelled after British laws due to its colonial affinities, the interpretation of the Nigerian company law has taken a departure from its British roots to embrace the American Contractarian model perspective. And to understand the concept of the Contractarian model perspective as applied here, and the implication of Nigerian law's subscription to that perspective, one must go to the basic conceptions of the corporation.

There exists a dichotomy in the use and deployment of corporate models. The company is viewed either from the perspective advanced by Adolf Berle (1932) as a shareholder focused entity, where "all powers granted to a corporation or the management of a corporation…are necessarily and at all times exercisable only for the ratable benefit of all the shareholders as their interests appear".[86] This is the **Contractarian model**. Or from the perspective offered by Dodd (1932) in countering Berle, where he construed a company as an entity with a wider array of interests to be met, which transcends the narrow and insular interests of the profit for the shareholders. His was a forceful argument for the stakeholder-society, where the directors of a corporation must become trustees not merely for shareholders but also for other constituents of the corporation such as employees, customers and particularly the entire community. This is the **Communitarian model.**[87]

To this end **contrarians** are of the view that corporations should serve the interests of their shareholders or maximize shareholders' value, while **communitarians** maintain that there should be a balance between shareholders and stakeholders. These are the two perspectives of construing a firm or company. One could see from the pedestals held by both that the contractarian model is narrow in its vision, while the communitarian possesses some interface that could act as

---

85 Ibid.

86 Berle, A. 'Corporate Powers as Powers in Trust (1931) 44 Harvard Law Review 1049. See also: Berle, A, 'For whom Corporate Managers are trustees: a note', 1932, 45 Harvard Law Review, 1365)

87 Dodd, E., 'For whom are Corporate Managers trustees? (1932) 45 Harvard Law Review 1145)

scaffolds for corporate social responsibility or ethical-ecological business culture.

It is important to note that though, as the U.K model from which the Nigerian model took its inspiration, has undergone some shifts in recent times to accommodate what could be termed ethical-ecological trends, by going the communitarian way, the Nigerian model has remained fossilized in the contrarian model, where a company exists only to maximize shareholders' value. In the British model, the conception of the purpose of companies moved to "enlightened shareholder value". This then requires companies to report on the impact of their operations on other stakeholders like employees, suppliers, communities and the environment. But there has not been any significant diffusion of these shifts in Nigerian company law.

In the Nigerian Companies and Allied matters Act (CAMA), which is the principal legislation on companies in Nigeria; the shareholders are still solely recognized as members of the company.[88] This testifies to the fact that the Nigerian law still retains and reflects shareholder supremacy and profit maximization for the shareholder; reminiscent of the contrarian model, as the raison d'être of a firm. And in this purview, companies are construed as private actors to be run exclusively in the interests of shareholders. And Nigerian courts have consistently followed this in their rulings and enforcement of case laws, as could be seen in the case of Kotoye v. Saraki (1994) 7 Nigeria Weekly Law Report (pt. 357) 414-467.[89]

One can see from the above recapitulation that the Nigeria corporate governance framework; due to its subscription to the contractarian view of firms and their purposes, is inherently incapable of generating the kind of theoretical ethos, which would have led to the germination and diffusion of an ethical-ecological orientation and consciousness, in the Nigerian business environment. Ethical-ecological rating has the communitarian conception of a firm as its scaffold. And the fact remains that the contractarian model creates some real challenges in the adoption and implementation of some Western notions of corporate social responsibility (CSR), like responsible employee relationship, in contexts like Nigeria.[90]

88 See: CAMA, 1990, Section 79

89 Amaeshi, et al., p.11

90 Amaeshi, et al., p.12

2.2 Microfinance as a New Sustainable Investment Vehicle for Poverty Alleviation

2.2.1 Introduction

Microfinance has joined the league of programs being considered globally in the fight against poverty. It has fascinated and attracted a wide and variegated range of attention and enthusiastic support across board. From wealthy philanthropists to global commercial banks like Citigroup and Deutsche Bank AG; to the topmost considerations of the UN, which went on ahead to declare 2005 the year of microcredit; this enthusiasm has equally attracted a lot of money to the industry.[91] Grameen Bank, one of the pioneers of the microcredit movement is reputed to have alone disbursed $4 billion in micro-loans over the last 10 years, and has a little over 7 million borrowers in Bangladesh. In India, about 1,000 microcredit organizations and 300 commercial banks lent $1.3 billion to 17.5 million people in 2006.[92] Worldwide, 3,133 microcredit institutions provided loans to 113.3 million clients.[93] These facts and statistics compelled some schools into construing microcredit as the newest silver bullet for alleviating poverty.[94] Mosley and Hulme captured this current of opinion thus;

> The idea of attempting to reduce poverty in developing countries through the provision of loans by specialized financial institutions to micro-enterprises, urban and rural, has in recent years generated enthusiasm bordering on hysteria (Rogaly, 1996). Politically, it appeals to the left as being redistributive and a direct approach to alleviating poverty, and to the right as facilitating the emergence of an independent, self-sustaining "penny capitalism". Financially, institutions such as the Grameen Bank of Bangladesh, the BKKs of Indonesia and BancoSol of Bolivia have often achieved higher loan recovery rates than those achieved by commercial banks in the same country in spite of lending to poor, uncollateralized individuals, making it appear that a reliable organizational technology for lending to the poor of developing countries now exists.[95]

This interest and enthusiasm for microfinance is accentuated by the perceived and actual role, which capital could, and have been historically known to play in economic development. Hernandez De Soto argued in the *Mystery of Capital,* that capital and access to it is the difference between the poor and wealthy econo-

91 Tom Easton, The Hidden Wealth of the Poor, The Economist 3rd Nov. 2005, cited in Aneel Karnani, op. cit

92 Cited in Aneel Karnani. Op. cit.

93 The State of the Microcredit Summit Campaign Report 2006

94 Aneel Karnani, op. Cit.

95 Mosley, P. & Hulme, D. Microenterprise Finance: Is There a Conflict Between Growth and Poverty Alleviation?, World Development Vol. 26, No. 5, pp. 783-790, 1998

mies.[96] Ross Levine, Thorsten Beck and Asli Demirgüc-Kunt equally found that financial development disproportionately boosts incomes of the poorest quintile and reduces income inequality. And that about 40 percent of the long-run impact of financial development on the income growth of the poorest quintile is the result of reductions in income inequality, while 60 percent is due to the impact of financial development on aggregate economic growth. Furthermore, financial development is associated with a drop in the fraction of the population living on less than $1 a day, a result which holds when conditioning on average growth. These findings emphasize the importance of the financial system for the poor.[97]

On a wider global scale and context, the rediscovery of microfinance[98] has been hailed in many circles as promising to be one of the practical responses to the poverty question. Its exploits in countries like Bangladesh, Bolivia and Indonesia account for some hope and fresh impetus into the global poverty alleviation practices; a situation that was hitherto increasingly characterized and clogged by donor fatigue, ideological inertia, bureaucratic confusion, corruption, and policy failure, especially in the African context. Its arrival in the anti-poverty arena changed the tone of the proceedings thus far witnessed in development economic theory and praxis. It is now a popular and fashionable tool in the war against poverty.[99] And it is being peddled as the newest darling of the aid community.[100] One of the things which make microfinance an appealing idea, according to Stanley Fischer, an erstwhile chief economist of the World Bank is that "it offers hope to many poor people of improving their own situations through their own efforts".[101] And this marks it out from other poverty alleviation policies like foreign aid and debt forgiveness, which are primarily top-down approaches, and have been part of the approaches that have failed the poor.[102]

If poverty is one of the most important global problems, the apostles of microfinance are seriously contending that the advent of microfinance is an "aggiornamento" that opened the windows to ventilate the dark stuffy room that was the development aid industry; which was stagnating into a museum of dysfunctional

96 De Soto, H. The Mystery of Capital,

97 Beck, T., Demirgüc-Kunt, A & Levine, R., Finance, Inequality and the Poor, 2007 http://www.econ.brown.edu/fac/Ross_Levine/Publication/Forthcoming/Forth_3RL_Fin%20Inequality%20Poverty.pdf accessed on Feb.4th, 2008

98 Our choice of words here is a tribute to the millennia of history from which modern microfinance took its origin. It was not invented in Bangladesh. See: Our chapter 2.2 for the history of microfinance.

99 Davis, L., Does Microfinance help the Poorest? What Programme design features might maximize impact on the poorest clients? http://def.acfid.asn.au/resources/sectors/microfinance/mf-poorest-lffd.pdf accessed on the 9th of February, 2008

100 Navajas, et al, 2000, cited in Davis, L., ibid.

101 Cited in Tom Eaton, The Hidden Wealth of the Poor, The Economist 3rd Nov., 2005

102 See: William Easterly, Op. Cit.

ideas; filled with the sepulchral bones of defunct ideologies, beneficial only in consolidating asphyxiating bureaucracies, and creating a cottage industry out of the aid business.[103] This industry[104] has been variously accused, not without justification, of trading more on people's philanthropy on the donor side, and creating odious debt burdens[105], than in serving the needs of the worlds' poor.[106] On the delivery/recipient side, the industry stands accused of furthering and financing corruption, rent-seeking, power-mongering and influence peddling in the recipient countries. In the light of these accusations and the donor fatigue, which the failures engendered, the advent of microfinance forced a review of the development aid dogma and praxis, which reigned supreme till the 1970s.

2.2.2 The Concept of Microfinance

Microfinance is about the poor and the alleviation of their predicament. It is about granting the poor access to microcredit. This enables them fund enterprises that will help them, as they work to overcome poverty. It encompasses what is "arguably the most innovative strategy to address the problems of global poverty"[107]. Built upon the presupposition articulated by Milton Friedman, with echoes in

---

103 Hancock, Graham. Lords of Poverty. London, Macmillan, 1991,p.xiii

104 This industry comprises of two arms described by Paul Collier "the Development biz" and "the Development buzz". Development biz is run by the aid agencies and the companies that get the contracts for their projects; while Development buzz is generated by rock stars, celebrities, and NGOs. See: Collier, op. cit., p.4

105 See: Adams, Patricia. Odious Debts: Loose Lending, Corruption and the Third World's Environmental Legacy. London, Earthscan.1991.

106 The debate on the effect of aids on third world economies has been fierce and controversial to say the least. The opponents of aid argue that aid inflow undercuts competitiveness of the export sector of the economic and hence growth; that high and volatile aid inflows compromise effective monetary and exchange rate management and puts excessive pressure on recipient governments' capacity to deliver their public expenditure programmes. Proponents of aid are of the view that if properly managed aid inflow could lead to economic growth. But the negative effects of aid like Dutch disease, the consequences of aid dependency for institutional development as well as the political costs of excessive reliance on non-tax revenues with its potentially adverse effect on domestic politics cannot be overemphasised. See: Graham Hancock, op. cit., who in the preamble to his book minced no words in stating as that his book, is an "attack on a group of rich and powerful bureaucracies that have hijacked our kindness. The bureaucracies he referred to are "those that administer the West's aid and then deliver it to the poor of the Third World in a process that Bob Geldof once described as a 'a perversion of the act of human generosity'". See also: DFID, The Macroeconomic effects of aid, Policy Paper, December, 2002.

107 Woodworth and Woller, 1999, p.6 cited in Schwiecker, S., The Impact and Outreach of Microfinance Institutions: The effect of interest rates, Tubingen, 2004, p.7

Hernando de Soto,[108] to the effect that the poor stay poor, not because they are lazy, but because they have no access to capital;[109] its importance is accentuated by the fact that there exists a consensus that among the economically active poor in the developing world, that a strong demand for small-scale commercial financial services for both credit and savings exists. And that where available, these and other financial services help low-income people improve household and enterprise management, increase productivity, smooth income flows and consumption costs, enlarge and diversify their micro-businesses, and increase their incomes.[110] Appraising microfinance in its journey so far, Beatriz Armendariz and Jonathan Murdoch in ***The Economics of Microfinance*** (2005) wrote with the same surprise that ambushed many development practitioners and economists, in the following words:

> Microfinance is one of those small ideas that turn out to have enormous implications. When Muhammad Yunus, an economics professor at a Bangladesh university, started making small loans to local villagers in the 1970s, it was unclear where the idea would go. Around the world, scores of state-run banks had already tried to provide loans to poor households, and they left a legacy of inefficiency, corruption, and millions of dollars of squandered subsidies. Economic theory also provided ample cautions against lending to low-income households that lack collateral to secure their loans. But Yunus vowed to one day make profits-and he argued that his poor clients would pay back the loans reliably. Today, Yunus is recognized as a visionary in a movement that has spread globally, claiming over 65 million customers at the end of 2002. They are served by microfinance institutions that are providing small loans without collateral, collecting deposits, and increasingly, selling insurance, all to customers who have been written off by commercial banks as being unprofitable. Advocates see the changes as a revolution in thinking about poverty reduction and social change, and not just a banking movement.[111]

Microfinance fills a gap in the formal banking system, which has for long paralysed the facility or ease of access of the poor to credit. Poor households or individuals cannot access capital from traditional banks because they lack collateral to secure and guarantee loans; and traditional banks are averse to risks and costs of making small, uncollateralized loans. Lacking this capital, the poor cannot rise above their subsistence existence. But microfinance rose, employing innovative contractual practices and organizational forms to reduce risks and costs of making loans, such as lending to groups rather than to one person,[112] thereby paving the way for those considered "un-bankable" to access finance, savings and con-

108 Hernando de Soto, The Mystery of Capital, Basic Books, 2000

109 Milton Friedman, cited in Schwiecker, op. cit. p.5

110 Robinson, M.S.: The Microfinance Revolution: Sustainable Finance for the Poor. Washington DC. The World Bank, 2001, p.6

111 Armendariz, B & Murdoch, J., The Economics of Microfinance, Cambridge, Massachusetts, MIT Press, 2007, p.ix

112 Karnani, A., Microfinance Misses its mark, Stanford Social Innovation Review, summer 2007,p.36

sultancy services from banks, instead of being abandoned to other economically inefficient sources of finance.

2.2.3 The Historical Evolution and Development of Microfinance

The concept of providing financial services to the poor or low income people is a much older phenomenon than is held in development economic circles.[113] Some accounts present microfinance as an innovation initiated as a ruse to keep Bangladeshi market women from the usurious and non-economical clutches of the moneylenders.[114] But contrary to these views many authorities are agreed that microfinance is not a recent development.[115] Neither is the development of regulation and supervision of microfinance institutions (MFIs). Almost every country that is now classified as developed has had its own peculiar history of what could be designated as microfinance. [116] Lending credence to the assertions above, Chowdhury et al, citing Mukherjee (1998) submitted as follows;

> although microfinance as it is practiced now was first experimented in the 1970s by BRAC, Grameen and others, lending for alleviating poverty was used in South Asia at least a half-century earlier by Rabindranath Tagore, the Nobel Laureate poet. To help his subjects (Tagore was a landlord) he promoted and organized co-operatives of poor villagers and provided loans to them for income-generating activities.[117]

Hans Dieter Siebel (2003) underlined the importance of situating the history and evolution of microfinance. He writes:

> Attributing the origin of microfinance to recent initiatives misses not only the historical depth and scale of microfinance, but also centuries of experience, which means: learning from trial and error, failure and success.[118]

To this end, microfinance is a concept with ancient roots. In many ancient traditional societies in Africa and all over the world, there existed ancient ties upon which credit initiatives orbited. Savings and credits groups have operated for centuries in various parts of the world under various names, and transactional conditions. Some of these include the credit concept of "mgbazi" in Nigeria, "isusus" of Gha-

113 See: Schwiecker, S., op. cit., p.5

114 Chowdhury, Mosley & Simanovitz., The Social Impact of Microfinance: Introduction; article in Chowdhury &Mosley (eds.) Journal of International Development, 16, 291-300 (2004) http://www.intersceince.wiley.com.DOI:10.1002/jid.1087

115 Hans Dieter Seibel: "History matters in microfinance", an article in Small Enterprise Development- An International Journal of Microfinance and Business Development, vol.14, no.2 (June 2003): 10-12

116 Siebel, op.cit.

117 Chowdhury, et al. (eds), ibid.

118 Hans Dieter Seibel, Ibid.

na, "chitfunds" in India, "tandas" in Mexico, "arisan" in Indonesia, "Cheetu" in Sri Lanka, "Tontines" in West Africa, and "pasanaku" in Bolivia, as well as many other savings clubs and burial societies found all over the world[119]. The emergence of informal financial institutions in Nigeria dates back to the 15th century.[120]

2.2.4 Microfinance, Sustainable Development and Socially Responsible Businesses

The Deutsche Bank, 2007 research titled *'Microfinance: An Emerging Investment Opportunity'* asserted strongly that Socially Responsible Investments (SRIs) ranks high on investors agenda today. This is underlined by the fact that SRIs rose sharply to 2.3 trillion Dollars in the US and 1.0 trillion Euros in Europe in recent years. Social responsible Investment according to report in essence strives to consider both the financial return of an investment and its social, environmental and ethical consequences. Basically, there are three overall investment strategies that include screening, shareholder advocacy and community investing. While the large majority of assets is held in socially screened investment funds or managed accounts, community investments such as microfinance currently enjoy strong growth rates.[121] To underline this, the report stated that:

> Among the SRIs, microfinance investments increasingly attract institutional and individual investors due to their double bottom line. While they allow investors to adopt a social investment strategy geared toward poverty alleviation they offer an attractive risk-return profile at the same time...Microfinance constitutes an emerging investment opportunity for institutions and individuals alike. Investors have barely started to explore its full potential[122].

One would be shocked to learn that corporate social responsibility consciousness exists in small scale ventures in traditional economies across the world. Ndidi Nnoli Edozien found in her 2005 study of ownership and management structures in the traditional Igbo economy that there is no clear separation of business from communal responsibility, which extends across economic responsibility to cover environmental, socio-economic (education, community development, peace building, job creation, training) and cultural factors.[123]

---

119 See: The history of Microfinance. http://www.globalenvision.org/library/4/1051/ accessed on the 20th of November, 2006

120 Siebel, 2003, p.12

121 Loc. Cit.

122 Loc. Cit.

123 Nnoli, Edozien: Ownership and Management Structures in the Economy: African Traditional Values Applied to Modern Issues of Sustainability and the Corporate Governance Function, Enugu, CIDJAP Publications, 2007, p.305

The contemporary clamour for socially responsible business could be understood against the backdrop of present realities. Contemporary globalization brought in its wake great gains to many nations, as well as confining many others to poverty. It brought progress on many fronts, as well as engendered the monumental erosion of cultural values across many societies.[124] It created rapid industrialization of fringe economies like that of China, but it also created scaffolds for the globalization of ecological crises, conflicts over strategic raw materials[125]. This is to the end that unbridled capitalism, the pursuit of economic growth, and an entrenched culture of consumerism have become an end in themselves, which are jointly and seriously threatening to embezzle the future of our world, by no longer serving the purpose of public welfare, human survival, or preservation of the natural environment.[126]

This square of contraries generated by the threats to human survival predicated on unbridled capitalism, created a dialectic, which questioned how development could be furthered, without compromising the ability of future generations to meet their own needs[127]. Out of this dialectic arose a synthesis which canvasses sustainable development, ecological and global justice[128]. According to Ndidi Nnoli-Edozien;

> The associated threats created include a growing impoverished majority in the face of plenty, and a reduced quality of life for humanity in the face of increasing ecological threats, among others. Not surprisingly therefore, the need for sustainability is increasingly recognized by governments, civil society and businesses alike. The challenges foreseen include establishing necessary conditions for business favourable to the pursuit of entrepreneurship and the acquisition of private goods without unduly compromising the common good.[129]

---

124 Project Group, Ethical-Ecological Rating/Oekom Research AG (eds.) Ethical-Ecological Rating: The Frankfurt-Hohenheim Guidelines and Their Implementation via the Corporate Responsibility Rating, Oekom Verlag, 2003, p.17
Brundtland Commission Report, http://www.un.org/documents/ga/res/42/ares42-187.htm accessed on the 31st of March, 2008

125 Sachs, W. & Santarius, T., (eds.) Fair Future: Resource Conflicts, Security and Global Justice, London, Zed Books, 2007

126 Project Group, Ethical-Ecological Rating/Oekom Research AG (eds.) Ethical-Ecological Rating: The Frankfurt-Hohenheim Guidelines and Their Implementation via the Corporate Responsibility Rating, Oekom Verlag, 2003, p.17

127 Brundtland Commission, op. cit.

128 Sachs and Santarius, Op. cit.

129 Nnoli-Edozien, N. Ownership and Management Structures in the Economy: African Traditional Values Applied to Modern Issues of Sustainability and The Corporate Governance Function, Enugu, CIDJAP Publications, 2007, p.15

2.2.5 Microfinance and Microfinance Banking in Nigeria

Microfinance in Nigeria is not a recent development.[130] Its practice in Nigeria is culturally rooted and dates back to several centuries.[131] In fact, informal financial solutions have existed for ages in Nigeria.[132] However, the Central Bank of Nigeria's 2001 survey indicated that the operations of formal microfinance institutions in Nigeria are relatively new, as most of them were registered after 1981.[133] The bulk of most microfinance institutions in Nigeria, true to its origins began as NGOs[134], that assigned themselves the task of promoting rural development and the welfare of women, as their mission and basis for their for their establishment.

In Nigeria, over 80 million people representing 65 percent of the population remain unserved by the formal financial institutions.[135] The aggregate micro-credit facilities available in Nigeria represents only 0.2% of the country's Gross Domestic Product (GDP). By the end of September, 2008, 815 microfinance banks, (MFBs) have been licensed for operation in Nigeria. And total credit to low income groups and entrepreneurs increased by 51.7% from 22.8 billion ($195 million) in December, 2007 to 34.6billion ($292 million) in July 2008.[136]

Although traditional sources of credit has been around in Nigeria for centuries; and informal sources of credit still exist side by side with the formal financial sector, formal Microfinance Banking operations is a very young industry dating back to the promulgation of the Microfinance Policy, Regulatory and Supervisory Framework for Nigeria in 2005.

---

130 Siebel, H.D., Does History Matter: The old and the new world of microfinance in Europe and Asia, a paper presented at The interdisciplinary workshop on Southeast Asia's credit revolution in Institutional, economic and cultural perspective, National University of Singapore, 7-8th October, 2005, http://www.uni-koeln.de/ew-fak/aef/10-2005/2005-10%20The%20Old%20and%20the%20New%20World%20in%20Europe%20and%20Asia.pdf accessed on the 4th of July, 2007.

131 Central Bank of Nigeria, Microfinance Policy, Regulatory and Supervisory Framework for Nigeria, p. 6

132 See: Felicia Ekejiuba, Currency Instability and Social Payments among the Igbo of Eastern Nigeria, 1890-1990, in Jane I. Guyer, (ed.) Money Matters: Instability, Values and Social Payments in the Modern History of West African Communities, London, James Currey Ltd. 1995, pp.133-161

133 Anyanwu, C.M., op. cit.

134 See: Shannon Bell, The Commercialization of Microfinance, Nicaraguan Developments; Vol. 22, No.4, Wisconsin Coordinating Council on Nicaragua, http://www.wccnica.org/node/206 accessed on the 7th of July, 2007

135 Bamisile, A.S., Developing a Long-term Sustainable Microfinance Sector in Nigeria: The Way Forward, presented at the Small Enterprises Educational and Promotion Network (SEEP) Annual General Meeting in Washington DC, October, 23-27, 2006.

136 Tradeinvest Nigeria. http://cms.privatelabel.co.za accessed on the 28th of January, 2009.

The poor need credit to unlock their entrepreneurial skills. And Hitherto now, their access to credit in Nigeria has been in most cases limited to the non-formal source, with its attendant risk and exposures to the usurious clutches of unscrupulous loan sharks and money lenders.

Prior to the formalisation of the microfinance market in Nigeria, the sector that could be identified as quasi-micro-credit sector saw players like:

a. Traditional and informal rotating savings and credit associations (ROSCAs): for instance "Esusu", "adashi"; Self-Help Groups (SHG); Moneylenders, pawnbrokers, friends, neighbours, etc.
b. Semi-formal institutions- E.g. Credit Unions; Savings and Credit co-operatives, multi-purpose co-operatives and NGOs
c. Universal Banks,
d. Community Banks (Which metamorphosed into Microfinance Banks at the instance of the Policy Framework
e. Development Banks

The importance of credit to the economic development and empowerment of the economic active poor has not been lost on the government. This is evidenced in the fact that this sector has consistently seen a myriad of government's attempts at laying down policy initiatives and guidelines to propel and regulate the sector as well as grant the poor access to credit. Some of interventions include:

1. The Rural Banking Programme which ran from 1977-1991
2. Lending as a percentage of Savings mobilized, which was implemented from 1977-1996
3. Sectoral Allocation of Credits which spanned 1970-1996
4. Concessionary interest rates which ran from 1980-1987
5. Agricultural Credit Guarantee Scheme, which was promulgated in 1977 and runs till date.
6. The Nigerian Agricultural Co-operative and Rural Development Bank Ltd (formerly named Nigerian Agricultural Cooperative Bank, which was established in 1972 and runs till date as well
7. Community Banks which came into existence in 1990
8. The Nigerian Agricultural Insurance Corporation (1996)
9. The National Poverty Alleviation Programme (NAPEP) which was launched in 1999
10. The Peoples Bank of Nigeria (PBN) 1990-2002
11. Family Economic Advancement Programme (FEAP) 1997-2001

2.2.6 Conclusion

Since microfinance is being touted as a new vehicle for sustainable poverty alleviation, we decided to use it in investigating the relevance or otherwise of the FHG in the Nigerian context. And to do this, we deemed it necessary to do a little expose on the concept of microfinance; how it all started, and its components. We equally cast a general look at the market for microfinance in Nigeria and what the situation is like. The aim of this is to justify our deploying sector for our investigations.

Insights gained over the years have shown the limitations of microfinance. It has equally shown its positive and negative effects on poverty. In spite of the hype about it, microfinance has in some cases led to deteriorated situations and debt equity ratio of the very poor.[137] To that end, the understanding that microfinance is not a magic potion leading automatically to better living conditions for poor people has led to specific questions on its efficacy as an anti-poverty intervention tool and ways to make it a better sustainable investment tool. And this has necessitated more focused questions like: "Under what conditions and with what mechanism can micro-finance programmes have a maximum effect on poverty "[138]?

On another pedestal, some critics fear that microfinance is increasingly being hijacked by global players driven by pure capitalistic motivations that have nothing to do with poverty alleviation or sustainable investment. This they contend changes the point of emphasis of microfinance from poverty alleviation to profitability. The fear is growing that this is radically changing the nuance of microfinance from its impact on the clients to its impact on the profit portfolio of the investors. But be that as it may, one of the cardinal bases for determining the success of microfinance remains its impacts on clients. Studies have been really inconclusive on the impact of microfinance on the clients. This lends credence to the contention, which we full subscribe to, that microfinance on its own, if not guided by ethical principles, would quickly fall into the same historical mistakes that other economic sectors and companies have fallen into.

Our dissertation therefore argues that ethical performance and social performance should be parts of any assessment of the impact of microfinance on the poor, the society and every other stakeholder, including the human environment. Our work supports the drive to introduce social performance assessment in microfinance assessment.

Social performance is a new and recent deal in microfinance evaluation or impact assessment. According to the SEEP Network;

137 Ibid.
138 Ibid.

> The starting point for many MFIs has been their mission and commitment to providing access to the poor and helping them improve their social and economic conditions. But while the microfinance industry over the years has adopted a set of financial indicators with clear reporting standards and guidelines to determine the financial health of institutions, there exists no corresponding set of social performance indicators.[139]

Since it is a new frontier in microfinance evaluation, it still entertains various viewpoints, producing a number of different tools for this purpose.[140] Many of the assessments tools developed here are still under construction; works in progress. Social performance deals with "the effective translation of an institution's social goals into practice in line with accepted social values"; these include sustainably serving increasing numbers of poor and excluded people, improving the quality and appropriateness of financial services, improving the economic and social conditions of clients, and ensuring social responsibility to clients, employees and the community they serve. Social performance assessment according to the SEEP Network "is the process by which an organization measures its social performance relative to its social mission and objectives, as well as to those key stakeholders. It can be administered as an internal or external process. When internal, it is a 'self assessment', and when external it is referred to as a 'social audit'

It is at this point that we intend to investigate if the FHG could be a complementary facility in this regard in the Nigerian context.

139 The SEEP Network, Social Performance Progress Brief, vol. 1 No.3., March 2007

140 Loc. Cit.

Part II Theoretical Framework

3. History and Stand of the Discourse and Praxis of Ethical Investment and Ethical-Ecological Assessment of Companies

3.1 General Introduction

Contemporary history is progressively witnessing the catastrophe mankind can engineer, when we squander our resources and/or ignore the warning signals our environment gives us. Environmental damage, climate change, erosion of values that conduce to sustainable handling of our resources all come together to brew the toxic cocktail of factors leading to the demise of doomed societies.[141] Ironically on the opposite end of the spectrum, the same history equally shows that ethical-ecological consciousness has been at the base of many cultures and has graced many human societies throughout history. And that most of those societies, where such consciousness was absent, all consumed themselves into extinction, as was the case with the societies on Easter Islands.[142] Human awe at the immensity of nature and profundity of our environment led primitive man into worshipping nature as deity.[143] The Igbos of Southeast Nigeria worshipped mother earth 'Ala' as the source of all good, and fructification. And to harm the environment in this conceptual scheme is an abomination against 'Ala'.[144] The relationship of man to 'Ala' is a symbiotic one, sealed with a lot of religio-ethical prescriptions and prohibitions, which one violates at his extreme discomfiture.[145] Spinoza's equation of God to nature in his *Ethics* 'Deus sive natura' can be construed as a philosophical articulation of this disposition present in many human societies. Societies since time began have had cause to confront the challenges, the demands and exigencies of its time rationally and responsibly or face the dangers of extinction.[146] Ethics have forever been a part of this navigation kit required by society in the turbulent and inclement sea of nature.

141 Jared Diamond. Collapse: How societies choose to fail or succeed. New York, Penguin Books, 2005, p.79

142 Cf. Easter Island-a Model of Non-sustainable Development in Brander, J. and Taylor S. (1998) The Simple Economics of Easter Island: A Ricardo.Malthus Model of Renewable Resource Use, in: America Economic Review, Vol. 88, p.119-138, cited in Hoffmann, Scherhon & Busch, Darmstadt Definition of Sustainable Investments, p.5

143 See: Carveath Read. Man and His Superstitions, Guernsey, Cambridge University Press, 1925 (1995 Edition).

144 See: V.C Uchendu, The Igbos of Southern Nigeria

145 Chinua Achebe, Things fall Apart, Ibadan, Heinnemann, 1958, p.

146 Cf. Diamond, Jared. Collapse: How Societies choose to fail or succeed op. cit.

Ethics is the product of a social structure. It witnesses to society at interaction.[147] This inheres in the fact that the Black-holes of solipsism can never produce the social equations necessary for the germination of ethics. To this end, egoism remains a very narrow pedestal for the construction of ethics. The view is a potent one that psychological egoism renders ethics useless.[148] Society as the human conquest of solipsism is witnessed by the fact that no man is an island unto himself.[149] Since we live in society, certain personal decisions and actions have social dimensions and impacts. And ethics recommends taking cognizance of others, upon whom our decisions and choices would impact. This is the ancient basis upon which ethical-ecological consciousness in a society as it relates to businesses came into being. This is why, "a society, which is interwoven by economic transactional relations, remains stable only as long as social rules and standards constitute a sufficient counterweight to the power and strength of economic relations."[150]

Progressively since the late 1970s, the clamour has been of increasing urgency for companies and enterprises to act in socially responsible way,[151] which would forestall the irresponsible manner in which we squander our resources and endanger our planet. Over and above this clamour, there is no doubt that the importance of responsibility-conscious social, ethical and ecological behaviour for companies grows by the day, as evidence of sustainable management philosophies that companies of today must either embrace or risk their existence. Scherhon brilliantly attempted an articulation of this movement

> On the financial markets we presently experience a sort of silent revolution. A small but steadily increasing share of investors are realizing that financial investments ought to not only fulfil economic criteria like being sufficiently safe from losses and promising fairly high returns, but that it should likewise satisfy ethical criteria in the sense that economic activities financed by the investments should not damage nature, not do harm to people, and not destroy culture. Apparently a different type of investor is entering the stage. He carries with him/her the idea that capital should no longer be focussed on its own expansion but should adopt ethical goals like "sustainability, human rights, and the vitality of communities".[152]

147 Schneider, Hans-Albert. Ethisches Rating: Begründung Bewertungsmoglichkeit Evaluation, Frankfurt am Main. IKO-Verlag, 2001, p.79

148 The Internet Encyclopaedia of philosophy. http://www.iep.utm.edu/e/egoism.htm accessed on the 11th of January, 2009

149 Cf. John Donne, Meditation, xvii

150 Eine Gesellschaft, die von ökonomischen Transaktionsbeziehungen durchwebt ist, bleibt auf der Grundlage sozialer Regeln und Normen nur so lange stabil, wie diese ein ausreichendes Gegengewicht zu der Kraft der ökonomischen Beziehungen bilden Wolfgang Meinig: Kollektiver Kollaps, In: Rheinischer Merkur Nr. 17, 24. April 1998, S15. Cited by Schneider, Hans-Albert: Ethisches Rating: Begründung Bewertungsmöglichkeit Evaluation, Frankfurt am Main, IKO Verlag, 2001, p.19

151 Schäfer, et. al, Who is Who in Corporate Social Responsibility Rating, Bertelsmann Foundation, 2006, p. 4

152 Scherhon, Gerhard., Will Globalization contribute to a World culture, in Reisch (ed) Ethical-ecological Investment: Towards a Global Sustainable Development, Frankfurt am Main, IKO Verlag, 2001, p.5

Reasons why companies of today and tomorrow must subscribe to corporate responsibility on both the social and ethical levels are not far fetched. In the United States of America for instance, a wave of corporate scandals engendered by the collapse of giants like WorldCom, Enron, and some others broke the dykes of regulatory complacency in this regard. These prominent scandals and other not so prominent ones gave rise to a wave of laws and tightening regulations designed to forestall future occurrence by incorporating the importance of corporate governance, responsibility and compliance with the law. To this end, the increasing criminalization of corporate conduct, which had led to an increase in propensity to sue companies, has equally led to an increase in the number of civil investigations and criminal prosecution of companies and their executives by authorities in various countries. An example of this could be seen in the United States of America, where new regulations like the Sarbanes-Oxley Act and Federal sentencing Guidelines, arose requiring codes of ethics, disclosures and internal controls, etc., for companies. In the face of all these, many companies across the globe are formalizing corporate ethics and compliance programmes. This helps to mitigate civil penalties, avoid criminal prosecutions, and deter class action complaints and so on.

Over and above the legal implications, there are economic motivations well. On the economic front, adherence to corporate social and ethical responsibility helps to prevent corporate scandals, burnish the image of companies and prevent reputational damage and a broad range of harm to business operations from preventable legal matters for instance, loss of customers, suppliers and alliance to plaintiffs, increased regulatory scrutiny, and diversion of management attention. Added to that; in many countries today, insurance companies are increasingly considering having an effective compliance and ethics programmes by companies as a factor in providing company insurance coverage and pricing insurance premiums for directors' and officers' insurance policies.[153]

When one adds all these to the fact that even in the present hard economic times, many and more people are staking their investment and shopping preferences with companies that behave ethically and care for the planet[154]; then the picture of its importance begins to emerge. Beyond all these, Scherhon rightly argues that "if ethical goals were generally followed along with the pursuit of profit, capital would take on responsibility for its ecological and social side effects; and the imbalance between capital and the two other factors of production-labour and

153 Cf. Thomas Matthews, Developing a Company's Ethics Program, http://www.nrf.com/Attachments.asp?id=22021&rid=843685 accessed on the 4th of January, 2009

154 Ruth Sunderland and Zoe Wood, Ethics still matter in hard times, The Observer, Sunday 16 November 2008 http://www.guardian.co.uk/business/2008/nov/16/observer-good-companies-guide-1 accessed on 4th of January, 2009

nature, would be reduced; economic development would then be sustainable; and the ongoing liberalization of capital transfers on the heels of globalization would then add to a genuine world culture"[155]

To that end, the movement, which canvasses that that companies are no longer to be evaluated based solely on the financial profits it makes for its shareholders, but also on the contributions they make to society has arrived into global consciousness. This led to the increasing demand for a completely new and different dimension of information, which conduces to companies being evaluated on the basis of the Triple Bottom Line principle, (TBL)which measures not only their economic or financial success, but also environmental and social performance, either in addition or in as an integral part of the economic evaluation.[156]

It is in this context that the Frankfurt-Hohenheim Guidelines rises and is gradually gaining dominance as one of the most comprehensive criteria for scientifically evaluating companies compliance to ethical criteria in their operations, policies and relationship. Before we explore further the concept and context of ethical investments and ethical-ecological rating, let's look at the relationship that has existed between economics and ethics in history; which engendered this call for companies to be responsible in their dealings

3.2 Ethics and Business: A Brief History of a Controversial Relationship

3.2.1 The Historical Paradox of Economics in the March of Civilization

There has been a historical paradox in the relationship between ethics and economics, which has been of a very ancient provenance. This is perceptible even in contemporary times. The contemporary manifestations or impacts of this rift may have been one of the inspirations of Ambrose Bierce when he, in the Devil's Dictionary defined a corporation as 'an ingenious device for obtaining individual profit without individual responsibility'.[157] In contemporary times equally, many have been questioning how ethics could ever feature in business decisions of the big companies and mighty corporations we have today,[158] when 'much corporate

155 Scherhon, G. loc. Cit.

156 Elkington (1990), cited in Schäfer, H., et al, Op. cit. p.4

157 Ambrose Bierce, The Devil's Dictionary, cited in Nick Webb, The Dictionary of Bullshit, Naperville-Illinois, Source Books, Inc., 2006,p.1

158 Cf. John Perkins, The Confessions of an Economic Hit Man, San Francisco, Berrett-Koehler Publishers, 2004. Cf. also Joseph Stiglitz: Globalization and its Discontents, Penguin Books,

language obscures any moral content'.[159] They cite the fact that simple things like management theory has been in many instances elevated to a quasi-ontological level of scientific orthodoxy, stripped of moral content. This they contend has only been a smokescreen for many companies to operate Darwinian processes to the point where it is as efficient as a freshly unwrapped razor blade,[160] deploying catchy phrases like 'Human Resources' which does not distinguish between human beings and pieces of office machinery; and 'downsizing', which masks the firing of workers to increase the company's profit margin for the share and stockholder to mask the cutthroat Machiavellianism, which happens to be the organizational blueprints running many major corporations in the global marketplace of today.

In spite of this historical rift, evidence abounds that economic processes and business enterprises have been some of the most ancient and universal drivers of progress native to human social history. They have seen to the march of civilization.[161] They have unleashed human ingenuity and enterprise; have underwritten human conquest of frontiers and pioneering into the furthest realms of reality; bringing a better condition of life, utility, value and satisfaction in its wake for humanity. Their effects on human progress predated the articulations of Adam Smith's Wealth of Nations. In fact, Smith's enterprise was a reflection on a phenomenon that was more ancient than his thoughts on them.

Economics as human relationship to ends and scarce means and their alternative uses; and its manifestation in business activities and enterprises have been of immense benefit to the human race. This relationship facilitated man's escape from the clutches of primitivity to the dawn of settled life. It underwrote man's voyage from the infancy of the industrial revolution to the new frontiers of space. It accompanied our journeys from the furthest reaches of the ocean to the deepest thresholds of the atom; from the teething problems of ancient equations of exchange to the sprawling complexities of the financial architecture of our day. This relationship has equally written the history of various civilizations. It has equally witnessed and attended the birth and demise of powers and empires. It has spawned political philosophies and ideologies.[162] It has underwritten theories and constructed anthropologies. It has powered revolutions and repressions. It has equally informed theologies and inspired movements and conceptual schemes. It has spawned wars and funded discontents. It has driven the dreams of discover-

2000. Cf. Also, Noreena Hertz: I.O.U, Penguin Books, 2005. See Naomi Klein, No Logo, Harper Row, 2001 and The Shock Doctrine, Penguin, 2007.

159 Nick Webb, ibid, p.5

160 Ibid, p.11

161 George Guest. The March of Civilization, Ibadan, Spectrum Books, 1979

162 Communism and Capitalism are footnotes to this.

ers, voyagers, inventors, merchants, pirates, even quacks and plunderers, conquistadores and bandits.

In the march of this history, economic processes and business enterprises used up natural resources to create utilities and markets for them. Many of them created new realities, utilities as well as the demand for them. Many in so doing sacked civilizations, plundered peoples, waylaid ships, raided kingdoms, and supplanted many cultural norms, which stood in their way to profit, or couldn't keep up with their demands for more materials.[163] They made values appear from nowhere and threw up processes to guide it. They equally annihilated so many social and autochthonous dynamisms and created new ones in their place. All in all, economic processes launched our race out of a nomadic hunter-gatherer existence to a –McWorld- so very interconnected in needs and aspirations; and so mature in our mutual dependence and ability to influence each other on a global scale. With enterprise and economic processes, mankind has profited greatly from the fruits of human labour, which in so many localities are been created and channelled to create global impacts.

On the other end of the scale, this powerhouse has also a cornucopia of misdeeds to its name. In spite of the fact that economic processes have facilitated human progress, various forms of economic growth and economic philosophies have attended the human socio-historical landscape, with varying impacts. It has in most cases acted as a metaphysic of exploitation of the weak by the owners of capital.[164] It has pulverised human communities, poisoned water bodies with chemicals and toxic wastes. It has decimated cultures and habitats in search for oil, and engendered ecological collapse of fragile ecosystems across the globe with oil spillages.[165] It has presided over wars[166], canonized piracies and plunder of peoples, countries and nations.[167] It has underwritten the sack of cultures and

163 The Inca civilization in Mesoamerica declined at the instance of the rapacious plunder of Pizzaro and the Spanish conquistadors' greed for gold. Congo has to bleed its heart out to satisfy the decimations of King Leopold II greed for rubber. The list is endless. In fact, the history of civilization happens is unfortunately the history of greed, treachery and decimations of peoples and cultures to satisfy the gods of profit. Cf. Jared Diamond: Guns, Gems and Steel. A Short History of Everybody for the last 13,000 years. London, Vintage Books, 1998

164 This is one of the insights of Karl Marx, upon which his harshest critic of capitalism was based. As Adam Smith goes as the architect of capitalism's orderliness and progress, Karl Marx goes as the greatest diagnostician of its disorders (See: Robert Heilbroner & Lester Thurow, Economics Explained, p.33)

165 Cf. Daniel Yergin. The Prize: The Epic Quest for Oil, Money, and Power, New York, Free Press, 1992.

166 The Opium War and the East Asian Company

167 Cf. Ogbunwezeh, E. F. The Evolution of a Hoax. http://www.kwenu.com/publications/ogbunwezeh/evolution_hoax.htm accessed on the 7th of January, 2009. See also: Jared Diamond: Germs, Guns and Steel, A Short History of Everybody for the last 13,000 years. London, Vintage Books, 1998

human heritages.[168] Thanks to the wastes and pollutants spewed by industrial products, our planet is showing serious strains at its ecological hems; all symptomatic of a planet in peril.[169] Our social systems and sources of sociocultural legitimacy are being dangerously eroded by a tsunami set-off by the global economic systems, which worships capital. It has equally eroded values that many societies cherish.[170] This same relationship which has underwritten progress ensured that humanity for instance, had a ringside seat as communism; the kind articulated by George Orwell in the Animal Farm, ripped the soul out of Soviet Russia and crowned itself an extravagant historical failure, after seventy years of consolidated dysfunctionality. In the early 1990s, we were equally witnesses as its polar opposite; 'predatory capitalism' rose from the ashes of a defunct empire at the expiration of communism; to bankrupt and auction off the Russian state to a few oligarchs at the expense of the Russian people.[171] We have equally witnessed on several occasions as white collar crimes in the highest echelons of Wall Street, has threatened many times to torpedo the global financial market and architecture. Need we recount MNCs exploiting the resources and peoples of the third world as cheap source of materials and labour to advance their profit margins?

In fact, assessing the impact of business or economics on the life of man, one witnesses the good, the bad, and the ugly. Corporate irresponsibility and outright criminality has been witnessed on so many fronts. Fraud and book cooking have been developed to fine arts in some companies. Businesses have been accused of creating commercial utopias, which raises human expectations beyond measure, ensuring that we as a race are in a race to consume ourselves out of existence.[172] Ponzi schemes designed to defraud unwary investors has refused to die, even at the thresholds of the 21st century. Many multinationals have also been guilty of supporting a socioeconomic superstructure, which 'far from levelling the global playing field with jobs and technology for all, are mining the planet's poorest back countries and neighbourhoods for unimaginable profits'.[173] To this end, 'the travels of Nike sneakers have been traced back to the abusive sweatshops of Vietnam.., Starbuck' lattes to the sun-scorched coffee fields of Guatemala, and Shell's oil back to the polluted and impoverished villages of the Niger Delta'.[174]

168 The Incan civilization of Mesoamerica has to be exterminated to assuage Pizzaro's greed for gold on behalf of her Most Royal Catholic Majesty, Queen Isabella of Spain.

169 Planet in Peril is a programme aired by the CNN detailing and bringing ecological issues to the fore. See CNN

170 Here we must bear in mind Amartya Sen's definition of development as freedom

171 See: Stiglitz, J. Globalization and its Discontent, 2000.

172

173 Naomi Klein. No Logo, London, HarperCollins, 2001, p.xvii

174 Ibid., pxviii

Add to this the fact that the amount executives of big companies have been paying themselves in recent times has been convulsively obscene in comparison to what many of their workers go home with; showing us the dark sides of capitalism.[175] Marx would be grinning "I told you so" in his grave, while Adam Smith would have pulled his Wealth of Nations off circulation, to include a chapter on ethics in it. If one is to invite Amartya Sen to mediate on this paradox, one would then see that it is thanks in part to business and economic processes and systems, that today:

> We live in a world of unprecedented opulence, of a kind that would have been hard even to imagine a century or two ago...People are living much longer, on the average than ever before... the different parts of the globe are now more closely linked than they have ever been...And yet we also live in a world with remarkable deprivation, destitution and oppression...persistence of poverty and unfulfilled elementary needs, occurrence of famines and widespread hunger...worsening threats to our environment and to the sustainability of our economic and social lives.[176]

Evidence shows more and more that as companies swim in profits, they grow more artful in dodging most of their social commitments to their employees and communities.[177] When they fail, predicated on administrative irresponsibility, mismanagement, and high level fraudulence, their rescue or bailout is socialized, but their profits are forever privatized. Evidence equally shows that business and economic systems and activities of companies predicated on this model are not sustainable. They impact negatively on all of us. According to the Authors of Fair Future, such an exploitative model of business predicated on a narrow definition of shareholder value, and profit maximization for the shareholders costs too much money and too many resources, and would completely ruin our biosphere.[178]

Over and above the depletion of our environment, such economic or business philosophy and praxis engender the destruction of our sociologies and cultural reinforcements, which has been the buffer preventing many societies from self destructing. In contemporary times, the facts are coming home to every diligent observer that the current form of economic growth is no longer of service to the public welfare or to the preservation of the natural environment, but has become an end in itself-one that primarily serves the purpose of increasing monetary, tending at the same time-properly calculated-to reduce prosperity rather than raise it.[179] This metamorphosis of the economic system from a means to an end in

175 Naomi Klein. No logo, p.231-257. See also: Galbraith, John Kenneth: The Economics of Innocent Fraud, op. cit. See also: O'Brien: Wall Street on Trial, op. cit.

176 Amartya Sen. Development as Freedom. Oxford, Oxford University Press, 1999, p.xi

177 Klein, op. cit., p.232

178 See Fair Future, p.ix

179 Project group Ethical-Ecological Rating/oekom research AG (eds.) Ethical-Ecological Rating: The Frankfurt-Hohenheim Guidelines and their implementation via the Corporate Responsibility Rating, Munchen, oekom Verlag, 2003, p.17

itself is not only a dysfunctional aberration, but a threat to human survival. This inheres in the fact that instead of furthering human progress and sustenance, it threatens it. These threats include a growing impoverished majority in the midst of plenty, and a reduced quality of life for humanity in the face of increasing ecological threats.[180]

If we are to summarize, it would emphasize the fact that the velocity at which so many animal and plant species go extinct; the speed at which global temperature rises and the polar ice cap melts; the volume of green house gases our industries and automobiles belch into the atmosphere; the volume of oil and other non-renewable resources that we consume; and the amount of toxic and radioactive wastes we produce in the process, as well as the danger such a trend portends to human survival is a frightening reason why we must consider alternatives or perish. Facts are emerging that the earth cannot for long sustain such prodigality. Many ecosystems are collapsing at our instance, and at a very fast rate. And our further dependence on them for our livelihood and their ability to shoulder human excess without replenishment is really questionable. The Easter Island example is a very real threat facing humanity today, if the present paradox is allowed to rampage unrestrained.

The issues at stake are global challenges with serious impacts at the local level. So many little successes are there witnessing to the need for local, contextual, and culture-specific initiatives directed towards returning sanity and moral credibility to the way we allocate our resources and do business. This is one of the things that justify any attempt at making companies and businesses act responsibly.

180 Nnoli-Edozien, N. Ownership and Management Structures in the Economy: African Traditional Values Applied to Modern Issues of Sustainability and the Corporate Governance Function, Enugu, CIDJAP Publications, 2007, p.15

Easter Island-A Model for Non-sustainable Development

In the 4th century a small group of Polynesians inhabited the Pacific Island. It was covered with a lush vegetation including palm trees, a basic resource. During the 11th century and 15th century, the population of about 10,000 people created a thriving society and economy; in this time most if the Moai statutes were carved. However, this economic pursuit resulted in the destruction of the vast majority of trees by the end of the 14th century. The Islanders were unaware of this fact as the growth period of a palm (40-60 years) exceeded the life expectancy of the people (app. 30 years.)

Easter Island was discovered in 1722 by European sailors. At this time the population had decreased to approximately 3,000 people. The islanders had depleted the natural environment hereby there was almost no vegetation on the island; therefore, it could not longer support the established population as well as their unique culture. Violent conflicts occurred collapsing the society, and even cannibalism emerged. By the end of the 17th century the population decreased even further, presently the mainland is supplying the island.

This example illustrates how non-sustainable and short-termed focused behaviour has the propensity to jeopardize the future.

Source: Brander, J. and Taylor, S. (1998): The Simple Economics of Easter Island: A Ricardo-Malthus Model of Renewable Resource Use, in American Economic Review, volume 88, pp. 119-139. Cited in Hoffmann, J., Scherhon, G & Busch, T. (eds.) Darmstadt Definition of Sustainable Investments, p.5

3.2.2 Business and Ethics: A Convergent Divergence?

The relationship between ethics and economics is a very ancient one. As philosophy raged in ancient Greece, Aristotle was on record as proffering the recognition that ethics and economics are inseparable. In fact for him, economics, ethics, and politics were parts of practical philosophy.[181] Adam Smith the father of modern economics one must realise was a moral philosopher. In his Wealth of Nations, he laid down the basis of economics, and in his Theory of moral sentiments, he developed important aspects of ethics, which shows that he has his foot in both conceptual worlds.

In spite of the fact that contemporary history has borne unholy witness to the totalizing imperialism of economics over ethics[182], business ethics; which since

181 Balz, Bernd-Christian, Ethisch-ökologische Geldanlage, Frankfurt am Main, IKO Verlag, 1998.

182 'The Imperialism of economics over ethics' is the title of an article dealing with the subject written by Jesus M. Zaratiegui and published in the Journal of Markets and Morality. It could equally be accessed online at this link: http://www.acton.org/publications/mandm/mandm_article_120.php

the divorce in Adam Smith,[183] was patronized with the same neglect, and relegated to the status of a pious irrelevance- like a wrinkled old maid, infertile and not recommended to our utility- seems to be finally making a come back to the attention of economists.[184]

The mediocrity of that split or the unbundling of economics from ethical themes and guideposts, predicated on the deficient assumption that a preoccupation with ethics in business, cannot construct an economics uninhibitedly capable of scaffolding the pursuit of self-interest in the presence of the invisible hand; is been witnessed today on so many fronts. It could be seen in the financial crashes, bubble busts, ecological crises, or the resource scarcity that threatens the human race with extinction. On the socio-economic domain, the trickle down effect or diffusion of profits, which such economics advocated as the rising tide capable of lifting all boats in the socio-economic waters has failed. It is not only that it failed to lift all 'boats', but that millions of 'boats' were ran aground by the tide, while hundreds of millions of others were not even touched, let alone being lifted.

Today, after over a century of dalliance with this economic metaphysic, which saw a discernible rift between ethics and economics, the results are in. Poverty has increased in the midst of plenty. Great economic tragedies are playing out before our eyes, like that seen in Africa and much of the global south.[185] Close to a billion people go to bed every night without food.[186] A whole range of countries, designated as 'The Bottom Billion' are increasingly diverging from the rest of the world economy, forming ghettoes of misery; creating large islands of chaos and discontent, characterized by extreme poverty of majority of their populations, mass ignorance and dysfunctional inequities.[187] The human species is using up the earth's resources at a faster rate than at any other time in history; so much so

183 The fact must be reiterated that Adam Smith, who incidentally was the father of economics, was primarily a moral philosopher. In spite of this, his work and ideas, which gave birth to the economics never, laid the accent on the cause of the wealth of nations on the social ethics of the individual, but on the individual drive to assert his interests over and above that of the others. The use of this word divorce is not intended to pass a moral judgement on the validity of Smith's methodology, it is simply a statement of the fact that ethics was not his primary preoccupation in the Wealth of nations.

184 See: Zaratiegui, J.M: The Imperialism of Economics Over Ethics, in Journal of Markets and Morality, Vol.2, No.2, Fall 1999. pp.208-219

185 Xavier Sala-I-Martin and his co-researchers found the over all African economic performance as the economic tragedy of the 20th century. See: Vila-Artadi, Elsa and Sala-i-Martin, Francesc Xavier, "The Economic Tragedy of the 20th Century: Growth in Africa" (July 2003). NBER Working Paper No. W9865. http://ssrn.com/

186 See: World Food Programme. http://wfp.org/aboutwfp/introduction/hunger_who.asp?section=1&sub_section=1 accessed on the 18th of October, 2008

187 Paul Collier, The Bottom Billion: Why the Poorest Countries are Falling and What can be done about it. New York, Oxford University Press. 2007.

that the rich countries are imprinting scandalous footprints per capita, than the rest of the world combined.[188] Many companies are behaving like robber-baronial principalities, while Many MNCs are yet to exorcise and purged themselves of "the rogue-army of occupation" mindset, which characterize their operations and relationship with the stakeholders especially in the poorer countries.

All these are testaments that an ethics-challenged economics is a dangerous anomaly, which dire consequences and festival of lessons have blotted history with their hues. This subsisting has been according to Singh, thanks to the fact that in a spirited 'effort to elevate economics into a science, economists across the years, adopted reductionistic approaches which divorced economics from ethics. And this ethically deprived economics became the foundation of a materialist civilization of infinite growth fuelled by the money-culture-the dominant capital-centred approach to development.[189] And this has never been healthy for human society. History has witnessed some of the consequences. The failures of Wall Street, the ecological devastations inflicted on the Niger Delta by Oil companies, the financing of war economies across Africa by multi-national corporations, the social injustice of sweatshops, child labour, and gender discriminatory practices in the workplace lends credence to the fact that removing ethics from economics tends to remove social responsibility, critical awareness, social justice and other safeguards that guarantee life and dignity to the human person as well as ecological integrity and the chance at sustainable development for all.

Economics, which represents the way we organize, use and allocate scarce resources, shapes the kind of civilization we construct or empower to flourish. Our institutions, technologies, livelihood practices and knowledge systems take their moments about our economics. Due to the limited nature and finite supply of resources at our disposal and their central importance in ensuring our livelihoods, issues and questions relating to the allocation of these resources then become intrinsically ethical in nature. [190] This explains the contention in many quarters that ethics is the soul of economics and that economics without ethics instead of underwriting human and social wellbeing, becomes an economics of greed, which canonizes avarice.

188 See: Sachs, Wolfgang, et al. Fair Future, Wuppertal Institute. Zed

189 Singh, Bishan, Economics without Ethics: The Crisis of Spirituality, PCDForum Column #80 Release Date June 1, 1996. http://www.pcdf.org/1996/80singh.htm accessed on the 18th of October, 2008

190 Bishan Singh, ibid.

3.2.3 On Capital versus Values

At the failure of Communism in 1989, capitalism rode on the back of the market-economy mantra to become the super eminent metaphysic driving the global economy.[191] This system which places accent on competition and the supremacy of capital and the markets was described by Homman and Ungethüm as the best of systems so far known to us, which conduces to the actualization of solidarity of all peoples under modern conditions.[192] This assertion is rightly not without opponents. In Johannes Hoffmann's view, the submission of Homman and Ungethüm is theoretically okay, but has fundamental deficiencies on the practical level. This is because of the fact that the market economy is dominated by capital. And capital by its very nature dedicates itself primarily to its own profit and multiplication; and is not obliged to consult ethical considerations, or lean towards sustainability in its drive for gains. In most instances, the resulting social and ecological costs issuing from the operations of capital are passed on to the public, while the investors go home with the huge and obscene profits. Here, the public go home with the pains, and the investors with gains.[193] When the pains come, it is socialized. But the gains are always privatized.[194]

In this regard according to Hoffmann, market economy becomes a smokescreen and a handmaid of rapacious capitalism. Expanding his views further in line with that of Ferdinand Braudel, he contended that capitalism, as the embodiment of this idolatry of profit, is not market economy, but a rogue economic ideology, which only battens on the market economy. This is because capitalism instrumentalizes the market-economy metaphysic, exploiting it to the advantage and privilege of capital.[195] In capitalism, money and profit assumes a quasi religious character, compelling people to make every other consideration in the social, cultural, and ecological realms, supremely subservient to it. In this metaphysic, everything is forced to take the backseat and genuflect subserviently to this assumption that capital and money represents the absolute measure of every value. To this end therefore, the capitalist market-economy canonizes capital, and grants it an effectively destructive privilege. And this privilege excludes

191 This is the kind of economic metaphysic which saw the rise of oligarchs in Russian and the bastardization of the Russian economy.

192 Homman, K. & Ungethüm, M., cited in Hoffman, J. Ethische Kritik des Wettbewerbsrechts, paper presented at the Symposium der Projektgruppe Ethische-Ökologisches Rating under the Theme: Sustainability als Gestaltungsprinzip für die Rahmenordnungen von Finanz-und Gütermärkten, 29-31st May, 2008, Frankfurt am Main.

193 Hoffmann, J. loc. Cit. p.20

194 This is one of the major critiques against the $700 Billion dollars Wall Street bailout passed by the American Congress in October, 2008

195 Hoffmann, J. loc. Cit.

every other consideration and spawns a self-consolidating protectionism, which can never be ethically justified.[196] To that end, Hoffmann rightly insisted that a capitalist market economy is not integral and hence destructive, since it takes no cognizance of other dimensions of human existence, which has a lot to do with the impact of business on human society and culture. To that end, any market-economy worth its name must in addition to capital (Wirtschaftskapital), include what he termed Naturkapital-**Land**-(which is all the free-gifts of nature geared towards production) as well as **Social Capital** (Sozialkapital) (which embosoms all the social and cultural furnished conditions and relations geared towards production).[197] The realization that sustainability transcends the profitability of capital (**Wirtschaftkapital**) to include other factors like Social Capital and Land is the rationale which justifies the ethical and ecological assessment of companies and enterprises to determine to what extent they are abiding to integral development, as well as to set down criteria for that assessment.

196 Ibid.
197 Ibid.

Can Big Business ever be ethical?

Big businesses were built by men well-endowed with ego and energy who were not noticeably inhibited by scruple. Cornelius Vanderbilt, the great robber baron of the railways, did not build his empire without dirty tricks. Capital was a weapon. Rivals were bought out or ruined. The workforce did what it was told; unions were repressed, and intimidation from mercenaries broke strikes. Robber barons ended many of the great nineteenth-century labour disputes by employing armed Pinkertons, the private detective agency that played such an ignoble role in intimidation and strike breaking.

For the British worker, conditions were unspeakable. Overseas, there was even more licence for employers. Before its power was finally handed over to the Crown, the British East India Company employed its own army. As recently as the mid nineteenth century, the Opium Wars forced the Chinese to grant trading rights by addicting their markets to a dangerous product. Money, power, and ambition drove these enterprises, and heaven help those who stood in their path.

The point is this: business has always been run by competitive killers. It's a process whereby you make your product as cheaply as you can and sell it for the very maximum the market will bear.

Although the great personal fiefdoms have, with some exceptions, been replaced by corporations, they or their successors still attract people with the same motivation as their nineteenth-century forebears. In a process rather akin to Queen Victoria's reinvention of royalty as the ideal family (a role at which the inmates struggle pitiably), in modern times corporations have tried to redefine themselves as pillars of the establishment-and thus deeply respectable. Foundations, sponsorship (of the right sort), concert halls covered in logos, and beautifully produced statements of "values and vision" abound.

This PR polish notwithstanding, those at the top are uninhibited by shame. The ratio between the lowest wage and highest are steadily increased to the point that it is possible for a CEO to be earning a thousand times more than a junior in the same corporation. In the last few decades, globalization has given corporations new opportunities for nifty footwork. Profits can be moved into low-tax economies; inter-company accounting allows the corporation to sell stuff to itself to boost turnover in key markets; and manufacturing flows across the world to whomever provides the cheapest and most desperate workforce.

Competition within and between corporations is feral, yet the language of corporations is reassuringly bland with a strong leaning towards the obscure, Latinate, and defensive. It is this disparity between the pretensions of corporate life and its savage reality that produces such a rich mother lode of Bullshit.

Source: (Nick Webb: The Dictionary of Bullshit, Naperville, Illinois: Source Books, Inc., 2006, p.2-3)

3.3 Corporate Social Responsibility in the Nigeria Banking System

3.3.1 The Concept of Corporate Social Responsibility

3.3.1.1 Introduction

Corporate Social Responsibility (CSR) has today become the rhetoric of every business enterprise.[198] It is increasingly assuming a vital role in the life and operation of businesses both nationally and internationally. With the march of globalization, we are increasingly witnessing a new wave of consciousness both at the corporate and individual levels, as people across board and across the globe recognize the importance of CSR. This wave of interest is thanks to the increasing recognition of 'its intrinsic value to the business bottom line and its ability to stave off social and reputation risks that may not only affect an enterprise's rate of returns or profitability, but also subject to questioning its 'social license' to operate'.[199]

The tremendous agitations over the last decade from so many quarters for companies to embrace Corporate Social Responsibility in almost all sectors of the economy, especially in the emerging markets. This is construed as a way of mitigating social risks associated with business operations like environmental degradation, human rights abuses, corruption, etc; as well as a way of encouraging sustainable development. On the strength of this, one can effectively say that CSR programmes now have a global reach.

These agitations as well as the interest by the international media and civil society softened the ground for the emergence of a more regulated and controlled business environment in relations to human rights, environmental rights, corruption, etc. This equally led to the emergence of a lot of several CSR voluntary codes of corporate conduct, declarations, MOUs, Good Neighbour Agreements (GNAs) etc. For industries like the extractive industries, one sees initiatives like the Publish what you pay campaign (PWYP), The Extractive Industries Transparency Initiative (EITI) and the UN Global Compact, which embosoms a broader framework of CSR and transparency principles.[200]

But the depth and diffusion naturally varies across countries and across the continents. The CSR as practiced in many industries most especially across the global south and most particularly in industries like the extractive industry 'has

198 Nwete, Bede. Corporate Social Responsibility and Transparency in the Development of Energy and Mining Projects in Emerging Markets: Is Soft Law the Answer? Part I of II, German Law Journal, Vol. 8 No. 4-1 April 2007.

199 Loc. Cit.

200 Loc. Cit.

failed to deliver measurable and sustainable benefit to both the people living along project corridors, and natural resource producing communities as a whole[201], as could be seen in the Niger Delta. This disparity has also been seen in instances of companies and businesses moving from areas or countries with strict regulations to regions with flexible business regulations.[202] This for instance scandalizes when one realised that some companies that mouth and show off their corporate social responsibility credentials in the Western world turn around to operate sweatshops, finance war economies, and other socio-cultural and ecological destructive practices in emerging economies.[203] The accusations are there and rife, that many companies and businesses line behind CSR[204] and the global compact, in an effort to hide their social and environmental sins under the blue cover of the UN logo.[205] These are some of the prospects and problems confronting the CSR.

3.3.1.2 What is Corporate Social Responsibility?

There is no universally accepted definition of CSR. Although CSR has been gained widespread attention since the early 1970s, it has defied a commonly accepted definition. Most of the frequently deployed definitions include the ones that construed CSR as: 'operating a business in a manner that meets or exceeds the ethical, legal, commercial and public expectations that society has of businesses. In this purview it transcends a mere collection of discrete practices or occasional gestures, or initiatives motivated by marketing, public relations or other business benefits, to embosom a comprehensive set of policies, practices and programs that are integrated throughout business operations and decision making processes that are supported and rewarded by top-management.[206] There is also the view describing CSR as a company's obligation to be accountable to all of its stakeholders in all its operations and activities. In this case socially responsible businesses are construed as those that take into account the full scope of their impact on communities and environment when making decisions, balancing needs of stakeholders with their need to make profit.[207]

201 Loc. Cit.

202 P. Raynard & M. Forstater, Corporate Social Responsibility, Implications for Small and Medium Enterprises in Developing Countries, report prepared for UNIDO, 2002, cited in Nwete, Bede. Op. cit.

203 Naomi, Klein. No Logo, London, HarperCollins, 2001, p.xvii

204 See: Christian Aid Report: Behind the Mask: the real face of corporate social responsibility

205 Nwete, Bede. loc. Cit.

206 Lamido Sanusi. Corporate Social Responsibility: A Challenge for Nigerian Banks, A paper presented to the Charted Institute of Bankers of Nigeria (CIBN), Kano Branch 2007 Annual Dinner, Nov. 24, 2007. http://www.triumphnewspapers.com/sunday/corl982008.html accessed on the 22nd December, 2008.

207 Macmillan, 2005, cited in Lamido Sanusi, op. cit.

The World Bank defines CSR as the commitment of business to contribute to sustainable economic development, working with employees their families, local community and society at large to improve the quality of life, in ways that are both good for business and good for development.[208] According to the ASCIO Policy Paper of June 2004, the term Corporate Social Responsibility is used 'interchangeably for other terms such as Corporate Citizenship and is also linked to the concept of Triple Bottom Line Reporting (TBL), which is used as a framework for measuring an organization's performance against economic, social and environmental parameters.[209]

The essence of the CSR is about building sustainable businesses, which need healthy economies, markets and communities. Its key drivers drawn from ASOCIO are identified as follows:

- **Enlightened Self Interest**-Creating a synergy of ethics, a cohesive society and a sustainable global economy where markets, labour and communities are able to function well together.
- **Social Investments-** contributing to physical infrastructure and social capital is increasingly seen as a necessary part of doing business
- **Transparency and trust-** Business has low ratings of trust in public perception. There is increasing expectation that companies will be more open, more accountable and be prepared to report punblicly on their performance in social and environmental arenas.
- **Increased public Expectations of business**-globally companies are expected to do more than merely provide jobs and contribute to the economy through taxes and employment.

In relation to its major components, the fact remains that CSR is conceptually large going by the level of the discourse at this time. But all participants in this dialogue focus as it were on few key issues, due to the unavailability of a commonly accepted definition or classification of the main components. Some of the main components we found across most of the definitions we considered include the following:

- **Environmental Protection:** The focus here is in constructing sustainable solutions for natural resource use and the reduction of the company's ecological footprint and adverse impact on the environment.
- **Labour security:** Here the accent is on freedom of association and the recognition of the right to collective bargaining; the elimination of all forms of

208 IFC-The World Bank, http://www.ifc.org/ifcext/economics.nsf/content/csr-intropage accessed on the 22nd of December, 2008

209

forced or compulsory labour; the abolition of child labour and the elimination of discrimination in respect of employment and occupation.

- Human Rights:
- Community Involvement
- Business Standards
- Marketplace issues
- Health Promotion
- Education and leadership development, etc.

3.3.2 Corporate Social Responsibility in Nigeria

In Nigeria, although corporate social responsibility practice by MNC is becoming well entrenched at least in theory, the absence in many cases of effective host state regulation scuttles and dampens the motivations of these companies to live up to their responsibilities.[210]

The theory and practice of corporate social responsibility in Nigeria can be traced to practices in the oil and gas sectors of the Nigerian economy, driven by Western multi-national corporations.[211] But most of these corporations deployed that as responses to their unpalatable image and are mainly focussed on remedying the effects of their extractive activities on local communities, to this end, these firms have often provided the communities with pipe borne water, hospitals, schools, etc. however, these provisions have been most times on an ad hoc basis and often not sustained. [212]

In the oil sector, due to the fact that oil is an international, politically-charged commodity, added to fact that most of the companies in the Nigerian oil sector are multi-national concerns, originating from countries where activists make life hell for such companies, when they go rogue even outside their home countries; the motivations to engage in CSR is at least there, even though it serves the companies purposes of attracting less bad press to themselves.

In other sectors of the Nigerian economy, the motivations to be engaged in Corporate Social responsibility are non existent. Most of the local companies have no international presence. For instance, no indigenous Nigerian firm has multinational operations even though some Nigerian banks are beginning to expand into the West African sub-region, and less than 20 percent of all registered

210 Amao, Olufemi O. Corporate Social Responsibility, Multinational Corporations and the Law in Nigeria: Controlling Multi-nationals in Host States Journal of African Law, 52, 1 (2008), 89–113 School of Oriental and African Studies. doi:10.1017/S0021855308000041.

211 Amaeshi, Adi, Ogbeche and Amao; Corporate Social Responsibility(CSR) in Nigeria: Western mimicry or indigenous practices?, p.16

212 Ibid.

companies in Nigeria are publicly quoted. Most of the firms are SMEs, family owned or privately held and operated companies.[213] Added to this, local consumer and civil society pressures are non-existent, and the government that is supposed to be the regulator of actions and corporate behaviour is itself dysfunctional and riddled with corruption. The law enforcement mechanisms are weak and compromised into inefficiency by institutionalised corruption.[214] Many companies to that end lack the motivations to live up to their social responsibilities when the possibility exists that it would task their profit columns a little bit or increase their operational costs.

3.3.3 Corporate Social Responsibility in the Nigeria Banking System

3.3.3.1 Brief Overview of the Nigerian Banking System

The Nigerian financial architecture is like that obtained in many parts of the world made up of the universal banks or the commercial banks and other finance institutions or houses like Discount Houses, Microfinance Banks (MFBs), Finance Companies (FCs), Bureaux-de-change (BDCs), Primary Mortgage Institutions, (PMIs) and Development Finance Institutions (DFIs). On top of this architecture sits the Central Bank of Nigeria, which is the apex bank, the regulator as well as the lender of the last resort.

The first bank to start operations in Nigeria was the Bank of British West African Limited, which is now known as First Bank of Nigeria Plc. It commenced operations in 1894. The enactment of the first banking ordinance was in 1952, which essayed to bring about the regulation of this sector. Since then, the Nigerian banking system has witnessed huge transformations in structure, size, number and diversity of participants as well as the basic thrust and dimension of their activities. Today, after a series of reforms, which reached its apogee in the 2005 Bank consolidation exercise undertaken by the Central Bank during the tenure of Governor Charles Soludo, 25 banks emerged as strong and viable with the minimum capital base of 25 billion Naira, compared to over 89 which existed before; and which were plagued by structural anomalies consequent on weak capital base.

On the heels of the consolidation, the banks embraced improved technology and started globalizing their operations. Four Nigerian banks are now operating in the United Kingdom, Six in Ghana, Two in Sierra Leone and One in Benin Republic. The consolidation equally facilitated easier access to credit. Banks' credit

213 Limb and Fort, cited in Ibid, p.17

214 Ibid.

to small and medium scale enterprises rose from 66.28 billion Naira in 2005 to 134.68 billion Naira in 2007, and 203.58 billion in 2007. The number of bank depositors increased from 13, 649, 000 in 2003 to 17, 662, 000. Today equally, the bank consolidation equally affected the Microfinance Banks, which were ordered to up their minimum capital base from 400 Million Naira to 1 Billion Naira in order to be licensed for operation. To date, there are over 800 registered Microfinance Banks operating in Nigeria in a market were over 80 million Nigerians are in need of micro-credit.

3.3.3.2 CSR and Nigerian Banks

The Nigerian banking system is not immune from the prevalent in Nigeria, which construes CSR from philanthropic perspectives. An instance of this could be seen in Submissions of Eddy Ademosu, the President of the Association of Corporate Affairs Managers of Banks in Nigeria, in presenting what he views as the practice of CSR in the Nigerian banking system contends as follows:

> A key indicator to determine the true worth and value of modern organizations is their ability to give back to the society part of their income through some mutually beneficial initiatives. These initiatives are encapsulated in the concept of CSR.[215]

Apart from the inhibitions of this narrow conceptualization, Joseph Achua contended that self-induced vices, regulatory laxity, inauspicious macro-economic environment, and endemic corruption in the economy as the major constraints to the discharge of CSR in the Nigerian banking system.[216] Apart from the structural issues he recommended: like the restructuring of the Central Bank of Nigeria to facilitate clearly separate the roles of bank supervision from fiscal policy management as to make the social, environmental and economic viability of Nigerian banking system more effective; he contended that the banking system as a whole should not only effect a redefinition of what profitability mean, but should 'focus less exclusively on shareholders and financial measures of success to include all stakeholders' relationships in their mission to sustain competitive success in the future. He equally saw it as imperative that external regulation should be blended with conscious self regulations by the banking institutions themselves for the reforms to effectively include the delivery of CSR, which should be anchored on effective corporate governance in the banking institutions.[217]

215 Ademosu, E. 'Corporate Social Responsibility: The Experience of the Nigerian Banking System'. A paper presented at the 2008 Conference of the Federation of African Public Relations Associations (FAPRA), April, 2008.

216 Achua, Joseph. Corporate social responsibility in Nigerian banking system. Society and Business Review Journal, Vol.3 Issue 1, 2008, pp. 57-71

217 Achua, Loc. Cit.

Suffice it to note that strides are being made in the positive direction in terms of CSR in the Nigerian banking industry. This could be seen in the fact that Nigerian banks spent a total amount of $5, 445,090.84 (Five million, four hundred and forty thousand and ninety dollars) on 19 CSR projects in 2002; and spent over $24,021,699.02 (Twenty four million and twenty one thousand, six hundred and sixty nine dollars) on 20 CSR projects in 2006. This shows a 341.16 percent increase between 2003 and 2006 in the total financial commitment of Nigerian banks to CSR projects.[218] Added to that, the regulatory authorities introduced regulations to guide ethical practices and professionalism in the Nigerian banking industry. In this regard, we have codes like The Code of Ethics and Professionalism for the Banking Industry, with a sub-committee on Ethics and Professionalism, which possess some quasi-arbitration authority.[219] We equally have The Securities and Exchange Commission (SEC) and Corporate Affairs Commission (CAC)'s Code of Best Practices on Corporate Governance in Nigeria; The Central Bank of Nigeria (CBN)'s Code of Corporate Governance for Banks in Nigeria Post-Consolidation (effective from April 3, 2006) and The Chartered Institute of Bankers of Nigeria (CIBN)'s Code of Ethics and Professionalism

3.3.4 Brief Overview of the Nigerian Microfinance Banking Industry

This has already been undertaken in chapter 2.2

3.3.4.1 CSR in the Nigerian Microfinance Industry

In the course of our investigation, we did not see any separate CSR codes or observation methods for the microfinance banking industry. The general presumption is that what obtains in the banking system as a whole generally applies to the microfinance banks in terms of CSR.

3.3.4 Conclusion

Our aim in this section is to expose what obtains as CSR in Nigeria as that is the nearest we can get to any formal presence of ethical-ecological awareness in the Nigerian banking industry as a whole and the microfinance banking sector in particular. We are able to see that the general conception of CSR in Nigeria is from the philanthropic angle, which in our view does not go far enough, in terms

218 Ademosu, loc. Cit.

219 Ademosu, loc. Cit.

of its ability to create the cultural pressures necessary to make companies internalise that responsibility has ethical implication, which transcends the financial handouts they presently throw at ethical-ecological issues in their sector. Their relationship to their workers and every other stakeholder is equally a relevant part of any serious consideration or subscription to CSR. This is what led us to the conclusion that the FHG is a more comprehensive framework for what the ideal should be based on the fact that we have the pedestals of those ideals already present in our cultural traditions, and which in our search for modernity, we relegated to the periphery of consideration in public and economic life in Nigeria. And we argue that we really need to rediscover that if we are not to destroy our environment, our culture and our relationships in the search for profit. And the FHG is a framework that could be of help in this regard.

3.4 Ethical Investment and Ethical-Ecological Rating

3.4.1 The Concept of Ethical Investment

Ethical investment is investment which explicitly seeks to take environmental, social and ethical issues into account. In this way investors are given the opportunity of aligning the power of their money with the direction of values, which are socially credible, environmental sustainable and ethical sound. Ethical investment makes the case that it makes financial as well as moral sense to invest in companies that are planning ahead to create a better environment. These are the kinds of investment where shareholders, investors, fund managers of stakeholders actively seek to invest in companies whose products and services are of long term benefit to the communities in which they operate and /or contribute to a better environment.

Ethical oriented companies that show a dedication and consistent evidence of the following considerations:

- A good safety record
- Openness about activities
- Pollution control
- Energy Conservation
- Production of recycling equipment
- Equal Opportunities

Ethical investment counsels avoiding investments in companies involved in such areas as

- Arms trade
- Nuclear power/ fuel
- Repressive regimes
- The tobacco Industry
- Anti-Trade Union activity
- Animal Experimentation
- Third World Debt/ Experimentation.
- Pornography, etc

Ethical investment encourages more responsible business standard.

3.4.2 The History and Evolution of Ethical Investment

The roots of ethical investment date back to the 19th century. It emanated from religious movements like the Methodists and the Quakers, who were concerned with issues such as fair employment conditions and temperance. At the dawn of the 1900s, the Methodist Church in North America overcame its inhibitions to invest in the stock market. Suffice it to note that they previously considered the Stock market as some form of gambling and hence an impure preoccupation or investment vehicle for a Christian. However, they did not invest arbitrarily. They wished to exclude certain types of companies, especially those dealing or involved in alcohol and/or gambling, which their faith discountenances. The Quakers were not long in following this trend, but were very keen to avoid companies that trade in or manufacture weapons.

In England, in the late 1960s and early 1970s, there were many groups that were looking at the possibilities of an investment fund that fulfilled ethical requirements. Charles Jacob, then an investment manager with the Methodist church was among the many that were in this search. He prepared a proposal that gave rise to the first ethical unit trust in 1973. But unfortunately at this time, his proposal failed to receive the approval of the Department of Trade. But it succeeded in being approved in principle a few years later. The 1980s saw an acceleration of ethical investments in the UK due to the concerns generated by the Apartheid Regime in South Africa. In 1983, EIRIS came into being as the first independent research service for ethical investors in the United Kingdom. In the same year, Friends' Provident, an outfit founded in 1832 to provide life assurance for members of the Society of Friends, popularly known as the Quakers, offered to manage an ethical fund with the investment criteria determined by a separate committee. This led to the birth of the Stewardship Unit Trust, Stewardship life fund and Stewardship Individual Pension Fund in 1984. Since this launch, this market has been expanding in the UK, with more than 90 ethically and socially responsible funds jostling for the market share. In the 20th century, more churches, charities and individuals began to take account of ethical criteria in their investment choices and decision. In the UK, it became a law in the year 2000 for occupational pension schemes to declare whether they took account of any social, environmental or ethical factors in their stock investment decisions.

Suffice it to note that this movement expanded into other countries around the globe. Many countries like Germany, Australia, and Sweden have towed the path of the UK's law for occupational pension schemes. This is vital muscle in favour of ethical investments in the sense that pension funds across the globe constitute by far the largest group of shareholders and could exert considerable influence over companies, and could be deployed as a great vehicle for effecting improvements in corporate behaviour.

Public clamour and demand for ethical investment vehicles took off in the United States in the early 1970s with the launch of the Pax Fund in 1971. This was a reaction against the Vietnam War. The discontent generated by the Vietnam War across America led some investors into querying how their money was been invested or used. Many investors were angry with the manufacturers of 'Agent Orange', the defoliant used by American forces against Vietnamese jungles and forests, which in turn caused deformation in the babies of the people who came into contact with it.

Around the world, ethical investments have been making inroads into the public consciousness in many economies. Asia has witnessed the launch of several ethical funds in countries like Singapore and Japan. Today, Europe boasts of over 280 ethical investment funds, while in the United States, the value of assets involved in some form of socially responsible investment has crossed the 2 Trillion dollar mark, and growing.

3.5 Ethical Assessment of Companies

3.5.1 The Concept of Ethical Assessment of Companies

Ethical assessment or rating of companies, like its counterpart the financial rating is an instrument for the assessment of companies. It is the assessment of companies on the basis of social, environmental, economic and ethical criteria. They are ratings which pay special attention to non-financial and often ethical criteria in evaluation companies and investments.[220]

220 Schäfer, H, et al. Who is who in Corporate Social Responsibility Rating?, Gütersloh, Bertelsmann Foundation, 2006, p.4

Some initiatives and principles rose to confront the growing clamour for ethical principles in business. The ISO 9000, the Global Sullivan Principles, the Global Reporting Initiative are all efforts attempts or efforts in this regard.

3.5.2 Characteristics of Corporate Ethical Responsibility

The common characteristics of Ethical or Corporate Social Responsibility Ratings are as follows:

- Production: Focus on the entire value chain;
- Product Range: an orientation on the life-cycle concept;
- A clear reference to stakeholder effects arising from corporate behaviour;
- The central role not only of economical, but also social (in part also cultural) and ecological macro and micro trends in the entire environment of a company;
- An integrated, methodical examination of social, ecological and economical effects of corporate behaviour
- An increasing assessment of sustainability /CSR along the management process in a company from the development of strategies, their implementation and applied control up to the actually achieved results, reporting and dialogue.

3.6 An Overview of Some Assessment Criteriologies

In this sub-chapter, we present in no particular order an overview of various criteriologies, policies platforms or frameworks that revolve around ethical-ecological criteria for companies. The aim is to show that there exist other frameworks other than the one we have chosen.

3.6.1 The UN Global Compact

The UN Global Compact launched in July 2000 is characterized both as a policy platform and a practical framework for companies that are committed to sustainability and responsible business practices.[221] The compact seeks to align business operations and strategies everywhere with ten universally accepted principles in the areas of human rights, labour, environment and anti-corruption. The Com-

221 http://www.unglobalcompact.org accessed on the 7th of January, 2009.

pact is not a regulatory instrument, but rather a voluntary initiative that relies on public accountability, transparency and disclosure to complement regulation and provide a space for innovation. It aims through a wide spectrum of specialized work-streams, management tools, resources and topical programs, to advance two complementary objectives, namely:

a. Mainstream the ten principles in business activities around the world.
b. Catalyze actions in support of broader UN goals, including the Millennium Development Goals (MDGs).

It is envisaged that by doing so, businesses as the primary drivers of globalization can help ensure that markets, commerce, technology, and finance advance in ways that benefit economies and societies everywhere and contribute to a more sustainable and inclusive global economy. The Compact seeks to combine the best properties of the UN, such as moral authority and convening power, with the private sector's solution-finding strengths and resources, and expertise and capacities of other key stakeholders. [222]

The Compact asks companies to embrace, support and enact within their sphere of influence, a set of core values in the areas of human rights, labour standards, the environment, and anti-corruption. The Ten principles are as follows:

1. HUMAN RIGHTS

Principle 1 Businesses should support and respect the protection of internationally proclaimed human rights; and
Principle 2 makes sure that they are not complicit in human rights abuses.

LABOUR

Principle 3 Businesses should uphold the freedom of association and the effective recognition of all the right to collective bargaining;
Principle 4 the elimination of all forms of forced and compulsory labour;
Principle 5 the effective abolition of child labour; and
Principle 6 the elimination of discrimination in respect of employment and occupation

ENVIRONMENT

Principle 7 Businesses are asked to support a precautionary approach to environmental challenges;
Principle 8 undertake initiatives to promote greater environmental responsibility; and

222 Ibid.

Principle 9 encourage the development and diffusion of environmentally friendly technologies

ANTI-CORRUPTION

Principle 10 Businesses should work against corruption in all its forms including extortion and bribery.

3.6.2 The Global Sullivan Principles

The Global Sullivan Principles of Social Responsibility (GSP) is a voluntary code of conduct that seeks to enhance human rights, social justice, and protection of the environment and economic opportunity for all workers, in all industries, in all nations. The Principles were designed to be adopted on a voluntary basis, by all types of organizations around the globe, with the spirit of exchanging ideas so that society as a whole can benefit.[223]

The Global Sullivan Principles prides itself as being 'a global framework for social responsibility for companies large and small'.[224] The principles are intended to be a catalyst and compass for corporate responsibility and accountability. The Sullivan Website referred to the principles as "aspirational, not apologetic… celebratory not punitive…advancing a development framework that enables businesses of all sizes and in all sectors to pursue their business objectives while being mindful and respectful of employees and the communities in which they operate.[225]

The objectives of the Global Sullivan Principles are stated as : to support economic, social and political justice by companies where they do business; to support human rights and to encourage equal opportunity at all levels of employment, including racial and gender diversity on decision making committees and boards; to train and advance disadvantaged workers for technical, supervisory and management opportunities; and to assist with greater tolerance and understanding among peoples; thereby, helping to improve the quality of life for communities, workers and children with dignity and equality.

Companies subscribing to or endorsing the Global Sullivan Principles (GSP) are expected to respect the law, and as responsible members of society apply the Principles with integrity consistent with the legitimate role of business. They pledge to develop and implement company policies, procedures, training and internal reporting structures to ensure commitment to these Principles through-

223 http://www.thesullivanfoundation.org/gsp/default.asp accessed on the 7th of January, 2009

224 http://www.thesullivanfoundation.org/gsp/default.asp accessed on the 7th of January, 2009

225 ibid

out their organization.[226] They are expected to maintain a continuous commitment to each of the eight principles, within the laws and customs of each country where they hold operations, including the implementation of internal policies, procedures, training and reporting structures. And they are expected to pledge to transparently implement the following principles, and provide information that demonstrates publicly their commitment to them. The principles are as follows:

- Express our support for universal human rights and, particularly, those of our employees, the communities within which we operate and parties with whom we do business.
- Promote equal opportunity for our employees at all levels of the company with respect to issues such as colour, race, gender, age, ethnicity or religious beliefs, and operate without unacceptable worker treatment such as the exploitation of children, physical punishment, female abuse, involuntary servitude or other forms of abuse.
- Respect our employees' voluntary freedom of association.
- Compensate our employees to enable them to meet at least their basic needs and provide the opportunity to improve their skill and capability in order to raise their social and economic opportunities.
- Provide a safe and healthy workplace; protect human health and the environment; and promote sustainable development.
- Promote fair competition including respect for intellectual and other property rights, and not offer, pay or accept bribes.
- Work with governments and communities in which we do business to improve the quality of life in those communities — their educational, cultural, economic and social well-being — and seek to provide training and opportunities for workers from disadvantaged backgrounds.
- Promote the application of these Principles by those with whom we do business.

3.6.3 Global Ethical Standard (GES)[227]

Global Ethical Standard, which was established in 1992, identifies itself as one of the most experienced agencies for SRI in Europe. It is the largest in Scandinavia, and belongs to the top three in Europe. It was previously named Caring Company (Independent research agency), but merged in 2002 with the company Etykana-

226 Ibid.

227 All the information presented here was based on the study: Who is Who in Corporate Social Responsibility and on the Global Ethical Standard website, which is http://www.ges-invest.com/

lytikera', and was renamed Global Ethical Standard in 2003, in order to establish themselves globally with trademarked products.

It is headquartered in Stockholm, Sweden and conducts research on over 4000 companies worldwide. Its self assigned mission and vision is to persuade companies and institutional investors of sustainability.

Its philosophy is that: maintaining international norms is vital, because authorities, NGO's and media use these norms to evaluate companies. Norms serve therefore as a reasonable foundation for evaluating companies

Services offered by GES include:

a. **'Global Ethical Standard'** as a basis examines the violation of international conventions on Human Rights, business ethics and weapons based on UN-information.
b. **'GES Controversial'** inspects activities in weapons, tobacco, alcohol, pornography, gambling.
c. **'GES Active'** developed as a tool for investors to exert influence on companies.
d. **GES Risk and Opportunity'** comprises ratings that deal with environment, Human Rights, Corporate Governance. Ratings are based on international norms (environmental management, industry specific key indicators for environmental performance, UN Universal Declaration of HR, **UN Convention on the Right of the child**, ILO Core conventions, and OECD guidelines for good Corporate Governance). Companies obtain ratings in each area from Aa to Cc. (Capital letters indicate general risk level in company industry, lower case levels indicate the risk level in particular company). Rating results are not publicized.

3.6.4 EIRIS[228]

EIRIS, which stands for Ethical Investment Research Service (EIRIS) is a charity set up in 1983 with the help of a group of churches and charities as a research organization to help them put their ethical principles into practice when making investment decisions. EIRIS Services Ltd, a subsidiary company of EIRIS, undertakes most of the research for clients and provides commercial services.

It is headquartered in London and has five international research partners, which are as follows: Centre for Australian Ethical Research (CAER, Australia), Fundacion Ecologia y Desarrollo (EcoDes, Spain), Institut für Markt - Umwelt - Gesellschaft (imug,Germany), EthiFinance (formerly Observatoire de L'Ethique,

228 Culled from 'Who is Who in Corporate Social Responsibility.

France) and Avanzi SRI Research (Italy). This enables the agency to offer an almost global research service. Their research covers companies from the UK, which is its base, continental Europe, North America and the Asia-Pacific region. EIRIS offers an independent research which covers almost 2,800 companies all over the world. It strives to promote the concept of ethical or socially responsible investment; providing clients with the information they need to put their own principles into practice when making investment decisions and provides a tailor-made service to match clients‘ social and environmental concerns. EIRIS does not promote any particular view on ethical issues. Rather, they provide clients with the information they need to put their own principles into practice. Clients of EIRIS can choose from a list of 350 indicators that refers to more than 40 analysis sectors (for example: protection of the environment and human rights), thus creating their own special 'ethical mixture' of sustainability criteria (so called 'à la carte-approach'). Besides the examinations by using positive and /or negative criteria EIRIS also offers an additional examination of activities in traditional exclusion areas. These include the topics concerning 'sin-stocks', as well as other criteria like gene technology, intensive agriculture and meat production. EIRIS emphasizes that the criteria list is constantly advanced through a 'constructive dialog' with clients, experts, companies, partner organizations and observation of competitors and other events of the day.

EIRIS sustainability assessment is not based on a specific criteria-catalogue, corresponding to the implicit sustainability-philosophy of EIRIS: Because of this a number of approaches according to ones personal investment perception is possible: a combination of positive and/or negative criteria, as well as the appliance of solely exclusive criteria, again with respective client specified weighting. Each company is analyzed against 350 environmental and social indicators, which cover over 40 areas of research, including the following:

Governance issues: Board practice, codes of ethics, social, environmental and ethical risk management, women on the board.

Environmental issues: environmental management, environmental policy, environmental performance, environmental reporting, ozone-depleting chemicals, pesticides, pollution convictions, tropical hardwood, various product/process impacts, water pollution.

Social issues: alcohol, community involvement, equal opportunities, gambling, health and safety, human rights, military production and sale, pornography and adult entertainment services, supply chains, tobacco, trade unions and employee participation, training.

Other issues: animal testing, disclosure, fur, genetic engineering, intensive farming and meat sale, positive products and service.

3.6.5 EthicSCAN Canada Ltd

EthicScan Canada Ltd. was established in 1989 by David Nitkin, the former president of Ethics Practitioners' Association of Canada. It is headquartered in Toronto Canada, and is one of the oldest and largest business ethics consultancy and CSR-research-clearing house in Canada. Its core business is ethical consultancy, sustainability research, social-and ethics audits, training, and publication. EthicScan identifies itself as an ethics consultancy, corporate responsibility research house, and educational resource centre. Its self assigned mission is to help organizations and individuals behave more ethically; which is extended to include social responsible consuming, managing, investing and partnering.

EthicScan is next to MJRA the most important agency in Canada. It also evaluates Canadian companies for EIRIS. It provides research, management tools, training and organizational analysis for executives, consumers, investors, civil society organizations, development officers and other stakeholders who want to enhance, benchmark and verify an organization's ethical standards, integrity practices and socially responsible behaviour. It compiles sustainability research for 1,500 corporations from 43 sectors using the Delphi-Method, together with 60 experts from stakeholder organizations for revising assessment criteria.

Its mission and vision are to support individuals, corporations and organizations with the realisation of their own values: training programs, acquisition, selection of business associates, ethical funds/consumption, etc. The company rejects a definition of CSR and adopts instead a Modified Delphi Process (MDP) which it enforces every three to four years for the definitions of its criteria and assessment. It has over 200 criteria for its evaluations. And the key evaluation areas include:

a. Equity and family issues
b. Community Responsibility
c. Ethical management practices and consumer relations
d. Environmental performance
e. Environmental management
f. Employee relations
g. Progressive staff policies
h. Sourcing and trading practices
i. Corporate governance
j. Candour

Its assessment occurs within the ten categories. An over all rating does not take place here and its audits place emphasis on performance and results, as well as systems on disclosure and reporting.

3.6.6 Johannesburg Securities Exchange SRI index[229]

The Johannesburg Securities Exchange (JSE) SRI Index was launched as a means to identify those companies listed on the JSE that integrate the principles of the Triple Bottom Line into their business activities, and to facilitate investment in such companies. In addition, the SRI Index identifies criteria for Corporate Governance as the foundation on which each of the triple bottom lines rests, as good Corporate Governance plays a major role in ensuring that sustainability issues are identified, managed and resolved.

The SRI Index is constituted from companies that form part of the FTSE/JSE All Share Index (consists of the top 160 companies listed on the JSE), and which participate in the SRI Index process voluntarily through submitting data in terms of a web-based questionnaire. The criteria are structured along the three pillars of the triple bottom line: environmental, economic and social sustainability. A company must address each of these pillars if it is truly to be said to have integrated sustainability into its business practices.

A company is classified in a high, medium or low impact category according to its JSE industry sector classification based on an assessment of a company's direct and indirect environmental impact as a whole. Corporate Governance is dealt with separately in the index as it is the foundation in which the triple bottom line is embedded. An Advisory Committee devises both the questionnaire and the criteria.

3.7 Ethical Assessment of Companies in Nigeria

3.7.1 Ethical-ecological Investment and Assessment criteria in Nigeria: A History of Absence

There are no there are no known ethical investments, investment-funds or ethical-ecological criteria for rating, evaluating or assessing companies and investments in Nigeria. Nigeria has no history of ethical-ecological or socially responsible investment as obtains in Europe or America today, although on a general level, Nigeria is an interesting case viewed from the perspectives of ecological governance[230] and its ethical implications.

229 Based on Schäfer, ,Who is Who in Corporate Social Responsibility, published by Bertselsmann Foundation and the website of the JSE

230 Hochachka, G., "Small Small"-Ecological Governance in Nigeria, http://www.polisproject.org PDFs/EcologicalGovNigeria.pdf accessed on the 25th of November, 2008

This absence does not mean that ethical or ecological issues do not feature in public discourse in the Nigerian public space and business environment. Ecological governance and its awareness happen to be strengthening in the country.[231] But in Nigeria due to the fact that the economy is poor, the politics fragmented along lines of anomie; the infrastructures dysfunctional and the public condemned to feeble reactions to particular issues of environmental or ethical violation, which impacts on their immediate environment or needs, ethical-ecological seems to have taken the backseat. It seems to have given way to other more urgent concerns faced by the people.

In the Nigerian context like everywhere else, ecological governance is equally about good governance as much as it is ecosystem viability. This inheres in the fact that lack of good governance in Nigeria is the single biggest barrier to sustainability in the Nigeria context.[232] This accounts for the lackadaisical attitude with which ecology and ethics in public life, institutions or business establishments are treated. Such issues receive from the government as well as from the general public a kind of lukewarm attitude in spite of the lip service paid to it in the government-controlled media. A public; majority of who, are struggling to survive gastronomic emergencies and other constraints imposed on them by poverty and a dysfunctional system cannot be expected to be philosophizing over such issues. Their poverty imposes on them pressures which they take out on the environment. These pressures equally make compromises in ethical principles more commonplace. This is the case in spite of the fact that Nigerians are witnesses to desert encroachment in the North of the country; erosion and landslides in the Southeast; oil-spillage, gas flaring, massive pollution and ecological collapse in the Niger Delta. This is also the case in spite of the fact that massive and pervasive corruption exists across all levels of government and public life. Companies have equally been known to cut corners, offering the unsuspecting public goods and services inferior in quality and most times dangerous to health. Examples of these could be seen in the explosive kerosene which was sold to the Nigerian public by oil importers, who cut corners to up their profits. This led to the death of so many Nigerians. And the government has not done anything in this regard to prevent future occurrence, and the Nigerian public has been about their normal business as if nothing happened. This is seen across all sectors of the Nigerian economic and public life. This is equally the case in spite of the fact that courses in business ethics are parts of the curriculum in different business schools and universities in Nigeria. But the concept and praxis of ethics in business and dealings with fellow men, which irrigated the conceptual universe of many Nigerian and African traditional systems like the Omenala; and which has

231 Hochachka, G., Op. Cit.
232 Ibid.

taken life in modern principles of CSR seems to have failed to engraft itself into the public consciousness in Nigeria. Its engrafting into the Nigerian body-politic or business practices of companies could be said to be wrapped in a cloud of unknowing, unconcern or postural apathy. Adedeji captures this vicious circle thus:

> Associated with the problems of environmental degradation is the deepening poverty, inequality and social marginalization which have also resulted in diminishing human security. In various parts of Nigeria especially among the rural dwellers, the pressure on the ecosystem and other natural resources is increasing, with growing rate of unsustainable exploitation of natural resources and pollution. Poverty and environmental degradation are linked in a vicious circle in which people cannot afford to take proper care of the environment (UNEP, 1999). Poverty has been and remains a major cause and consequence of environmental degradation and resource depletion.[233]

The government, media, and the academia on the other hand do not seem to be helping matters. Desertification, Soil erosion and landslides have been recurring issues in the Nigerian experience and public space, but there has never been an official initiative towards tying it to the abuse of our environment in modern times, neither has there been a public outcry in that regard.

The government sometimes seems to encourage environmentally harmful policies through actions like massive cutting down of trees and deforestation, which has led to near ecological collapse and loss of flora and fauna in many parts of the country. These are done sometimes to make way for structures and buildings which are abandoned half way to their completion.[234] In other instances, government has been known to conspire with its inaction; and government officials with active collusion in the rapacious use of the Nigerian forest and other natural resources, where loggers engage in unsustainable lumbering practices, which takes no cognizance of the long term impact of their action on wildlife, flora and fauna, let alone the ecological stability and integrity of our environment. Adedeji lends credence to our assertions here. He speaks his observations thus:

> Government policies of economic growth and the collaboration with multinationals have encouraged rapid decline in the state of the nation's ecological system. The past military governments have constantly depressed environmental activities and many activists even suffer attacks from the government and armed militias often sponsored by multinationals especially in the Niger-Delta region of the country. The governments in the country are often intolerant about any public outcry or expression of dissidence towards government operations towards rapid economic growth. Many of the ecological problems in the country are part of what Seager (1993:5) called 'the progeny of a very particular clusters of powerful institutions acting in particular ways. These clusters are the military, multinationals, governments and environment

233 Adedeji, Hakeem. Oludare., Op. cit.

234 A case in point here could be seen in Independence layout of Enugu State, where the government of Chimaroke Nnamani destroyed a pine forest very close to Okpara square in the name of building judiciary quarters. This pine forest has maintained some ecological sanity and stability around independence lay out for sometime prior to the advent of his administration.

movements. The aggressive and competitiveness of the nation's economy coupled with long years of military rule and mismanagement have increase the neglect for the good management of the environment. The political economy has emphasised uncontrolled economic growth which neither worry about efficient energy use or conservation of natural resources. Much energy is wasted during the production process and nature's diversity was relegated to the back and the plants that occupy the lands are generally of lower quality and usefulness.[235]

This supports the conclusion that in Nigeria, there seems to be a pervading social amnesia or erosion of memory to the historical fact that ecological awareness, governance and management have been ontologically enshrined in the cultural principles of many human societies. Man has always depended on his environment for his sustenance. Studies have shown that wherever human beings destroyed the ability of their eco-systems to support life, extinction or near-extinction of that race has always been the fallout.[236] This inheres in the fact that our environment has always been an essential arena where our lives play themselves out. Our cultures, our governance structures and systems are themselves situated in our ecological systems. And our economic and social systems are built upon this as well.

The observations to the effect that the Nigerian ecological systems are deteriorating dramatically at all levels are most apparent today. According to Oludare Hakeem Adedeji,

> Environmental degradation problems such as pollution, erosion (soil erosion, coastal and river erosion), gas flaring and oil spillage, acidification and flooding are occurring at rampant rate and with varying degree of impacts in many parts of Nigeria. For example the tropical rainforest (TRF) destruction has imperilled the forested regions near the equator with countries such as Nigeria facing huge soil loss, siltation of rivers and streams, loss of biodiversity etc. Nigeria, particularly the southern region have very sensitive soils and the region is classified as a potentially problem area which acidification is likely to become a problem. Acidification may cause much damage to sensitive components of the ecosystem e.g. the soil and vegetation which forms the base resources.[237]

Nigeria is an essential arena where poverty, corruption and bad governance are conspiring to sire a very looming threat of ethical and ecological collapse. Gail Hochachka brilliantly articulated this situation thus:

> Nigeria is representative of sustainability issues in Sub-Saharan Africa, in which poverty and corruption are intermingled, both adding to ongoing ecological degradation. In this context

235 Adedeji, op. Cit.

236 Diamond, Jared, Collapse: How Societies Choose to Fail or Succeed, New York, Viking Books, 2005.

237 Adedeji, Hakeem. Oludare., Political Economy and Ethics of Ecological Problems in Nigeria: Challenges to Environmental Management and Sustainability in the New Millenium, http://www.hicsocial.org/Social2003Proceedings/Oludare%20Hakeem%20Adedeji.pdf accessed on the 25th of December, 2008

of overpopulation and poverty, any environmental intervention quintessentially includes human communities. Environmental sustainability is impossible without addressing the socio-economic needs in the villages. Poverty is in turn exacerbated by declining natural resources, and vice versa calling for an integrated approach to any intervention.[238]

The country's recent history over and above been marred by its infamous environmental and social injustices in the oil and gas industry,[239] has been tainted and laid prostrate by corruption in governance and public life. This canker is so pervasive and has degenerated into a social pathology upon which no functional structure could ever be built or sustained; both on the social or economic domains. The Nigerian authorities seem less keen on a blanket law against corruption. This could be seen in the fact that the Nigerian senate refused to ban 'gifts' as a part of its new code of ethics, which is been advanced as a part of Nigerian culture,[240] as well as the refusal of the lower house of parliament to pass the Freedom of Information Bill, which would grant citizens access to government records, where most of the corruption are sired.

That is on the demand side of corruption. On the supply side, many companies construe Nigeria as a paradise for their obnoxious and ethically and ecologically-challenged practices. For instance, Pfizer, the American pharmaceutical giant stands accused of shipping its risky medical experiments down to Nigeria. Using human beings as guinea pigs, these experiments drew widespread condemnation in Nigeria, where federal investigations is underway and two class action law suits still pending.[241] We are yet to know the results of that trial. Siemens, the German electrical giants were involved in the bribery of Nigerian government officials to the tune of 10 million Euros to gain government contracts in Nigeria. Many Chinese companies are flocking to Nigeria driven by their great financial muscle. Their march across Africa and Nigeria in particular has witnessed some scandalous disregard for ethical practices in business.[242] These are some examples attesting to the tough business context and socio-economic landscape in which ethical-ecological consciousness as a concept and a canvass for making rational and informed business and socio-economic decisions, which would impact on sustainable development, must be appraised in the Nigeria of today.

238 Hochachka, G. "Small Small"-Ecological Governance in Nigeria, See: http://www.polisproject.org/PDFs/EcologicalGovNigeria.pdf accessed on the 29th of December, 2008.

239 Ibid.

240 See: Ethical Corporation, Business Briefs 2005, http://www.ethicalcorp.com/content.asp?ContentID=3741

241 See: Joe Stephens, "American Congress Pursues Legislation to Limit Risky Overseas Drug Trials" art. in Washington Post of Saturday August 4, 2001, p. A05. http://www.washingtonpost.com/wp-dyn/articles/A29545-2001Aug3.html)

242 See: Nigeriasolidarity.org: Chinese firms dehumanizing treatment of Nigerian workers, http://www.nigeriasolidarity.org/art047.htm accessed on the 29th of December, 2008

3.7.2 Factors Explaining the Absence

There a lot of factors that can account for the absence of ethical or ecological criteriology or praxis in the Nigerian business environment. One must not lose sight of the fact that ethical and ecological issues receive from the government as well as from the general public a kind of lukewarm attitude. It could be said to be wrapped in a cloud of unknowing, unconcern or postural apathy.

One of the major factors that could be suggested to explain this absence is the fact that Nigeria has not been a manufacturing society in the class of Europe and America. The traditional economic base was basically agrarian until the colonialists came to Nigeria. This advent changed the social dynamic in so many ways than one and led to the emergence of a mercantilist class, which adopted the colonial exploitative mentality, thereby displacing the age long traditional conceptual scheme, which underwrote business interactions and relations in the traditional set up. This had far reaching consequences for the society, in that business and mercantilist decisions were divorced from ethical considerations, which has been its base in the African traditional society. From then onwards till this moment, Nigeria has failed to exorcise this influence, which militates against the emergence of an ethical-ecological awareness in her business environment.

In addition to that, since there are no criteriologies or frameworks for assessing that in the Nigerian context, there is no way one can measure or ascertain whether companies or individuals respect or subscribe to any code of ethics in their investments or business dealings in the Nigerian context. Many companies have the principles of Corporate Social Responsibility hoisted on their mission statements, company papers, adverts and websites. But due to the fact that CSR is construed from a philanthropic point of view in the Nigerian context, the activities of most of these companies does not go far enough. In the Nigerian banking industry, there are codes of ethics and corporate governance that banks and their employees are required to subscribe to. But none of these can qualify as evidence of ethical criteria of action or a tendency thereto.

The situation is equally not helped by the socio-economic situation. As reiterated earlier, in a socio-economic embrace where the economy is poor, the politics fragmented along lines of anomie, the structures dysfunctional and the public is condemned to piece meal reactions to particular issues of environmental or ethical violation which impacts on their immediate environment or needs we cannot hold out much hope for the germination or operation of these frameworks as motivations to action.

3.7.3 An Overview of the Ethical Pedestals of Nigerian Pre-Colonial Society

Before the advent of colonialism, Nigeria was a large mass of land, populated by quasi-isolated tribal pockets, and ethnic nationalities. These constructs interacted with each other through trade, intermarriage, and even wars. There were no states so to say in the contemporary sense. There were villages, kingdoms, empires and republican democracies. , the Kanem Bornu, and Oyo empires, the Benin Kingdom and other Yoruba Kingdoms were empires in their own rights. Ndiigbo of Southern Nigeria had already fashioned a functional republican and egalitarian democracy in antiquity, while ancient Greece slumbered in primitivity, which archaeological evidence dating back to 450BC excavated by Thurstan Shaw in Igboukwu showed.[243]

These social embraces were characterized by singular political and culture centres within their sphere of influence. This gave rise to common identity, both lingual and cultural. They ran their societies on their own terms, save naturally, when conquered in wars. In spite of this, the cellular political unit of African life was the tribe. It was so basic, and yet so primordial. It transcends the clans, composed of families, to embrace a wider collection of clans. This presupposed common ancestral or cultural ties, dating to time immemorial. Most of these tribes pay allegiance to one heritage. It was a basis of social bonding. It was the influential factor in the political, socioeconomic and cultural matrix of the Nigerian tribal communities. This could be seen today, in the fact that politics in Nigeria, despite its affinities to Eurocentric-Judaeo-Christian vision of modernity, and to modern conceptions of democracy, still conjugates the tribal verb.

On the level of socioeconomic interactions, many African traditional societies, including the various culture groups across Nigeria operated a very developed hybrid of functional constants which cuts across their society, ethics, religion and culture. This tradition shows a very developed sense of respect for the human person, his society and his environment.[244] And these values were configured to bear on the socio-economic and cultural life and processes of the traditional society.

Most of them have quasi-religious character, as taboos are used to enforce adherence and general application. For instance, in Igbo traditional society, 'Omenala'-meaning ***'the law of the land'*** …offers an important principle and philosophy in understanding the interplay between community and individual; forces of nature and forces of nurture; religion and business; the environment and humanity; and generally helps us better understand various factors and values

243 Ogbunwezeh, Emmanuel F. Africa: The Ontology of Failed States. http://www.dawodu.com/ogbunwezeh1.htm accessed on the 29th of December, 2008

244 See: Mbiti, J.,African Religions and Philosophy, (1969) Onwubiko Oliver, African Thought and Culture, Enugu, Snaap Press, 1994.

that ensured sustainability and stakeholder participation among the traditional Igbo people.[245] In this purview, it is elevated to the level of an ***'aru'***-abomination or violation of the land,[246] for one to cut a tree in the communal forest, or fish in the river during the season, when it was forbidden to do so. It is equally an 'aru' for one to produce, package, and sell poisonous, damaged, or rotten goods or food in the market, no matter how it is packaged.[247] But most of these cultural values failed to cross the threshold of their traditional ambience to stamp their impress on the post-colonial, urban Nigeria business life and environment. In fact, they failed to transcend the socio-cultural flux provoked by the colonial and post-colonial dynamic, into the modern/urban business culture in many sectors of the Nigerian economy. To this end, there was no broad, comprehensive or coherent transplantation of these cultural values into the policy environment of modern Nigerian, post-colonial cash economy.

3.7.4 The Socio-cultural Impact of Nigeria's encounter with the Colonial Dynamic

At the advent of the White man was sociologically a tsunamic experience for Nigeria. Chinua Achebe captured this well in his novel of the same title: *Things fall apart!* Nigeria and her centre could no longer hold. She became embroiled in a dynamic, which would change her structure, her culture and her future forever. At the instance of colonialism, the former league of tribes coagulated into pseudo-states. Strange bedfellows became fellow citizens over night. Consanguinal relatives found themselves facing each other as citizens of different countries.

245 Nnoli-Edozien, N., Ownership and Management Structures in the Economy: African Traditional Values Applied to Modern Issues of Sustainability, Enugu, CIDJAP Publications, 2007, p.20

246 Ala-the Land in Igbo cosmology is the mother goddess that owns us all. A violation of Ala or her ordinances is a great crime that requires not only cosmic restitution, but also a social restitution that is costly in the extreme the offender. Offences that constitute this violation include incest, stealing yams, killing someone at a funeral, swearing falsely while calling 'Ala' as your witness, and so on. 'Aru' is any act that violates the ordinance or the sanctity of 'Ala'. And punishment for this violation include banishment, ostracism, exile and in extreme cases death. 'Ikpu aru'-Placating 'ala' is the restitution imposed by ala for such violations.

247 Most of these prohibitions were time-tested methods with which these societies sought to protect their environment by giving it time to recover from the yields it gave the community in the previous season. In these practices, one can see a highly developed sense of respect for the environment, for nature and nature's gifts. For the traditional Igbo, nature is so holy that to violate her is a crime attracting the highest repulsion from the community. (See:V.C Uchendu: The Igbos of Southeast Nigeria. See also: Nnoli-Edozien, Ndidi; Ownership and Management Structures in the Economy, Enugu, Cidjap Publications, 2007, p.228)

The African psyche, society and culture were ripped apart. The changes were too radical, as his culture was demonized and labelled as inferior. He had to forfeit his language in so many cases. He was equated to dogs, when he seeks admittance into drinking parlours, because dogs were not admitted. There arose what Chinweizu characterized as a "mis-education" on the socio-cultural level, which deformed the collective psyche of the natives, from which it is yet to recover.

To carve up Africa to the various spheres of influences, drawing boards were built in 1885 Berlin. Africa was scrambled up among the occupying powers. The aim was to ensure each power an unimpeded and unmonitored freedom to loot as much as they could in their area of influence. At this configuration, the Belgian-Congo became an abattoir, where King Leopold's polymorphous perversity, sought and obtained unrestrained ventilation. For the sake of rubber, Leopold's men sacked villages, decimated cultures, and harvested a pyramid of chopped hands, in an orgy of brutality, unmatched even by Hitler's men. Congo bled, and haemorrhaged her resources into Belgian coffers. The Germans tried the annihilation tactics on the Herero of Namibia. British piratical treachery blossomed in Nigeria and her other territories. All in Europe, Africa bled, so that Europe could have a river of wealth flowing through her.

To effectively continue this when their various suns must have set, they created states; which were simply neo-colonial dependencies. And to run these states, they mass-produced a semi-literate, middle-class of yes-men, to complement the paucity of men they have on the ground. This crop of creatures became the collaborative vehicle of colonial exploitation. Hatred for them, which was a rampant phenomenon, sometimes took deadly proportions, as was mirrored in Achebe's Things Fall Apart, where Okonkwo had to kill a court messenger, to vent his anger on an invading establishment that has despoiled the land of his fathers, and decimated his culture. Almost all the Modern states in Africa today were built on socio-political ontologies, oozing from this engineered political metaphysic. The people never dialogued their differences as a basis for federating. They never talked to each other about a political union. They woke up one morning, and saw themselves conscripted into geopolitical constructs they neither chose nor bargained for. For the natives, it was a bazaar of unfunny jokes, and for the colonial officers; a duty for country and queen.

These states were created to facilitate and ease the efficiency of rapid colonial exploitation. That was their raison d'etre. They were never designed to be independent, or cease being a source of cheap raw materials, and slave labour for colonial industries. They were equally meant to be a cheap market to cushion the inflationary effects of mechanised mass production. The colony was a laboratory of caprice. Every socio-economic, geopolitical or cultural hypothesis was subjected to clinical trials on the hapless colonies. This accounts for the fact, that every discredited socio-political, economic or eugenic theory was once tried out in Africa.[248]

The fact must be reiterated that colonialists were excited by profit and seduced by adventure. To satisfy these greedy gods, they engendered chronic chaos, advertised brutality and consulted their avarice, more than their humanity. Their governance, nay maladministration of their colonies was vulgar in its opulence, convulsively ugly and malodorous in its negative flamboyance. In many instances a grand racist and supremacist ideology, as well as a denigrating anthropology of their colonial subjects informed colonial policies.[249] Imperialism is synonymous with mindless exploitation. It is a psalm of oppression composed by a powerful rogue nation against a militarily weak and technologically inferior country. In this relationship, an arrangement is hewed out of the dark crooked woods of imperialistic deceit, which ties the colony to the pseudo-legal apron strings of the colonialist. Here, the resources of the colony are the primary and only factor informing whatever the colonialist does in the colony. The resources and labour of the colonies are recklessly exploited to cause rivers of wealth to flow in the mother country, while the colony reels in underdevelopment and poverty. The colony is regarded as a massive laboratory for colonial experiments in socio-political engineering. Examples of these experiments include the warrant chieftaincy introduced in Nigeria, eugenics and genocide, like the lot of Herero tribe of herdsmen of Namibia, whom their German colonial masters nearly exterminated in 1904. A German official that took part in that pogrom committed to his diary one of the most convulsively wicked thoughts and judgment ever passed on a race of people. He wrote of the Herero tribe; "I believe that the nation should be annihilated"[250] Other examples include social correctional practice, like Australia, which the British used as a penal colony for the dregs of the British society and the pyramid of human bones and skulls left by the Belgians in Congo[251]

British Imperialism is eloquently unique in that it succeeded more in reducing almost all their colonies to comparative nothingness. A clinical look at the Commonwealth of Nations reveals an assemblage of retrogressive and dependent economies, whose growth has been basically sabotaged and compromised by British plunder. Nigeria, which incidentally we would turn to shortly, is a colossal testimony to this. Of this Jean Paul Sartre wrote that "united by profit, the

248 Cf. Ogbunwezeh, E. F. Africa: The Ontology of Failed States, http://www.dawodu.com/ogbunwezeh1.htm accessed on the 29th of December, 2008

249 Ogbunwezeh, Emmanuel Franklyne. The Tragedy of a Tribe (Book readied for publication) p.21

250 Gen. Lothar Von Trotha, Cited in Newsweek of August 21,2000,P.36

251 Chinweizu, The West and the Rest of Us, London, Nok Publishers, 1978, PP. 61-71

peoples of the mother countries baptized their commonwealth of crimes, calling them fraternity and love".[252] What obtains in Nigeria is what obtains across Africa in varying proportions. We captured it well on another occasion, when we wrote:

> The African continent is littered with failed states. Most of these states are economic backwaters, social apologies and political ruins. This landscape runs from the Casablanca to the Cape Town and from The Horn of Africa in the East to the Island of No Return in the West Atlantic. Most of these states true to type were the creatures of imperial convenience. To that end, they were meant to serve a purpose after which their ontological legitimacy or raison d' etre would then expire. At this expiration; the states, naturally not designed for self-propulsion; were condemned to tether on the brink, and finally implode upon the inglorious weight of their inherent contradictions. Colonialism designed and inspired the problems. But the decadence was then driven along by a horde of native pirates; trained in the fine art of piracy. These set of political actors were rogues personalities, weaned on selfishness. They were brilliant students of kleptocracy and political perversity. In about four decades they completely outclassed colonial perfidy and bested them in thievery. They did an inglorious job of mismanaging Africa, so much so that she is today the laughing stock of the world.[253]

This was the situation which made the germination of ethical-ecological awareness an uphill task. Although ethics as a currency of operation in business and social life has an ancient and august pedigree in African culture, the advent of colonialism sacked this sociocultural dynamic and attempted a quack replacement of it with an alien narrative, which was allergic to everything African. Colonial conceptual schemes attempted a quack reconstruction of African reality in the exploitative image and likeness of colonialism, in the name of civilizing Africans. Being a metaphysic of exploitation,[254] it labelled African values and realities, which were beyond its narrow epistemic schemes as paganistic and savage.

This exploitative conceptual scheme was never exorcised from our societies. It was rather compounded by decades of bad governance, which created a culture of contempt for the rule of law by both individuals and businesses. This led to the cultivation and consolidation of tolerance for business and political misconduct.[255] Little wonder that in a clime like this, an ethical-ecological awareness never gained the requisite prominence in the life and conduct of the affairs of companies. These were some of the historical factors why Nigeria did not have a history of ethically or social responsible investments, and why the primal Nigerian business environment could not generate such consciousness.

252 Frantz Fanon, Op. Cit., P.23

253 Ogbunwezeh, E. F, ibid

254 Ogbunwezeh, Emmauel Franklyne: The Evolution of a Hoax,

255 Ethical Corporation. 'Nigeria's corruption' http://www.ethicalcorp.com/content.asp?Content ID=3319 accessed on the 2nd of January, 2009

In order to make it clearer, let us analyse the context in which businesses operate in Nigeria and round off with what corporate social responsibility has come to mean in contemporary Nigerian business climate. This is to help us situate and make the case for the necessity of an ethical criteriology for assessing and evaluating companies in Nigeria

3.7.5 Situating the Omenala Principles as an Example of the Contextual Interface for the Introduction of the FHG into the Nigerian Context

Although our work took cognizance of the major business and socio-cultural currents in Nigeria, our examination of a cultural tradition that could act as the interface for the introduction of the FHG in the Nigerian context took particular attention of the Omenala principles of the Igbos of Southern Nigeria. This is informed by the fact that the Igbos are one of the most unusually-driven, enterprising, and business oriented peoples in Nigeria and Africa as a whole. And Igbo sub-communities dominate key economic sectors in Nigeria.[256] And they are the most diffused tribe in Nigeria. They could be found almost all over Nigeria much more than any other tribe. They carry their heritage and tradition with them, although highly adaptive to their environment. This does not mean that Omenala is the only traditional-ethical principles. The Yorubas for instance have the 'Omoluwabi concept'. But the reasons we situated above was what recommended our choice of Omenala.

The 'Omenala' is the principles, source and foundation of Igbo values of community and sustainability.[257] Among the Igbo people of Nigeria; lacking a literary tradition, the Omenala which is the whole gamut of their culture, customs, worldview, morality and laws of the land embodied the heritage of the ancestors handed over by oral tradition from one generation to the next.[258] To this end, 'Omenala or Omenani' literally translated as ***"what obtains in the land or community"***, is the construed as the best concept or word that captures Igbo philosophy.[259]

The Omenala has five key principles, which could be rendered as follows; namely: *preservation, guidance, direction, continuity and equity (reconciliation).* These principles are the believed to guarantee the rationality behind the

256 Chua, Amy. World on Fire: How Exporting Free-Market Democracy breeds Ethnic Hatred and Global Instability. London, Arrow Books, 2004, p.108

257 Nnoli Edozien, Ndidi. Ownership and Management Structures in the Economy: African Traditional Values Applied to Modern Issues of Sustainability and the Corporate Governance Function, Enugu, CIDJAP Publications, 2007, p.129

258 Loc. Cit.

259 See: T.U Nwala, Igbo Philosophy, 1985, p.26 and following. Cited in Nnoli Edozien, loc. Cit.

actions, values, norms and beliefs.[260] According to Ndidi Nnoli-Edozien, the Omenala as the basis of traditional law in Igbo society expresses those communal values with potential to protect the community and enhance solidarity as a way of life. Thus Omenala becomes a central thread guaranteeing the protection of life and property, the harmony for members of society among themselves and with nature, as well as their linkage to the divine through the ancestors and the deities. Omenala provides a proper foundation for a sustainable economy where the preservation of the environment, the enhancement of the principles of equity and fair-play and the promotion of an economy in which individual prowess was encouraged alongside communal values, existed.[261]

The principles of subsidiarity and solidarity are the intrinsic pillars of Omenala. Nnoli-Edozien articulated this well:

> Self-reliance, understood as subsidiarity was strongly promoted among the Igbos through the Omenala: 'Onye kwe chi ya ekwe' (literally: if you agree, your chi will agree) meaning 'God helps those who help themselves'. Nonetheless the inherent values of the Omenala linked the success of the individual to, the entire progress of the community (solidarity), understood as the individual in a communal context.[262]

In Igbo societies, the economy, law, and religion are very closely interlinked. And the Omenala is the point of this linkage between religion, culture, morality, law and socio-economic realities. And the enforcement of Omenala is anchored in the religious worldview of the Igbo.[263]

According to the findings of Nnoli-Edozien, the Omenala is the regulator of socio-economic factors. It through the 'Nso ala' (Sacred Laws) guides four areas of human behaviour in society, namely:

a. **Life**: Here, human life especially that of a clansman is regarded as sacred so that homicide, murder, suicide and other unnatural forms of death (all referred to as 'ochu') are regarded as a breach of the 'Nso ala'.
b. **Communal Harmony:** Here interpersonal relationships are regulated and include such areas as marriage ceremonies, naming ceremonies, initiation rites, title taking, death rituals, burial rites, economic and social activities of various sorts, such that it was important for community members to be present at communal events, even if it were their enemies celebrating, so that reciprocity was accorded them on their own events.
c. **Respect for the Past (Ancestors):** Here the past ancestors were regarded as those who received the laws of the land (Omenala) from the earth deity, 'Ala'

260 Loc. Cit.
261 Nnoli Edozien, op. Cit., p.131
262 Loc. Cit.
263 Ibid., p.135

and passed these on to future generations. In observing the laws and customs of the Omenala, one was said to be in union with the socio-spiritual head of the visible community, hence one is undoubtedly linked to its invisible segment-the dead 'Ndichie' (ancestors). To that end, it is a taboo and a great crime to speak against the ancestors-the living dead- or show irreverence or disrespect towards them. This is the principle from where the Igbo understanding of sustainability took its cues.

d. **Economy and Property:** Here, one sees that the economic life of the Igbo, who were primarily agrarian, was built upon and revolves around their land. To this end, stealing staple foods like yams, destroying the earth especially in the cutting of old trees, surreptitiously altering the boundary of a piece of land and claiming an unmerited title to it, or offending the ala by quarrelling during the 'Sacred week' (all referred to as 'Aru') are all punishable offenses against Omenala. This is what underlines the fundamental respect the Igbo people have for nature proving and underlying tendency to ecological sustainability.

The Omenala constitutes a great base for the FHG to touch down in the Nigerian context because of the ontological similarity that both share. Spirituality, which is a great character of both pedestals, remains the basic impulse and motivation for ethical-ecological investments.[264] This extended, lies in the fact that 'the context for all human activitiy is the totality of creation. Faithful action requires that we use our power to live in harmony with creation and affirm the independence of everything on earth and the dignity of all parts of creation. And to do less is to sow seeds of our own destruction. In this purview, the global economy is measured not only by what it produces and its impact on the environment, but also by how it touches human life and whether it protects or undermines the dignity of the human person. To this end, economic decisions possess human and moral consequences.[265]

3.7.6 Summary and Conclusion

Our aim in this section was to show that although there are no ethical-ecological criteriology or rating agency in Nigeria deploying the ethical criteria, there exist cultural pedestals that could help in the downloading of a foreign criteriology, which possess core similarities with the Nigerian reality. Among many of these

264 Claus Lücker. Spirituality: A Basic Impulse for Ethical-ecological Investment. In: Reisch, Lucia (ed.) Ethical-ecological Investment: Towards Global Sustainable Development. Frankfurt am Main. IKO-Verlag, 2001, p.31.

265 Loc. Cit.

cultural pedestals, the Omenala is one of those that rise to prominence became it is an ancient tradition, which embodies the life and aspirations of the Igbo people, and shares some deep connections with the pedestals of the Catholic social teaching, upon which the Frankfurt-Hohenheim Guidelines took its basic inspiration.

4. Introducing the Frankfurt-Hohenheim Guidelines as a Framework for our Examination

4.1 Introduction

The Frankfurt-Hohenheim Guidelines (FHG) is a set of guidelines or criteriology developed for the ethical assessment of companies. Ethical rating or assessment of companies, as reiterated earlier, is the assessment of companies on the basis of social, environmental, economic and ethical criteria. These are ratings which pay special attention to non-financial parameters, and often ethical criteria in evaluating companies, institutions, and investments.[266]

The FHG was developed within the framework of an interdisciplinary project, which could be seen in the depth of the criteria it encompassed. It was among others designed to bring the influence of moral reasoning to bear on the movements of capital in order to focus normative moral understanding, such as reflected in the ecological movement, and make it fruitful for the structuring of socio-economic life and for cultural development. This is in lieu of the belief that technological developments, economic systems, and monetary structures are not celestial constructions that dropped down from heaven. They are products of processes at work within the human society and culture; with all its imperfections and shortcomings. To this end, they are capable of changing culture as well as being influenced to change by the culture. Culture by virtue of the inherent moral understanding it possesses within it, is capable of changing any system or structure whether economic, technological or monetary, if these structures become destructive to the people it is meant to serve.[267] This is the basis of the effort of the FHG.

In order words, the guidelines are scaffolded by the conviction that economic activity is functionally dependent on the general recognition of moral standards. Such standards, which happen to be the conditio-sine-qua-non for economic activity, are neither products nor creatures of the economic system. These indispensable prerequisites upon which economic activity is based, lie outside the economic system; and are solidly anchored in the moral understanding of the social culture and its normative contents. But these standards can be adversely

266 Schäfer, H, et al. Who is who in Corporate Social Responsibility Rating?, Gütersloh, Bertelsmann Foundation, 2006, p.4

267 Hoffmann, Ott & Scherhon. Ethische Kriterien für die Bewertung von Unternehmen, Frankfurt am Main, IKO Verlag, 1997, p.109

affected, undermined, impaired or even destroyed by the economic system in extreme cases.[268]

The importance of criteria such as the FHG is underlined by the fact that many companies in contemporary times have gone rogue on their social responsibilities.[269] The increasing narrow conceptualization of profit canonized "shareholder value" as the Holy Grail, which companies and their directors must achieve over and above every other consideration. It was considered in many instances, their fiduciary duty. But ethical criteriologies arose as the gadflies who ask the question: Is shareholder value the only measure of worth for a business? Should it rightly and morally be considered the only legitimate aspiration for a company that operates in a society we claim to be human? What about the impact of business operations on our environment? What about ecological integrity consequent on manufacturing and business processes? What about the staff? What about the customers and their social relationships; which are all impacted upon by business processes and operations of companies? What about the safety of the product? Such criteriology aims to hold companies to their responsibilities, which should not be only the subject of legalisms, but from a deeper appreciation of our common nature and future.

4.2 A Brief History of the Formation and Development of the Frankfurt-Hohenheimer Guidelines

The FHG for the ethical assessment of companies was the product of interdisciplinary co-operation. Building on a comprehensive and integral approach to the concept of sustainable development, the interdisciplinary project group "Ethical-Ecological Rating, headed by Professors Johannes Hoffmann and Gerhard Scherhon, developed a scientifically-based criteriology for the ethical assessment of companies. This criteriology named the Frankfurt-Hohenheim-Guidelines conduces to the evaluation of business activities for their contributions, either positive or negative; to social, cultural and environmental sustainable development.

The FHG was constructed upon the quest for a fundamental change to the economic system at various levels, both global and local.[270] To this end, it hopes

268 Ibid., p.24

269 Cf. Naomi Klein, No Logo. Op. cit.

270 Cf. Ries, Simeon. Intercultural Assessment of Sustainability: Intercultural adaptability of oekom research AG's Corporate Responsibility Rating (CRR) according to the criteria of social and cultural responsibility, MBA Management Project Report Submitted to NIMBAS Graduate School of Management, 2001, p.19

and advocates that funds should be channelled or directed into channels, that lead to gradual changes in the everyday world, in the direction of encouraging innovation that are socially, environmentally, and culturally compatible.

The initial thesis of the FHG contends that development, systems and structures are not alien inventions that dropped down from space to us below, but are the results of social processes within a culture.[271]

4.3 The major pedestals of the FHG

The FHG methodology is based on the Renns Value-Tree Analysis (VTA), which emphasizes moral and evaluative parameters instead of technical and economic criteria. And based on a rational choice model of decision making, it reflects a dynamic approach, which does neither define sustainability nor the outcome of the process:

The Value tree of the Frankfurt-Hohenheim Guidelines' methodology is made up of three levels of criteria.

The first level sets a distinction between the normative structuring concepts; namely:

- ❖ Cultural Sustainability
- ❖ Social sustainability and
- ❖ Environmental sustainability

The second level analyses the spheres of action, such as "internal groups with special interests" in the branch of social sustainability.

The third level encompasses the concrete groups, such minorities, women, etc.

With this approach, over 200 criteria comprise a framework for the analysis of potential factors and questions for the assessment of a company from ethical-ecological perspectives.[272]

4.3.1 Social Sustainability

We have five areas of social compatibility, namely:

---

271 Hoffmann, Johannes, op. Cit, 1997, op. Cit.p.21

272 Project group Ethical-ecological Rating, EER (2000), Essays presented to the symposium "Intercultural responsibility of the ethical assessment of enterprises according to the criteria of cultural, social and environmental sustainability, Frankfurt, p.22, cited in Ries, S. op. cit., p. 21

A. Social Compatibility of company organization.

Here, the guideline measures factors like

- Management principles
- Hierarchy
- Organization strategies
- Work council, codetermination bodies
- Unions; collective agreements
- Codetermination in workplace
- Suggestion-box system

B. Internal Interest groups: general interests

In relation to this, the guidelines considers issues like

4.3.2 Working-hours regulations
4.3.3 Job security
4.3.4 Working atmosphere, mobbing
4.3.5 Humanizing of work conditions
4.3.6 Hiring and firing policies
4.3.7 Remuneration, bonuses, profit sharing
4.3.8 Health
4.3.9 Personnel development
4.3.10 Social Services

C. Internal interest groups: special interests

In this regard, issues considered include:

- Older employees
- Semi-skilled employees
- Foreign employees
- Trainees
- Handicapped employees
- Women
- Free-lance workers.
- Marginal employees
- Adolescents

- ➢ Children
- ➢ Sick persons
- ➢ Long-term unemployed
- ➢ Temporary employees

D. External Interest groups

In this regard, the guideline considers the companies relationship to the following

- Customers
- Foreign countries (esp. LDCs)
- Investors
- Competitors
- Suppliers
- Neighbourhood and neighbours
- General Public
- Sponsoring

b. Products.

Here, the guideline considers the following:
- ➢ Particular product areas
- ➢ Planned obsolescence

4.3.2 Environmental Sustainability

The environmental Compatibility Criteria has eight areas, namely:

1. Practices with respect to environmental institutions
2. Practices with respect to environmental information
3. Living beings
4. Energy
5. Materials
6. Transport
7. Emissions
8. Environmental Technology.

4.3.3 Cultural Sustainability

The basic requirement of cultural sustainability is that a company should respect the culture of its host nation or society, and should not interfere to change the culture simply for the sake of maximizing its profits.[273] And the classical dilemma is the question of whether in this purview should be construed valid the issue of a company adopting practices that are ethical questionable like bribery and corruption because they are common in the host country.

The Cultural Compatibility criteria have four areas of considerations, namely:

1. Anthropologically given motivational Structures

Under these structures, the Guidelines measure factors like

c. Responsibility vs. the right of the stronger (aggression vs. social welfare)
d. Close mindedness vs. Openness
e. Self-glorification vs. low profile
f. Competition vs. solidarity
g. Unlimited expansion vs. self restrain

2. General Moral Principles

The general moral principles are like a 'Decalogue'. They are moral principles which a company must observe in order to be deemed ethical in their practices. They are as follows:

a. You shall observe the fundamental bio-cultural norm in all spheres of activity
b. You shall not cause or inflict pain
c. You shall not render anyone incapable
d. You shall deprive no one of their freedom or opportuinities
e. You shall deprive no one of their pleasure in something
f. You shall not deceive or defraud
g. You shall keep your promises
h. You shall respect the property of others
i. You shall obey the law
j. You shall subject no one to moral obligations beyond their ability to fulfil them.

273 Hoffmann, Johannes, 1997, cited in Ries, Simeon, Intercultural Assessment of Sustainability, 2001, p.11

3. Value Concepts

The value concepts measures whether companies or investments are involved in or furthers

a. Unrestrained action:
b. And whether companies **accept limits in coexistence with others**

4. Virtues

Under virtues we have:

a. Cardinal virtues
b. Secondary virtues.

4.4 FHG's Implementation through Corporate Social Responsibility Rating (CRR)

The CRR is a product of the rating agency, *oekom Research AG*. The Rating, which subjects international companies from a wide variety of sectors of the economy to a scientifically-based analysis, was developed or based on what is considered by many as the most comprehensive set of criteria for ethical assessment of companies, namely: The Frankfurt-Hohenheim Guidelines (FHG). It was developed by oekom AG in conjunction with the Project Ethical-ökologische Rating; an academic interdisciplinary project group in Germany, led by the social ethicist, Prof. Dr. Johannes Hoffmann, and the economist Prof. Dr. Gerhard Scherhon. According to Dr. Simeon Ries, the FHG is a public good, only protected by copyright. This inheres in the fact that there can be no monopolistic use of the FHG. Any individual or institution can use the guidelines to develop a FHG-based rating system. And one of the companies to have been able to do this is the oekom Research, AG, Germany, who now own the CRR. [274]

The CRR assesses companies' responsibility towards the following:

1. The natural environment (Environmental Sustainability)
2. Persons affected by Corporate activities of the companies (Social Sustainability)
3. And Society and Culture (Cultural Sustainability)

274 Loc. Cit.

The basic structure of the CRR

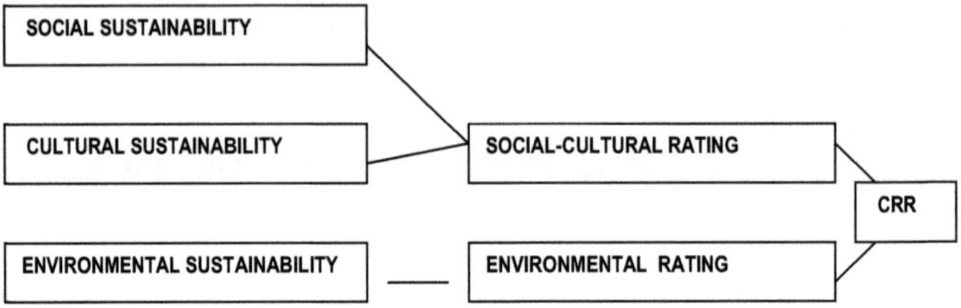

Part III Empirical Work

5. Examining the Relevance of the FHG Cultural Compatibility in the Nigerian Context

At this point, it is important once more to reiterate that our work employed the same questionnaire developed by the oekom research, AG on the basis of the Franfurt-Hohenheim Guidelines, and successfully adopted by Dr. Agi James Makil for the Indian context.[275]

The questionnaire which was used by Dr. Makil in the Indian context was modified to suit the Nigerian context and the case study, which we applied it to.

Dr. Makil's work, for which he earned a PhD, investigated if the ethical-ecological criteria developed off the Frankfurt-Hohenheim Guidelines and the corporate responsibility rating, offers a suitable basis for the assessment of companies in the Indian context. He equally sought to see the relevance or otherwise of the FHG in the measurement and promotion of sustainable development in India.

It is the same ideas that we have for Nigeria. But while Dr. Makil used companies quoted in the Indian stock exchange for his case study, we used microfinance banks, which are supposed to be in the frontlines, in the battle against poverty in Nigeria.

Pointing out this difference is important because of the fact that even though we applied a derivative of the FHG in examining the contemporary problems faced by the various societies we investigated, the socio-economic and cultural contexts of India and Nigeria varies tremendously. And this is the beauty of the FHG; which is that it could with modifications, be made to speak to the socio-economic and cultural realities of different environments.

275 See: Agi, James Makil, Ethisch-okologische Bewertung von Unternehmen in Indien auf Basis des Frankfurt-Hohenheimer-Leitfadens und des Corporate Responsibility Ratings-Prufung der interkulturellen Brauchbarkeit vom Frankfurt-Hohenheimer-Leitfaden und des Corporate Responsibility Ratings fur die Messung und Forderung von Nachhaltigkeit im Indischen Kontext: Doctoral dissertation submitted to the Faculty of Catholic Theology of the Johann Wolfgang Goethe University, Frankfurt am Main, 2008

5.1 Cultural Compatibility/Sustainability Survey

5.2 Hypothesis

The hypothesis we formulated, which our empirical research sets to validate or otherwise is in relation to the Cultural compatibility rating of the Frankfurt-Hohenheim Guidelines is as follows:

Over all, the Cultural Compatibility/sustainability rating of the Frankfurt-Hohenheim Guidelines is relevant in the Nigerian context.

5.3 Questionnaire Evaluation and Results

5.3.1 General Moral Principles

5.3.1.1 Principle 1: You shall Observe the Fundamental Bio-cultural norm in all spheres of activity (FHG 3.2.1)

As a matter of principle, people should help protect the natural resource base, on which the lives of future generations will depend

One could readily see that Question 1 is the conversion of criteria 3.2: (General Moral Principles), sub, 3.2.1 (You shall observe the fundamental bio-cultural norms in all spheres of activity) into a question. The respondents were asked if in an ethical-ecological criteria designed to rate companies in Nigeria, whether this question to companies should be a relevant inclusion into the list of criteria, which companies must possess or pass in order to be declared ethical-ecological compliant in their views.

There were various admixtures of reasons for their positions. Most of the respondents did not give single reasons for their positions; they gave reasons that could be grouped under so many different headings. For instance, some of the respondents, who listed *"the fear and respect of God*" as their reasons for feeling strongly that we should protect our natural resource base as a matter of principle, including in the same sentence, *the fear not to attract the curse of our ancestors*, as another reason for their positions. Untangling these reasons, the major recurring reasons include:

1. The respect and fear of the creator (84%)
2. The respect and fear of attracting the curse of our ancestors 42 %
3. The need to avail the future generations the chance at life (49%)

QUALITATIVE ANALYSIS	
This first principle: "*As a matter of principle, people should help protect the natural resource base, on which the lives of future generations will depend*" sets the tone and the groundwork for the whole questionnaire on cultural sustainability. The results post a remarkable concern for the environment across the spectrum in Nigeria quite oblivious of religious affiliation or area of the country that the respondents come from. This shows that 100% of the respondents felt strongly that as a matter of principle that the natural resource base should be protected; and that all and sundry should be involved in this. Surprisingly on this score, there were no dissents. It was a unanimous portrayal of an ecological consciousness, which though strongly present across board in Nigeria, has hitherto failed to percolate into the business mainstream, or find lucid expression in corporate policies of so many firms and enterprises, as could be gleaned from the actions of some levels of government, companies and multinationals, most especially in the oil sector. This could be strongly interpreted to mean that Nigerians, especially those at the receiving end of the economic process are strongly in favour of seeing the protection of our natural resource base, as a matter of principle. And one must bear in mind that those in this class represent over 70% of Nigerians whom the World Bank claimed are living below the poverty line.	Strongly yes (+2) 100% Yes (+1) 0% Undecided (0) 0% No (-1) 0% Strongly No (-2) 0%

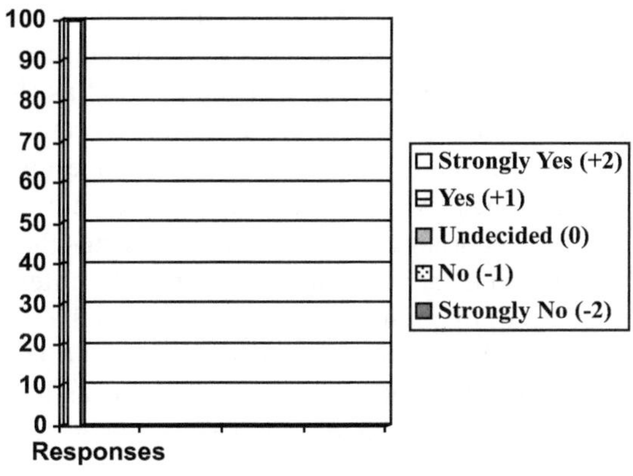

4. To avoid Catastrophes like drought and desertification (20%)
5. No reason listed (16%)

These reasons advanced by the respondents show that God/ancestors are major players in the consideration of Nigerians when it comes to ecological issues bordering on the natural environment. This portrays a religious bent, which could be used as a vehicle for sensitizing Nigerians on the dangers of not protecting their natural environment. God and the ancestors play a role in the consideration of Nigerians. Some non-African observer may be forced to gloss over this important factor, or dismiss it as a reflection of a society fossilized at a socio-economic anomie, still clutching to some outdated mental schemata populated by fear of the unknown. But over and above the Nigerian social space being saturated with God-talk[276], this may not be unrelated to Africa psyche being emblazoned with religious sentiments. Mbiti was on record as reminding us that to be an African is to be religious. And the response elicited by this question seems to drive home that fact. In a similar development, Ndidi Nnoli Edozien, in her work designed to shed some insight into the ownership structure of Igbo businesses discovered a similar trend; where about 83% of respondents to her questionnaire responded that their businesses belonged to God, over the 99% who responded that their businesses belonged to them.[277]

Across the responses, one notices that all elements of African cosmology are represented, though in varying dimensions and intensity, as reflected in the percentage of those who gave those as their reasons, which one sees reoccurring throughout most of the responses. This sits well with the African conception that all natural resources belong to God, as well as to the community; [278]as could be seen in 84% of the respondents citing respect for God as the reasons for their strong feelings that the natural environment should be protected. 42% listing the respect and fear of attracting the displeasure of their ancestors is reflective of the African holistic cosmology, where time and existence are one continual tapestry of cyclic import; comprising the world of the living-(the present) the living dead-(Past; ancestors) and the unborn(the future). The inference could equally be drawn here that traces of communal ownership could be established. Africans agree that the world and all in it belongs to God and to the community. This agrees with the findings of Obiora Ike and Nnoli-Edozien (2001), that in Africa, "...communal ownership existed and is understood as a way to connect people

276 God-talk is used to depict the fact that Nigerians are massive adherents to religions of various faith expressions.

277 Nnoli-Edozien, Ndidi., Ownership and Management Structure in the Economy: African Traditional Values Applied to Modern Issues of Sustainability and the Corporate Governance Function, Enugu, CIDJAP Publications, 2007, p.276

278 Ibid., p.203

to their Creator, to their economy, to their community, to their workplace and to each other". And ownership, understood in a sustainable manner, was such that the interests of the ancestors, the future generations and the present living members of society were considered integrally and concurrently.[279] In line with thinking about the present, 20% of the respondents cited the need to avoid catastrophes like drought and desertification that could jeopardize the ability of the present to sustain life and livelihoods.

In lieu of cultural sustainability, defined as the compatibility of economic activities with the progressing cultivation of society's potential for social change with respect to the individual's chance of development and self-realisation; the community's integrating abilities; the natural environment's and the future generations' abilities to survive and the chances of indigenous cultural development, we can see that an interpretation of the views of our respondents are in perfect agreement with these tenets. This could be well appreciated when one takes FHG's definition of "potential for change", as it applies in the definition of cultural sustainability. Here potential for change is construed as referring to the general consensus on the culture specific outlooks on life, the cultural arrangements, and the way societies symbolize their view on time, experience their visions and forward their perspectives for human development in community.

The responses to Question 1 transcended its statistical implication to show a pattern of internalized perspective on life, or what the "potential for change" (vide, Supra) denotes as 'culture-specific outlooks on life' and 'the way societies experience their visions and forward their perspectives for human development in community". And the way Africans forward these views as could be seen from the patterns established by our responses, which is that all nature environing us belongs primarily to God; and that in respect to the supreme deity, we should pay our respects to his creation and not abuse it. This view agrees with FHG's Cultural sustainability interpretation of "cultural arrangement", which is construed to consist of 'manifest perspectives, institutions and rules; and also deals with symbols, rituals, myths all of which give orientation for interpreting the world and shaping people's life in harmony with nature.[280]

By overwhelmingly voting for this criterion, our respondents are in effect sending a clear message that no company should be rated as culturally sustainable, if its activities, policies and operations stand in violation of the natural environment. Under this purview, so many Multi-national concerns operating in the Niger Delta, who are responsible for gas flaring, oil spillage and environmental pollution, will never qualify as culturally sustainable firms.

279 Ike and Nnoli Edozien, Understanding Africa, 2001, p.106

280 Ethical-Ecological Project/oekom Research AG (eds.), op. cit., p.28

5.3.1.1.1 Question 1.1: Is it relevant to ask; whether companies profit from executions and the displacement of ethnic groups

QUALITATIVE ANALYSIS	
This second question, which is an adaptation of criterion 3.2.1.2 of the FHG was in keeping with the over all component of Cultural sustainability rating. Here we see some extremes in the responses submitted by our respondents. 69% of the respondents view this question as totally relevant, and should be a major question or hurdle which every company must overcome, in order to be declared culturally sustainable. In between stands no one as could be seen in the fact that none of the respondents see it as relevant. The majority saw it a totally relevant, indicating that they feel strongly about it. 25% of the respondents were undecided, while 6% see it as irrelevant; and no one saw it as totally irrelevant. Here, there were no overriding reasons advanced for their responses. Some contend that this question should be a major furniture of any ethical-ecological rating for Nigeria because of the fact that the respect of human dignity is an important right, which companies should not be allowed to violate, even if they are microfinance banks.	Totally relevant (+2) 69% Relevant (+1) 0% Undecided (0) 25% Not Relevant (-1) 6% Totally not relevant (-2) 0%

Is it Relevant to ask whether Firms profit from Execution and Displacement of Ethnic

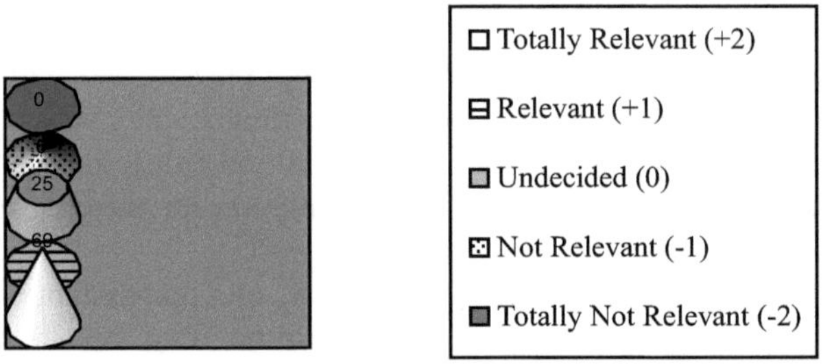

Without any intention of reading meanings into indices that were not given in the responses, one must realise that capital punishments are recognized under the Nigerian law. It is equally.pertinent to note that even after the civil war, when human rights were at their nadir, and death clouded the sky, years of military dictatorship have brutalized the psyche of Nigerians and seems to have inured them to offering a kind of pathological apathy to human rights issues. That 25%

are undecided on this score may be thanks to such pathological acquiescence. We could add that to the fact that extra judicial killings by the Police and the military and political assassinations have been commonplace in the Nigerian social space to warrant a huge outrage. This situation may be due to the wider fact that human rights have taken a huge battering in the Nigerian public space. That 69% saw that as relevant may be thanks to a lot of factors which our questionnaire was not designed to elicit. Over and above the basic decency of much of humanity, the African believes that life is the supreme good: Ndu bu isi- (Life is the greatest good) as the Igbos of Southern Nigeria would have it. And this could be inferred from the responses, which transcended religious boundaries.

That a significant number-25% are undecided equally speaks of the fear that accompanies freedom of expression in Nigeria, as could be seen in the Ken Saro Wiwa's case, who was executed by the State for protesting the destruction of the cultural and ecological basis of life and livelihood of his people in the Niger Delta. That this percentage subsisted in spite of the fact that many communities have been displaced by oil prospecting activities in Niger Delta, may be thanks to the economic hardship facing Nigerians which makes them susceptible to caring and relating to their basic Maslownian needs against the broader picture, which equally affect their lives radically, when the factors are counted.

5.3.1.2 Principle 2: You shall not Cause/Inflict pain (FHG 3.2.2)

As a matter of principle, people should not cause or inflict pain

QUALITATIVE ANALYSIS	
On the third question, which queried whether the respondents believe that companies striving to be classified as ethical-ecological compatible; or whether they as investors would love companies especially microfinance firms and banks to eschew inflicting pain on others as a matter of principle; for them to be considered an ethically sound portfolio for investment; there were quite some interesting observations. 75% of the respondents are strongly of the opinion that firms should eschew inflicting or causing pain on others as a matter of principle. 13% believe that should be the case, but not as strongly as the 75%. 6% were undecided; standing on the middle. Another 6% are of the opinion that that shouldn't be included in the criteria that companies must fulfil in order to be deemed ethical.	Strongly Yes (+2) 75% Yes (+1) 13% Undecided (0) 6% No (-1) 6% Strongly No (-2) 0%

People should not not cause or inflict pain

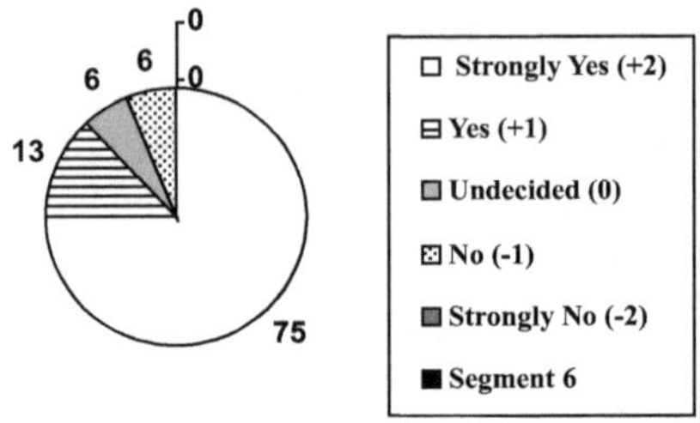

Most of our respondents did not offer reasons for their answers. We can only guess at what their inspirations are in this case. I am compelled to think that every ethical tradition begins with the fact that not inflicting pain on others is a self evident basis upon which every interaction between human beings at whatever level should commence. Our respondents seem not to be left out of this ethical foundation. The Igbos of Nigeria articulated this in their "Egbe belu ugbo belu" philosophy", as well as in their "Nwa mmuo emegbuna nwa mmadu, nwa mmadu emegbuna nwa muo", attitude to relationships both at the interpersonal or business levels. Like earlier reiterated, this is conjectural at worst.

This may have inspired the inability of our respondents to articulate their reasons why companies should eschew from inflicting pain, although they overwhelming voted that it is totally relevant to ask whether companies are involved in actions, products or processes that inflicts or is capable of inflicting pain on others as a matter of principle. That is for the majority. 6 percent of our respondents contend that it is not relevant to ask whether companies inflict pain or not, as a part of the criteria to measure ethical compatibility. One recurring reason advanced was that what pain may mean here is ambiguous. Some respondents contended that no matter what one does, there is someone who is at a disadvantage or pain. Some other respondents contended that some pain administered to attain an end that is of benefit to the whole community is not ethically wrong. Here one respondent gave the instance of government destroying some houses with the aim of build roads that will benefit the whole community, or in respect of adhering to the master plan of the city.

5.3.1.2.1 Question 2.1: The behaviour of International Companies in a local context

Is it relevant to ask, whether International companies supply dangerous products that are prohibited in the home country to Nigeria, where the products are considered "harmless" (Toxic waste)

QUALITATIVE ANALYSIS

This question which is to elicit the responses of the respondents on what ethical standard international firms or multinationals should be subjected to, in order to determine their ethical compatibility, was like all other questions, a recast of the criterion 3.2.2.2 of the FHG.

69% of the respondents are of the view that the question is totally relevant to any such criteria that would be valid in the Nigerian context. That is the simple majority. No other position attracted such a massive vote. 6% view the question as simply relevant. 6% were undecided. They were neither concurred nor disagreed with any of the positions. 12% thought the question irrelevant to any such criteriology.

Coming to reasons submitted for the various positions, some of those who thought the question irrelevant were of the opinion that the regulation of what foreign firms do in the Nigerian business space is the province of the government. And that if the government does its job well, the criteriology will be freed from such concerns in order to face other issues that most urgently need to be included.

QUANTITATIVE ANALYSIS

Totally Relevant (+2) 69%

Relevant (+1) 6%

Undecided (0) 6%

Not Relevant (-1) 6%

Totally Not Relevant (-2) 12%

Opinion on what International Companies are allowed

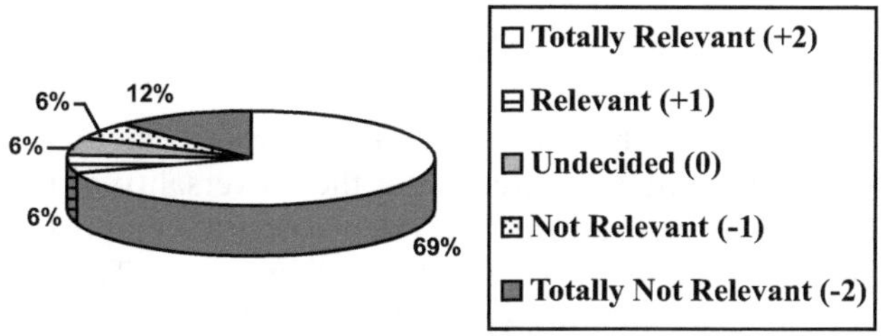

5.3.1.3 Principle 3: You shall not render anyone incapable (FHG 3.2.3)

As a matter of principle, people should not constrain the capability of others

QUALITATIVE ANALYSIS	QUANTITATIVE ANALYSIS
This question which was constructed from criterion 3.2.3 of the FHG falls under the ten commandments of general moral principles. 88% of the respondents strongly feel that asking the question that people should as a matter of principle not constrain the capability of others, is relevant to any criterion invented for the sake of rating companies in the Nigerian context. No votes were recorded for those who feel simply that it is right. The same goes for the undecided and those who said "No". But those who said a "strong no" were 12% of the respondents. That over 80% of the respondents is in favour of that shows the relevance of it to the Nigerian context.	STRONGLY YES (+2) 88% YES (+1) 0% UNDECIDED (0) 0% NO (-1) 0% STRONGLY NO (-2) 12%

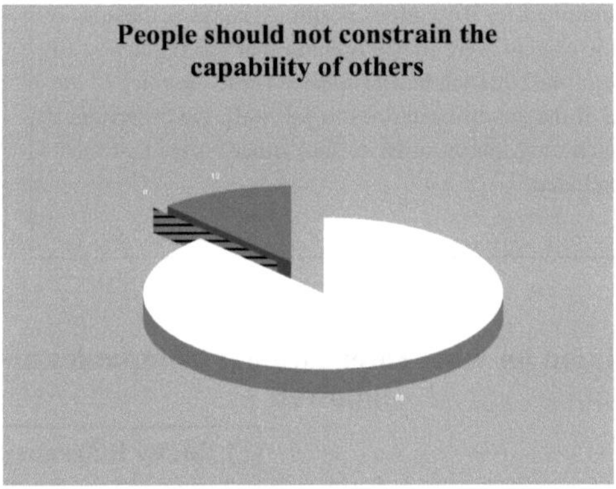

The reasons advanced by the respondents for their answers are not significant enough as to create a pattern or trend. But the universality of the golden rule could be a path of the explanation to that. The respondents simply feel that it is not good to constrain or destroy the capability of other people. There were no great philosophical reasons for their answers; which could mean that it is a norm that they live by, even if they cannot articulate great philosophical treatises to buttress or support their answers. And that they were ready to see this translated into the business environment speaks to the eternal yawning of all men for some moral order in the course of the events environing their lives. This is akin to what is seen in the very next question, which reads like a follow-up on this one.

5.3.1.4 Principle 4: As a matter of principle, people should deprive no one of their freedom or opportunities (FHG 3.2.4)

QUALITATIVE ANALYSIS

This question, which is seems to flow from the preceding one, is in actual fact an expansion of the content of the former. This at least seems to be the understanding of our respondents as the filled in their opinions without any of them listing any reasons for their answers. On this question, 94% of the respondents are strongly in support of the question and only 6% were undecided. These were the only two values that were filled in. This shows a very broad support of this point. And this attests to its relevance in the Nigerian context.

STRONGLY YES (+2)	94%
YES (+1)	0%
UNDECIDED (0)	6%
No (-1)	0%
STRONGLY NO (-2)	0%

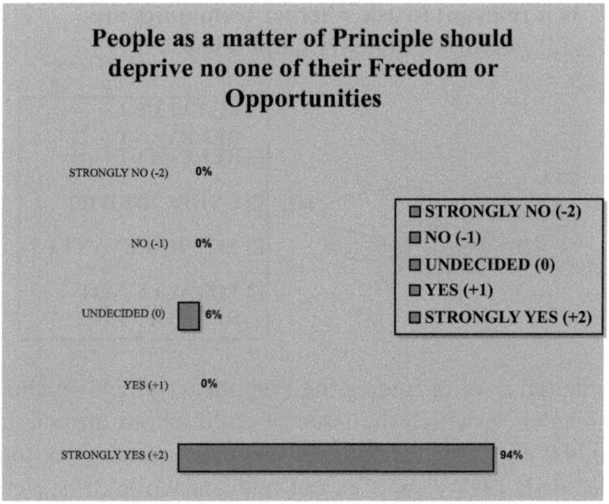

5.3.1.4.1 Question 4.1: Is it relevant to ask whether companies tolerate heavy child labour?

QUALITATIVE ANALYSIS	
This question, which is a reworking of criterion 3.2.4 of the FHG was intended to elicit responses which would reflect the opinions of Nigerians on child labour as it holds and applies in their context, and whether that should make its way into any criteriology designed to shoulder or show the cultural compatibility of companies in the Nigerian context. 44% see the question as totally relevant. 12% of the respondents were undecided. 19% viewed it as not relevant, while 25% see it as totally irrelevant. A variety of reasons were advanced for the various stands taken. But majority of them reflect a cross-cultural conflict between two conceptual schemes, which has defined Nigeria socio-cultural evolution in the present time.	Totally Relevant (+2) 44% Relevant (+1) 0% Undecided (o) 12% Not Relevant (-1) 19% Totally not Relevant (-2) 25%

Is it relevant to ask whether companies are involved in heavy child labour?

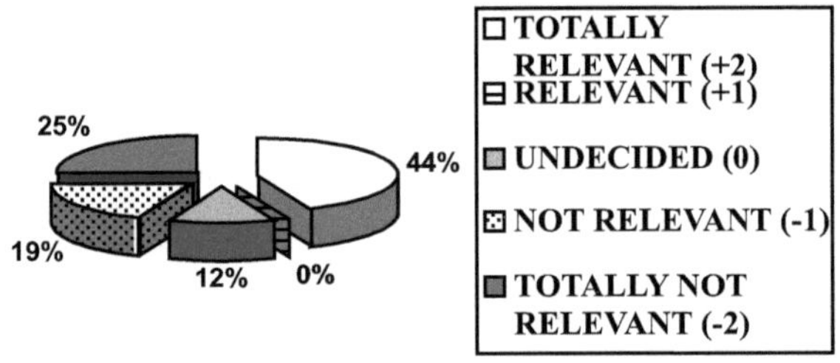

This question elicited a lot of interesting responses, which we can conclude; attests to the ambivalence, which the issue of child labour attracts in the African social embrace. 44% of our respondents view the question as totally relevant. 12% were undecided. 19% view it as not relevant while 25% view it as totally not relevant. This is a reflection of the conflict between what many term western conceptual schemes and African traditional pedestals of socio-cultural import. In Africa, since time immemorial children have been parts of the family structure, where everyone has had his own share of work, and is expected to contribute his own labour in the family farm, right from the earliest ages when he could function as an individual entity. This labour according to Chinua Achebe in Things Fall Apart is what in idiomatic terms helps, "a child to wash his hands, as to be able to dine with the elders". A child is supposed to learn how to work and to cut his teeth in household chores before ascending the social pedestal of responsibility as he grows up. In most parts of Africa, labour even for kids is a norm of socialization and not deemed exploitation. But the cultural fluidity and contact with western civilization challenged this traditional conceptual scheme and sought to impose western conceptual standards on African sociological themes. This seems to be what generates this ambivalence. One could see from the responses and the table, that the sum total of the respondents who see it as irrelevant; that is adding those who say it is not relevant, which is 19% and those who say it is totally not relevant, which is 25%, it equals the number that says it is totally relevant. And if we add the people, who are undecided-12%-; or who are caught in between those who see it as not relevant, we would have a majority-56%-,who are unconcerned about that as an issue, or who see it as a non issue altogether.

Child labour in Nigeria is a very touchy issue. This is understandable in spite of the efforts of the authorities to make laws prohibiting the exploitation of the child. But the problem commences, when one questions what should be included in child labour or child exploitation. Do we classify the domestic labour performed in one's own household, the household of relatives or of other families as child labour? Do we classify farm work on the family farm as child labour, or do we classify begging, petty sales and services performed by urban children managed by their own households as child labour? All these are the touchy areas, which from the reasons advanced by our respondents happen to be the factors informing their opinions on this point. Added to this ambiguity is the excruciating economic situation in Nigeria. With over 70% of the population living below poverty line, one could understand the hesitations of families subsisting on meagre resources, in closing all doors to some extra income, which their kids no matter their ages, could bring into the family. With the high illiteracy rate, many families are peopled by parents with low skills to market, who are forced by their situation into various kinds of dependencies, even depending on their kids to bring in some income, either from street hawking or begging, which exposes these kids to a lot of social, health and psychological dangers.

All in all, this is one other veritable example that ethics is really culture specific. And we argue that if this point is to make its way into any criteria designed for the Nigerian context, it must be radically examined and reworked as to reflect local normative systems and structures. If this is not done, its validity for the local context may be seriously questioned as has been reflected in the opinion of our respondents.

5.3.1.4.2 Question 4.2: Is it relevant to ask whether companies create working conditions detrimental to the family?

QUALITATIVE ANALYSIS	
In reaction to this question, 56% of our respondents are of the view that it is totally relevant as a part of the questions that must face Microfinance banks operating in the Nigerian environment if they are to be considered ethical in their policies and operations. 13% were undecided. 6% found it not relevant while 25 percent found it totally irrelevant. Many of the reasons advanced showed no pattern that could support a conclusion that there is a common refrain among the respondents. One thing noticeable here though is a trend that runs through the entire responses given. Nigerians are as variegated as there are persons in the country. To this end, one may not be surprised if one finds 4 different people holding four different and parallel ideas on the same subject. That is the ideological beauty of Nigeria, and this extrapolated to another level may be the reason why consensus both at the social and political levels are pretty difficult ends to achieve.	Totally Relevant (+2) 56% Relevant (+1) 0% Undecided (0) 13% Not Relevant (-1) 6% Totally not Relevant (-2) 25%

Whether Companies should create working conditions detrimental to the family?

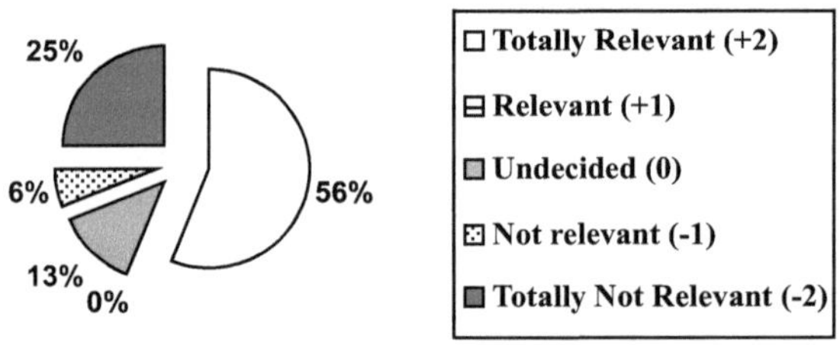

A look at the results here shows that 56% is not an overwhelming majority. Does this point to a trend that African family values are eroding, or are in regress in the face of economic downturn which Nigeria has been experiencing for quite some time now? This question is important because if a society changes radically, the cultural basis upon which its ethics could be based is equally affected. For instance, in a state or social construct where the sources of social legitimacy is violently overthrown, or where the chains of authority is replaced in a very radical way, the people may come to subscribe to new sources of social legitimacy which has no respect for the long cultural basis upon which the people have made their moral decisions and choices all through their history. This is a poor example, but when Hitler overthrew the Weimar republic in Germany, it introduced a radical shift in the source of social legitimacy from the society to the Fuhrer. And people were compelled to do anything for the sake of the Fuhrer, even when those courses of action defeat their reason, or do violence to their moral codes and principles. The same may be the case with the Nigerian family situation, which as can be observed from the fact that 25% of our respondents view taking companies to task over their fidelity to family welfare programmes as totally irrelevant, in an ethical-ecological criteriology designed to confer a badge of ethical compatibility on companies in Nigeria. This is further compounded by the fact that 6% see it as not relevant, while 13% are comfortably sitting on the fence; undecided. One could see that the sum total of those who are either undecided or who view it as irrelevant-44%-is very close to the majority that see it as relevant-56%. And in such a multivalent social embrace, the voices of the minority, especially a simple minority that has a 44% stake should not be easily swept under the carpet.

There were no compelling reasons, which aggregated to create a trend as to why the respondents answered the way they did. A sprinkling of respondents, who viewed the question as irrelevant to the criteriology; when their reasons are taken apart, seems to have bought the contractarian model of companies, which is operational in the Nigerian business environment. Their views that companies are simply there to maximize profit for its shareholders, and that making policies that would benefit families remains the reserve of the government seems to have informed their responses. We therefore argue that if this criterion is to be brought into a criteriology, which is rightly its place, a deconstruction of the contractarian model need to be undertaken to sensitize Nigerians on the import of not losing their families values to the onslaught of commercial interests of the few. Recapturing and propagating family values in the Nigerian business environment should be of the highest priority. The family happens to be the basis of every society. Whatever goes wrong in the family is reflected in the whole society. To this end, no ethical consideration that bypasses this foundation of all socio-economic, political and cultural relationship is worth any serious consideration or thought. This fact is what vouches for the validity of this question, and validates its inclusion in the FHG.

5.3.1.4.3 Question 4.3: Is it relevant to ask, whether companies cooperate with countries in which ethic, political or religious minorities or women are systematically oppressed?

QUALITATIVE ANALYSIS	
Here 44% of the respondents deemed the question totally relevant. 6% are of the opinion that it is relevant. 31% chose to stay on the fence. Another 6% deemed it not relevant, while 13% of the respondents feel that the question is totally irrelevant. Here the sum of the respondents who are undecided and those who think that the question is irrelevant are equal to the simple majority that deems the question as relevant. This is to say that the opinion here is evenly divided, though not on the same intensity.	Totally Relevant (+2) 44% Relevant (+1) 6% Undecided (0) 31% Not Relevant (-1) 6% Totally not relevant (-2) 13%

Co-operation with countries that systematically oppress minorities and women

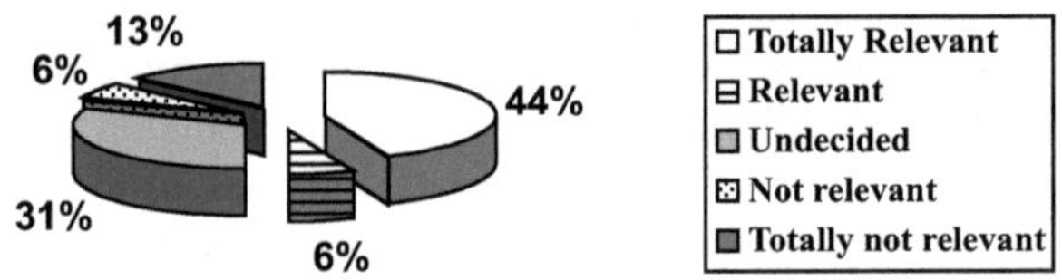

This criterion recasts our attention to the toxic fallouts that has attended the relationship between business and power centres. History has dutifully recorded that business, mostly construed in the contractarian sense, has this great facility of succumbing to the temptation of choosing success over conscience.[281] In the Nigerian example, Big Oil concerns have chosen profit over the ecological integrity of the environment where they prospect for oil. To this end, the Niger Delta ecology has been ripped asunder. This ecological collapse deprives the people of this riverine community of their means of survival and livelihood.

History's face has been darkened by business collaborating with ethically leprous regimes and power centres, to create monumental havocs and abominable atrocities that have grown to haunt human memory. A perfect example of this was seen in Nazi Germany, where the big businesses and heavy industry collaborated in creating the most monstrous military might and evil regime known to 19th cen-

281 See: Guido Knopp, Hitler's Managers, München, Goldmann Verlag, 2007, p.7

tury mankind. Hitler was supported by brilliant managers and business conglomerates like Albert Speer, Ferdinand Porsche, Fritz Thyssen, Gustav Krupp, Hjalmar Schacht, Alfred Jodl, Werner von Braun and so many others. This regime enjoyed the patronage and support of great companies like IG Farben, the chemical giant, which created and manufactured the zyklon B gas, used in the extermination of Millions of European Jewry. Reviewing the case of these men and that of all such historical scoundrels, Guido Knopp posed serious moral questions: *"Waren sie willige Helfer der Nazis, dachten sie nur an den eigenen Erfolg? Konnten sie sich der Vereinnahmung durch Hitlers Diktatur nicht entziehen? Hatten sie es tun können, wenn sie es gewolt hätten?"* (Were they willing helpers of the Nazis, were they thinking only about their own personal successes? Couldn't they extricate themselves from Hitler's dictatorship? Would they have done it, even if they had wanted to?).[282]

Finding answers to these questions are pretty tough. But Knopp was right about a point, which could be extrapolated to every other inglorious regime, be they in the past, present and in the future. This is to the effect that evil regimes desperately need the employment of good managers to proliferate unchallenged. About the Nazi regime, Knopp writes:

> Das NS-Regime brauchte Manager, wenngleich es dieses Nachkriegswort nicht selbst benutzte: Ohne sie, die >>Meister<<ihres Fachs als Banker, Unternehmer, Konstrukteure, Ingenieure oder Militärs, wäre Hitlers Reich nicht effektiv gewesen.[283]

This translated means that the National Socialist regime needed managers, even though the regime itself never used this word, which could have been anachronistic based on the fact that this word gained currency after the Second World War. Without these men, who are masters and experts in their fields as bankers, entrepreneurs, constructors, engineers and military strategies, Hitler's Reich would not have been effective.

The FHG is aware that the relationship between companies doing business in countries where rogue regimes are in power raises a lot of moral dilemma. Back to our example as eruditely articulated by Knopp. During Hitler's regimes, many of these talented men and great industrialists, who did not march with the regime or did not go on exile, were sucked into the vortex of the regime. Sight must equally not be lost of the fact that many others considered their personal success more than their consciences. This according to Knopp is the reason why the history of these men, whom he called Hitler's managers, remains a lesson for us all and for all times.[284]

---

282 Guido, Knopp., Op. Cit. P.7

283 Loc. Cit.

284 Ibid.

That 44% of our respondents deem this totally relevant and 6% deem it as relevant making up 50% of the positive scale gives room for worry. One would have expected that in a multi-ethnic nation like Nigeria, people would worry about the survival of their ethnic nationalities and other primeval allegiances much more than so many other considerations. But the responses show that 31% of the respondents are undecided. This may be construed to mean that they deem other things of central importance than the rights of minorities, especially women; or that systematic oppression of minorities is not on the front burner in a country where almost every section is screaming of being marginalized in the larger scheme of things or in the share of the national cake. We can adduce from the responses and from other sources that this is reflection of the fact that Nigerians are still struggling with their basic Maslownian needs as to pay heed to other factors on the Maslownian scale of human needs.

5.3.1.4.4 Question 4.4: Is it relevant to ask, whether international companies attempt in an aggressive manner to impose their own methods and values on the Nigerian people?

QUALITATIVE ANALYSIS

To this question, 56% of the respondents viewed the question as totally relevant to such a criteriology in the Nigerian context. 6% were undecided. 19% viewed it as not relevant, while another 19% were convinced that it is totally irrelevant as a constituent of such a criteriology.

Many of the respondents here offered various reasons for their answers, as has been the case throughout the questionnaires. But majority of those who viewed the questions as totally relevant were of the opinion that protecting local banks and industries will help the Nigerian economy grow and create jobs for millions of young Nigerian school-leavers, who due to lack of jobs wander the streets and are susceptible to falling into nefarious activities like armed robbery, 419 (Advanced Fee Fraud) and other ugly activities that are socially reprehensible.

There is no steady pattern created by the reasons given by those who viewed the question as not relevant. A few gave the reasons that the question is not relevant to such a criteria because there are not too many foreign companies in the microfinance banking sector in Nigeria, and that the control of international companies and whatever line of action they choose is the exclusive preserve of the government.

Totally Relevant (+2)	56%
Relevant (+1)	0%
Undecided (0)	6%
Not Relevant (-1)	19%
Totally Not relevant (-2)	19%

International Companies aggessively imposing their methods and Values on the Nigerian People

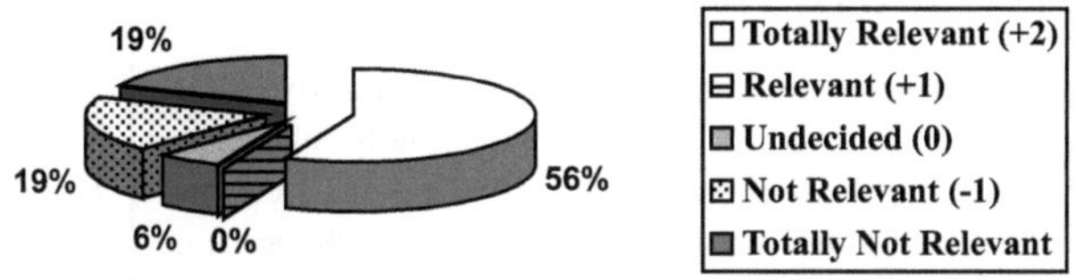

5.3.1.4.5 Question 4.5: Is it relevant to ask, whether companies in Nigeria buy patents not to use them but to keep competitors off the market?

QUALITATIVE ANALYSIS	
In reaction to this question, 44% of the respondents view the question as totally relevant, while 6% see it as merely relevant. 38% of the respondents were undecided. And 6% apiece were of the view that it is not relevant and totally not relevant. From the table, one could see that the sum of half of the respondents were either undecided or in disagreement with the relevance of the question as a constituent of such a criteriology. One of the major trends running through the reasons submitted by those who were undecided was that they cannot determine the relevance of this question in the sense that in the area of banking and finance, patents are not the order of the day. Some of the stated that on a wider scale, which would apply to other industries that deal on goods, methods, and productive processes, that the question would then adopt another character altogether, which would have bought a switch of their opinion from their inability to make a decision to the "totally relevant" column.	Totally Relevant (+2) 44% Relevant (+1) 6% Undecided (0) 38% Not Relevant (-1) 6% Totally Not relevant (-2) 6%

Buying Patents to keep competitors off the market

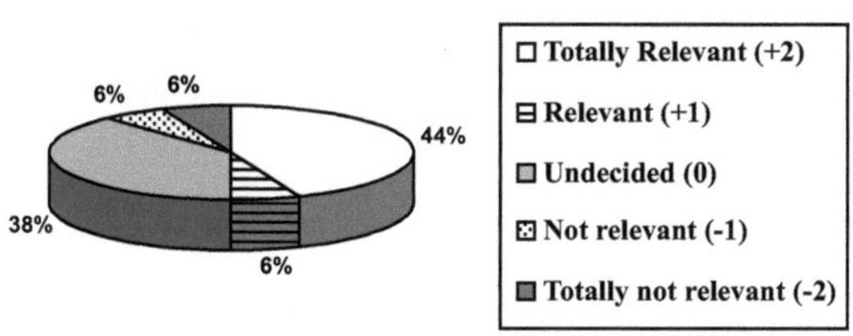

5.3.1.5 Principle 5: As a matter of principle, people should deprive no one of their pleasure in something? (FHG 3.2.5)

QUALITATIVE ANALYSIS	
This question elicited a response that was strong on the positive scale. 68% of the respondents construed the question as totally relevant to any such criteriology for the Nigerian context. 13% saw it as relevant, while another 13% were sitting on the fence; undecided. 6% saw it as totally irrelevant. Majority of those who viewed it positively cited the freedom of an individual to engage himself in any thing legitimate, as a fundamental human right, which no construct or business should help to destroy or be seen to collaborate in denying the people. The majority who marked it totally not relevant did not offer reasons for their response.	Totally Relevant (+2) 68% Relevant (+1) 13% Undecided (0) 13% Not Relevant (-1) 0% Totally Not relevant (-2) 6%

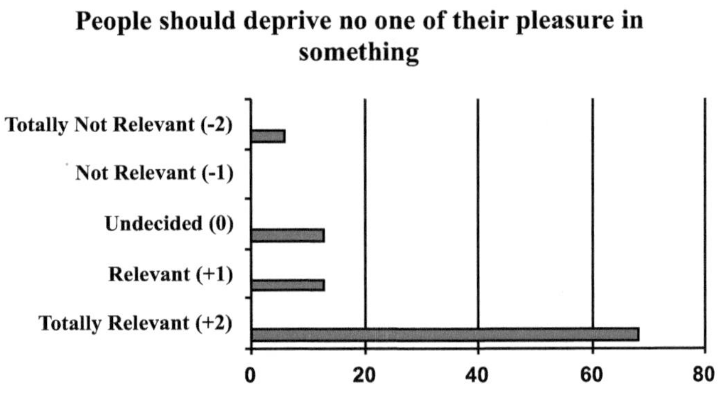

5.3.1.5.1 Question 5.1: Is it relevant to ask whether companies show respect for indigenous traditions, rites and festivals

QUALITATIVE ANALYSIS	
In response to whether this question is relevant to any ethical-ecological criteria in the Nigerian context under the FHG cultural compatibility rating, 50% viewed it as totally relevant. 25% viewed it as relevant. 19% were undecided, while only 6% saw it as not relevant.	Totally Relevant (+2) 50% Relevant (+1) 25% Undecided (0) 19% Not Relevant (-1) 6% Totally Not relevant (-2) 0%

Is it relevant for Companies to show respect for Indigenous traditions, rites and festivals?

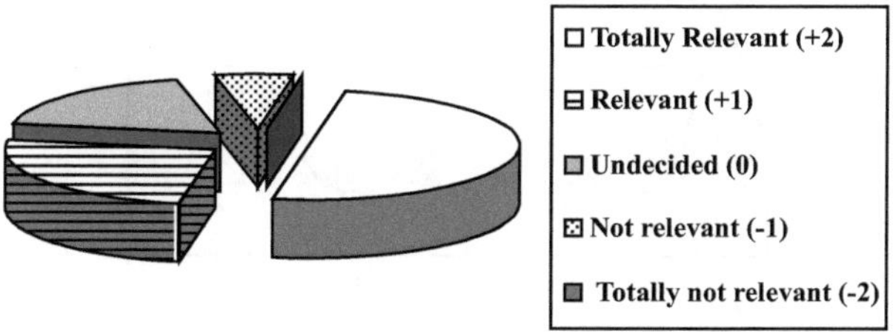

5.3.1.6 Principle 6: As a matter of principle, people should not deceive or defraud? (FHG 3.2.6)

QUALITATIVE ANALYSIS	
This is one of the question in which all the respondents are agreed upon. 100% of the respondents view the question as totally relevant. There were no equivocations in their answers. The decision here was unanimous. Some of the trends as it relates to the reasons advanced include that it is against the commandments to defraud people or deceive them. This attests to the fact that many Nigerians are religious conscious and that over and above the basic decency of the human person, they owe allegiance to their religious traditions and derive the legitimacy of their ethical positions therefrom.	Strongly Yes (+2) 100% Yes (+1) 0% Undecided (0) 0% No (-1) 0% Strongly No (-2) 0%

As a matter of principle, people should not deceive or defraud

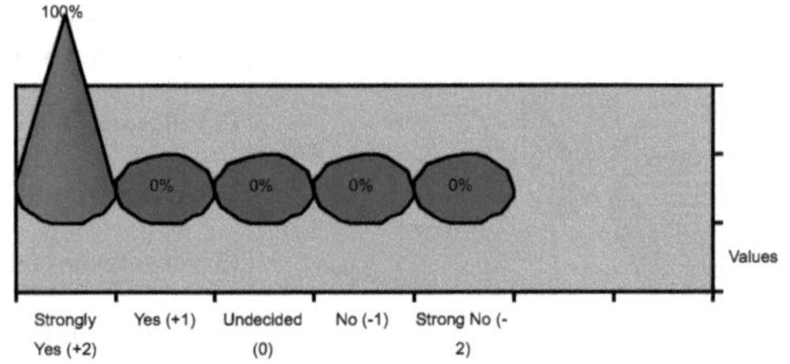

In the Nigerian business environment, fraud is a protean juggernaut. At all levels of society, politics, and business, there have been serious financial misappropriations, embezzlements and outright thievery recorded. Companies and banks have in most case helped politicians or conspired with public officials to defraud the people. It is the light of this that the unanimous agreement of our respondents here, becomes an interesting observation in a social situation were corruption in public life is legendary.[285] This unanimous response sounds like a vote of no

285 See: Ogbunwezeh, E.F., Religion and the Socio-economic Realities of Nigeria: A critique of Religion in a corrupt Social Milieu, in Theophilus .I. Okere (ed.) Religion in a World of Change: African Ancestral Religion, Islam and Christianity, Owerri, Whelan Research Academy, 2002, pp.60-71

confidence on the pervasive corruption, fraudulence and perfidy in social, public and business life in Nigeria.

Corruption in Nigeria to say the least has enjoyed an unchallenged reign. The country has consistently ranked very low on Transparency International ratings. Corruption may explain why poor leadership, which is a conspiracy of bad leadership and an emasculated followership, has essayed to sire a corrupt and dysfunctional state. This may equally explain why Nigeria husbands a compromised socio-economic architecture that has been sabotage to impoverish the poor and confer unmerited privileges on the elite.[286] To this end, the inference from this is that the man on the Nigerian streets has some allergies to been defrauded. This is a universal aspiration of mankind. No one likes to be duped in business, even the fraudster himself never likes to be defrauded. We argue then that this is a basis to build the relevant sanctions that protects the individual and the public from fraudsters, who have overran the Nigerian public space with gimmicks like Advanced Fee Fraud, popularly called 419. Many corrupt banks officials have been known to have aided and abetted the trade and unholy vocation of fraudsters. And this taints the reputation of the industry and engenders a loss of public confidence. Banks on the other hand should be made aware of this general aspiration of the Nigerian people. To this end, any bank which wishes to keep the respect and confidence of the people should be made to realise that the people do not like being defrauded and that they believe that as a matter of principle, banks and financial houses should not be privy to business transactions designed to defraud people in any form or shape.

286 See: Ogbunwezeh, E.F., The Church as a Catalyst for Development in Africa, in Ike, Obiora (ed.) Eternity is Love: Africa and the Legacy of Gaudium et Spes, 40 years after. Enugu, CIDJAP Publications, 2006, pp.227-246

5.3.1.6.1 Question 6.1: Is it relevant to ask, whether companies create with their products a higher impression on quality than they actually possess?

QUALITATIVE ANALYSIS	
To this question which is an adjunct to the preceding one, on fraudulence 69% of the respondents are of the view that the question is totally relevant. 13% remained undecided. 6% saw it as not relevant, while 12% saw it as totally irrelevant. Here one notices a departure from the unanimity recorded on the preceding question (Vide, Supra: Question 6). From the reasons submitted to this question, one cannot determine whether this question was not clearly tied to fraudulence which it is and which was spelt out in clear unequivocal terms in the preceding question.	Totally Relevant (+2) 69% Relevant (+1) 0% Undecided (0) 13% Not Relevant (-1) 6% Totally Not relevant (-2) 12%

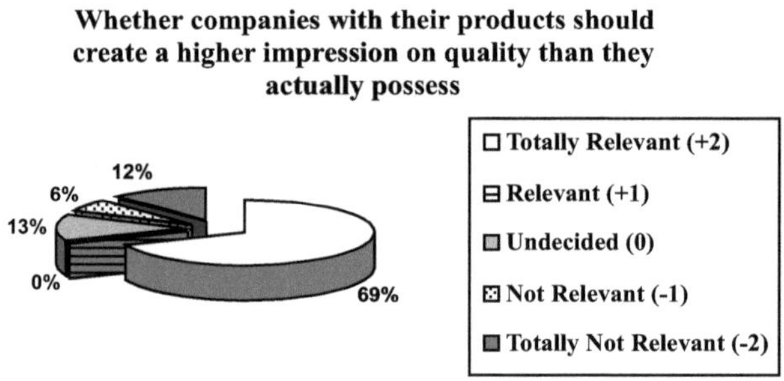

5.3.1.6.2 Question 6.2: Is it relevant to ask, whether bribery of politicians and decision makers in companies exists?

QUALITATIVE ANALYSIS	
In response to this question, 70% of the respondents were of the view that the question is totally relevant to such a criteriology. 18% were of the opinion that it is relevant. 12% were undecided. None of the respondents deemed it irrelevant. Synthesizing the reasons adduced for their answers, most of those who deemed it totally relevant viewed bribery of politicians as a sin against God and a crime against the country. Others viewed it as economic sabotage when a company pays politicians to be favourable to them.	Totally Relevant (+2) 70% Relevant (+1) 18% Undecided (0) 12% Not Relevant (-1) 0%

Is relevant to ask, whether bribery of politicians and decision makers in companies exist?

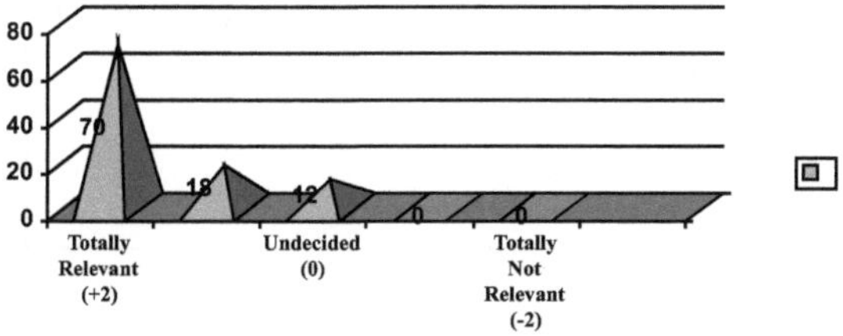

Bribery and corruption of politicians and public officials, though a universal problem even in the developed democracies,[287] has been unfortunately the major furniture of the Nigeria socio-political environment. The country has consistently fallen among the lowest in the Transparency International annual corruption index. One of the most notorious cases where a company was caught bribing Nigerian government officials, was that of the German engineering giant Siemens, which bribed Nigerian government officials to the tune of 10 million Euros. [288]

287 Governor Blagejovic stands accused of the attempt to auction off Barack Obama's seat for a fee. See: Time Magazine, http://www.time.com/time/nation/article/0,8599,1868074,00.html accessed on the 21st of December, 2008

288 Dionne Searcey, "U.S Cracks Down on Corporate Bribes" in Wall Street Journal of May 29th, 2009, http://online.wsj.com/article/SB124329477230952689.html accessed on the 11th of October, 2010.

That our respondents view corruption as seriously in bad taste, is attested to by their response as to the validity of the question. An overwhelming majority viewed the inclusion of this question in any ethical-ecological criteriology for companies as relevant. We are of the view that this is a basis upon which to fight corruption in Nigeria. The people are tired of it, because they are living testaments to its effects in public life.

5.3.1.7 Principle 7: As a matter of principle, people should keep their promises! (FHG 3.2.7)

QUALITATIVE ANALYSIS	
This is the 7th general moral principle upon which the cultural compatibility rating of the FHG is based. Like all the principles which stipulated the general direction of the question; or which is the base out of which the follow-up questions took their relevance, this set out the general rules of conduct, which as it were limit the unrestrained indulgence of anthropological drives. This is another of the cases where our respondents posted unanimity in their response. There were no dissenting voices here. 100% of our respondents were of the opinion that promises are sacred, which should be kept as a matter of principle.	Strongly Yes (+2) 100% Yes (+1) 0% Undecided (0) 0% No (-1) 0% Strongly No (-2) 0%

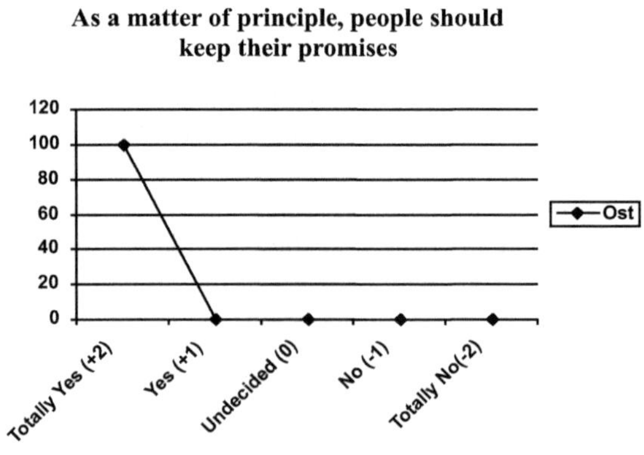

5.3.1.7.1 Question 7.1: Is it relevant to ask whether companies honour contracts and guarantees even though a situation of economic dependency of the country exists?

QUALITATIVE ANALYSIS	
Reacting to this question, 68% of the respondents viewed the question as totally relevant. 21% followed construing the question as relevant. 6% were undecided. 3% viewed the question as not relevant to any such criteriology while 2% viewed it as totally not relevant.	Totally Relevant(+2) 68% Relevant (+1) 21% Undecided (0) 6% Not Relevant (-1) 3%

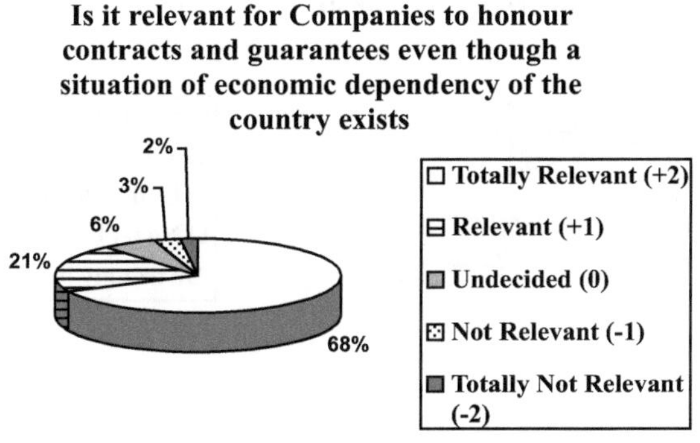

5.3.1.8 Principle 8: As a matter of principle, people should respect the property of others! (FHG 3.2.8)

QUALITATIVE ANALYSIS	
In reaction to this principle, 88% of our respondents answered strongly yes to confirm their agreement with it. 6% answered yes. None filled the undecided column. The same went for strongly no. 6% answer simply no to show their disagreement with the principle.	Strongly yes (+2) 88% Yes (+1) 6% Undecided (0) 0% No (-1) 6% Strongly No (-2) 0%

Principle 8: As a matter of Principle, people should respect the property of others.

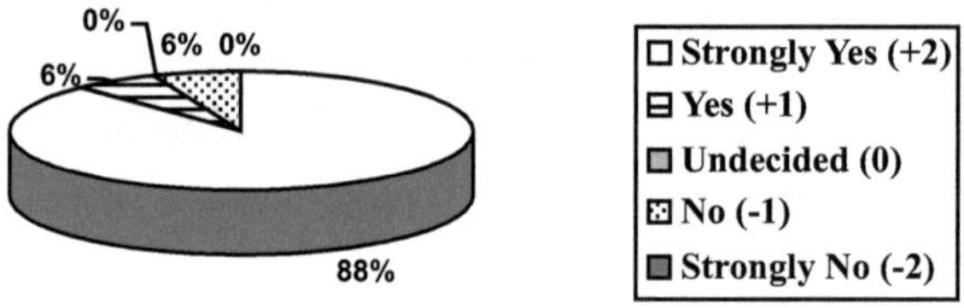

5.3.1.8.1 *Question 8.1: Is it relevant to ask, whether local products are displace from the markets by international companies?*

QUALITATIVE ANALYSIS	
44% of the respondents viewed the question as totally relevant. 13% saw it simply as relevant. 12% were undecided. 12% viewed it as not relevant and 19% saw it as totally not relevant.	Totally Relevant (+2) 44%
	Relevant (+1) 13%
Many of the respondents especially those who were undecided viewed foreign products as of superior in quality than most locally made ones. This may have informed their indecision. Standing between patriotism and economic realities is really not a very comfortable position to be in as could be seen in the 12% that stood firmly on the fence, neither agreeing nor disagreeing to the relevance of the question as a part of a criteriology designed to measure the ethical-ecological compatibility of firms and banks in the Nigerian context, especially in the microfinance sector.	Undecided (0) 12%
	Not Relevant (-1) 12%
	Totally not relevant (-2) 19%

Is it relevance to ask, whether local products are displaced from the market by international companies?

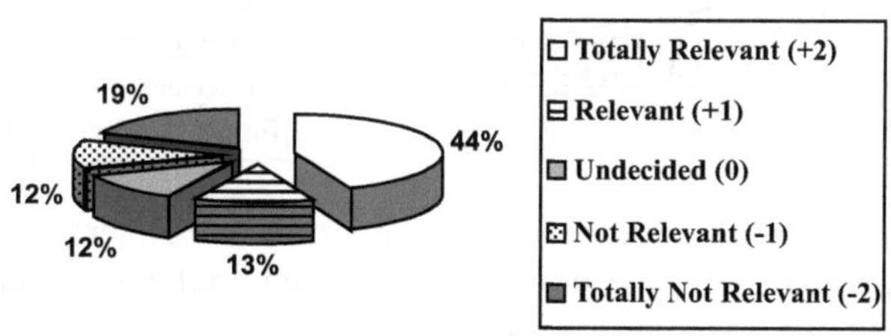

5.3.1.8.2 Question 8.2: Is it relevant to ask, whether there is any protection of nature and biological diversity by companies?

QUALITATIVE ANALYSIS	Totally Relevant (+2) 35%
To this question, 35% of the respondents viewed it as totally relevant. 13% see it as relevant. A whooping 31% are undecided, sitting on the fence. 7% view it as not relevant, while 14% view it as totally not relevant	Relevant (+1) 13% Undecided (0) 31% Not Relevant (-1) 7%

Is it relevant to ask, whether there is any protection of nature and biological diversity by companies?

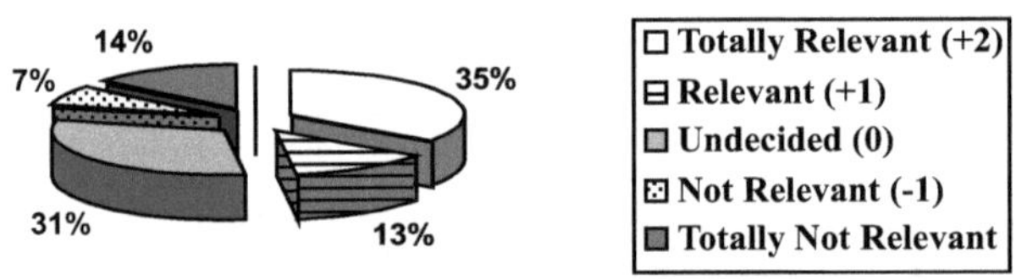

To this question, which should be of great importance to Nigerians, our respondents showed a marked unconcern than was expected. In the Nigerian Niger Delta, militants are involved in a war with the government, establishing a flourishing kidnapping enterprise designed to bring their plight to national and international awareness. The ecology of the Niger Delta has to a great extent being compromised by the prospecting, exploration and exploitation activities of the international oil concerns like Shell BP, ExxonMobil and ChevronTexaco. That is in the southern part of Nigeria. In the north, the threat of desertification grows by the day.

That 35% of our respondents view the protection of nature and biological diversity by companies as totally relevant to any ethical-ecological criteria applicable in the Nigerian context is really a dangerous sign. It is either that their socio-economic situation is so dire that any other consideration outside their daily bread is an unaffordable luxury or that they lack the awareness of the connection between their environment and a sustainable future for themselves and their posterity.

5.3.1.8.3 Question 8.3: Is it relevant to ask, how companies react to questions concerning personal property that was annexed in the past and given to companies?

QUALITATIVE ANALYSIS	
Here, half of the respondents construed the question as totally relevant, while 12% viewed it as relevant. 31% sat on the fence, undecided and 7% saw it as totally not relevant.	Totally Relevant (+2) 50% Relevant (+1) 12% Undecided (0) 31% Not Relevant (-1) 0%

Is it relevant to ask, how companies react to questions concerning personal property that was annexed in the past and given to companies

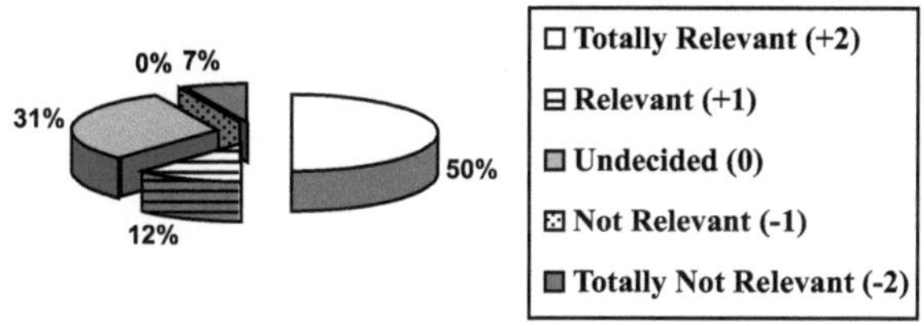

5.3.1.9 Principle 9: As a matter of principle, people should obey the law (FHG 3.2.9)

QUALITATIVE ANALYSIS	
On this principle, we experienced the very same patronage by the respondents. Here 94% of the respondents are strongly in favour of the principle. Here many of the respondents are convinced that without the law, anarchy will be the other of the day in Nigeria. Various reasons advanced here leads to the inference that Nigerians hunger and thirst for the rule of law, although many of the reasons show a marked distrust of the state as capable of maintaining law and other, or ensuring that the law rules over caprice.	Strongly yes (+2) 94% Yes (+1) 0% Undecided (0) 6% No (-1) 0% Strongly No 0%

Principle 9: As a matter of principle, people should obey the law!

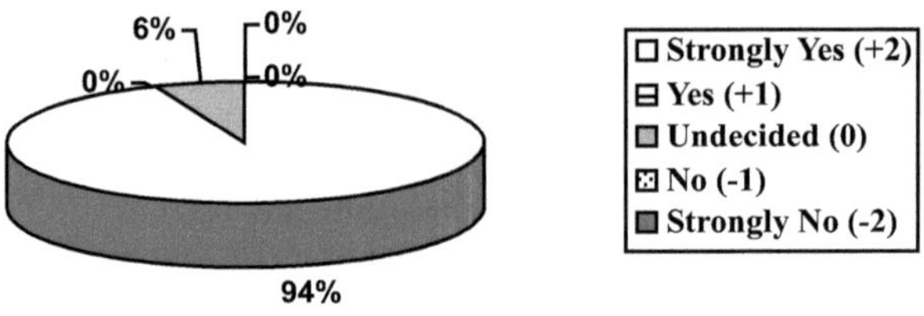

5.3.1.9.1 Question 9.1: Is it relevant to ask, whether companies respect the code of ethics prevailing in the specific industry?

QUALITATIVE ANALYSIS	
To this question equally, we witnessed the same trend as was recorded on the preceding principle. 94% of the respondents viewed the question as totally relevant. 6% were undecided. The reasons advanced ranged from each profession or sector having a code or set of ethics, which facilitates the smooth operation of that particular sector. Others opined that without certain code of ethics, no sector would function effectively.	Totally Relevant (+2) 94% Relevant (+1) 0% Undecided (0) 6% Not Relevant (-1) 0% Totally not relevant 0%

Is it relevant to ask, whether companies respect the codes of ethics prevailing in the specific industry?

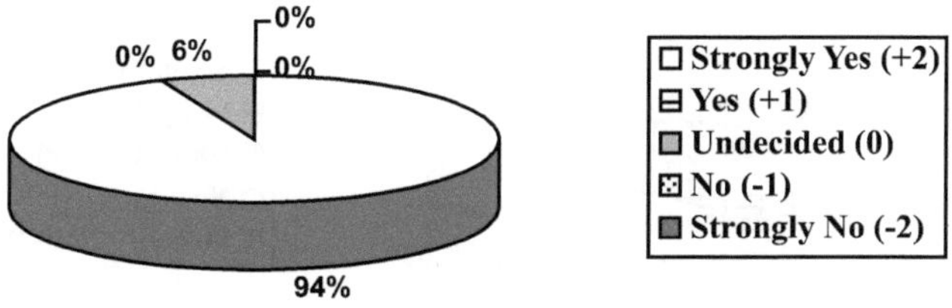

5.3.1.10 Principle 10: As a matter of principle, people should not subject anybody to moral obligations beyond their ability to fulfil them (FHG 3.2.10)

QUALITATIVE ANALYSIS	
Here equally, like we witnessed on all the other principles, the majority were strongly in support of its relevance in any criteria designed to appraise companies for ethical-ecological compatibility in the Nigerian context. 63% said strongly yes to the principle, 25% were undecided. 12% said strongly no.	Strongly yes (+2) 63% Yes (+1) 0% Undecided (0 25% No (-1) 0% Strongly No 12%

Principle 10: As a matter of principle, people should not subject anybody to moral obligations beyond their ability to fulfil them

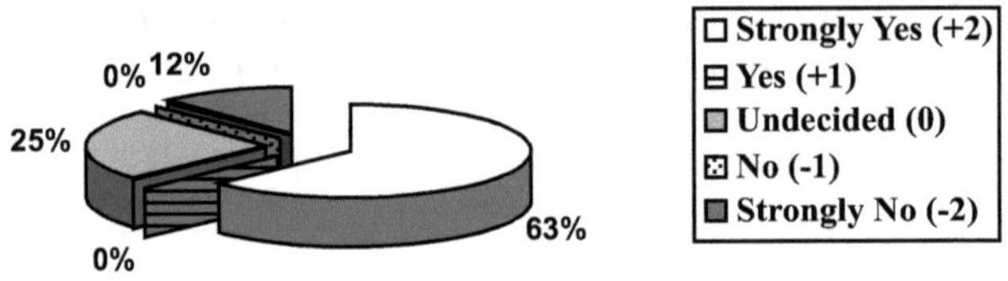

5.3.1.10.1 Question 10.1: Is it relevant to ask, whether companies show consideration for employee groups requiring protection (handicapped, children, and women)?

QUALITATIVE ANALYSIS	
To This question flowing from principle 10, 75% of the respondents viewed it as totally relevant to any such ethical-ecological criteriology designed for the Nigerian context. 12% saw it as relevant. 6% of the respondents were undecided, and 6% viewed it as totally not relevant.	Totally Relevant (+2) 75% Relevant (+1) 12% Undecided (0) 6% Not Relevant (-1) 0 Totally not relevant 6%

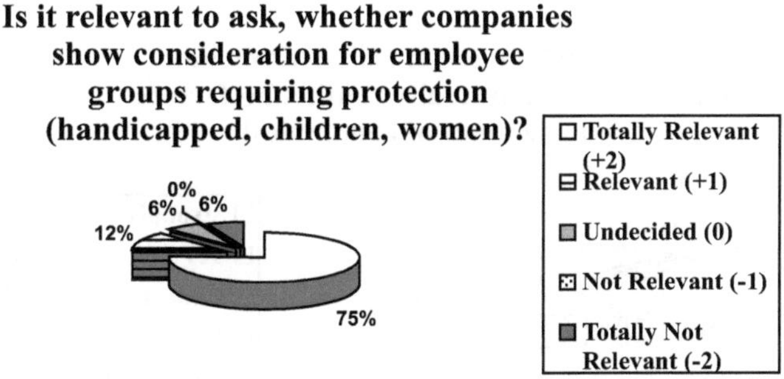

5.3.2 Anthropologically Given Motivational Factors

5.3.2.1 Motivational Factor 1: Competition and Solidarity are two mutually conflicting factors driving actions of companies!

QUALITATIVE ANALYSIS	
On this score, 56% of our respondents showed their stand to the question by answering "strongly yes", while 25% were undecided. 6% viewed it as not relevant and 13% construed it as totally not relevant.	Strongly yes (+2) 56% Yes (+1) 0 % Undecided (0 25% No (-1) 6% Strongly No (-2) 13%

Motivational Factor 1: Competition and solidarity as two mutually conflicting factors driving actions of companies!

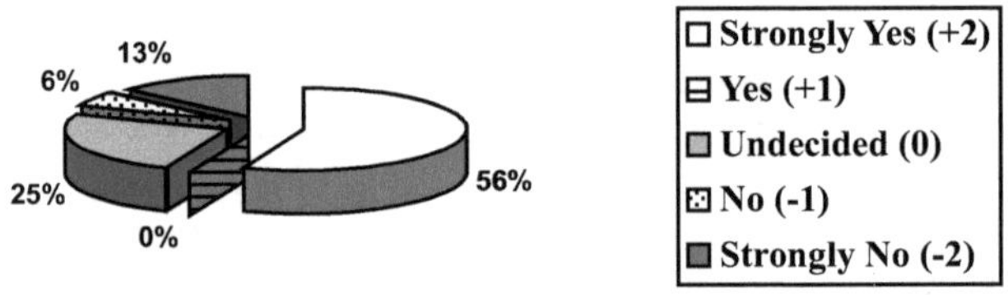

5.3.2.2 Motivational Factor 2: Unlimited expansion and self restraint are two mutually conflicting factors driving actions of companies!

QUALITATIVE ANALYSIS	
On the second motivational factor, 56% were strongly in favour, 25% were in favour. 13% were undecided and hence took no stance. And 6% were strongly opposed to it.	Strongly yes (+2) 56% Yes (+1) 25% Undecided (0) 13% No (-1) 0% Strongly No (-2) 6%

Motivational Factor 2: Unlimited Expansion and Self Restraint are two mutually conflicting factors driving actions of companies!

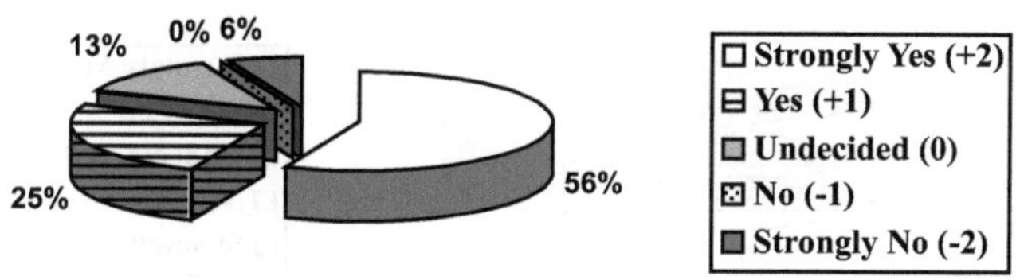

5.3.2.3 Motivational Factor 3: Self-glorification and low profile are two mutually conflicting factors characterizing the image of companies to the society!

QUALITATIVE ANALYSIS	
The third motivational factor elicited a more diversified response. 44% of our respondents strongly supported it. 19% simply supported it, while another 19% remained undecided. 6% disagreed with the factor and 12% totally disagreed with it.	Strongly yes (+2) 44% Yes (+1) 19% Undecided (0) 19% No (-1) 6% Strongly No (-2) 12%

Motivational Factor 3: Self-glorification and low profile are two mutually conflicting factors characterizing the image of companies to society!

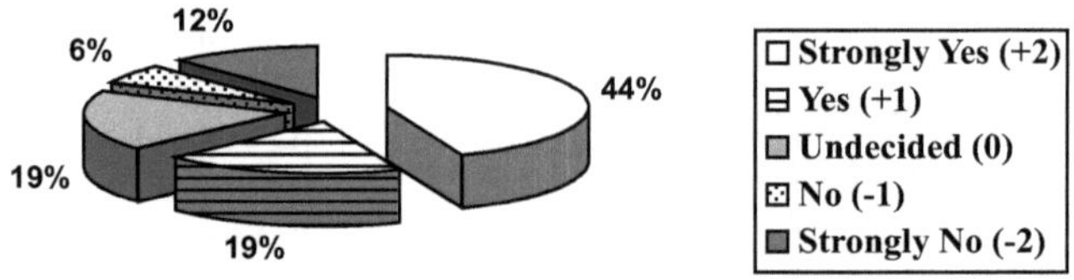

5.3.2.4 Motivational Factor 4: Close-mindedness and Openness are two mutually conflicting factors driving the action of companies!

QUALITATIVE ANALYSIS	
On this factor, 31% were strongly in favour, while another 31% simply supported it. 19% of the respondents were undecided. 7% were not in agreement, while 12% were strongly in disagreement with it.	Strongly yes (+2) 31% Yes (+1) 31% Undecided (0) 19% No (-1) 7% Strongly No (-2) 12%

Motivational Factor 4: Close-mindedness and openness are two mutually conflicting factors driving the actions of companies!

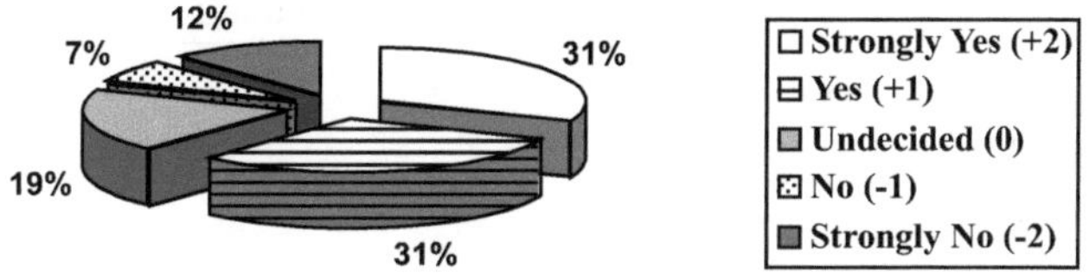

5.3.2.5 Motivational Factor 5: Responsibility and right of the stronger are two mutually conflicting factors driving the actions of companies!

QUALITATIVE ANALYSIS			
Here we recorded 25% of our respondents being strongly in support, while 19% were in support. 31% were undecided on this point. 6% were in disagreement and 19% were strongly in disagreement.	Strongly yes	(+2)	25%
	Yes	(+1)	19%
	Undecided	(0)	31%
	No	(-1)	6%
	Strongly No	(-2)	19%

Motivational Factor 5: Responsibility and right of the stronger are two mutually conflicting factors driving the action of companies!

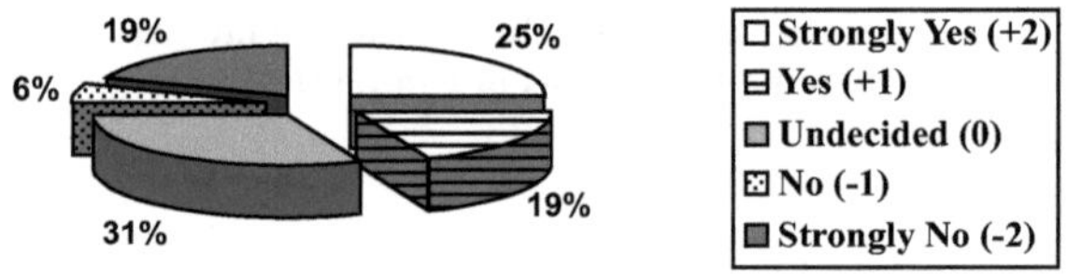

5.3.3 Orientations and Virtues

5.3.3.1 Orientation 1: Is it relevant to ask, whether companies impose moral constraints on their actions?

QUALITATIVE ANALYSIS	
On this first orientation, 50% of our respondents viewed it as totally relevant. 13% followed suit viewing it as relevant. 18% remained undecided while 6% of our respondents viewed it as not relevant. It was capped off by 13% which viewed the orientation as totally not relevant.	Totally Relevant (+2) 50% Relevant (+1) 13% Undecided (0) 18% Not Relevant (-1) 6%

Orientation 1: Is it relevant to ask, whether companies impose moral constraints on their actions?

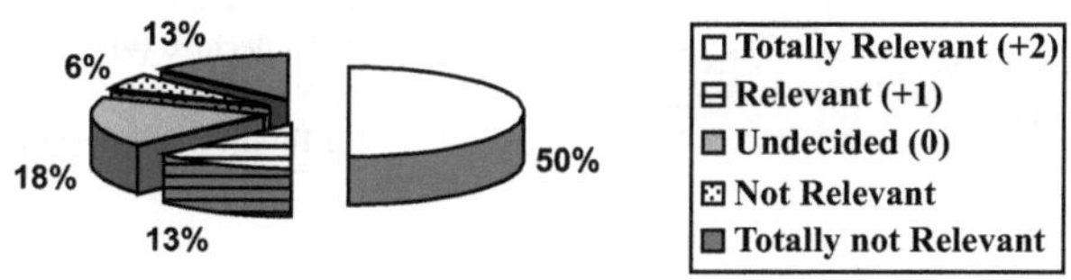

5.3.3.2 Orientation 2: Is it relevant to ask, whether companies impose limits on their actions, which are conducive to a harmonious co-existence with others?

QUALITATIVE ANALYSIS	
On the second orientation, 44% construed it as totally relevant. 50% were undecided. 6% construed it as not relevant.	Totally Relevant (+2) 44% Relevant (+1) 0% Undecided (0) 50% Not Relevant (-1) 6% Totally not relevant (-2) 0%

Orientation 2: Is it relevant to ask, whether companies impose limits on their actions, which are conducive to a harmonious co-existence with others?

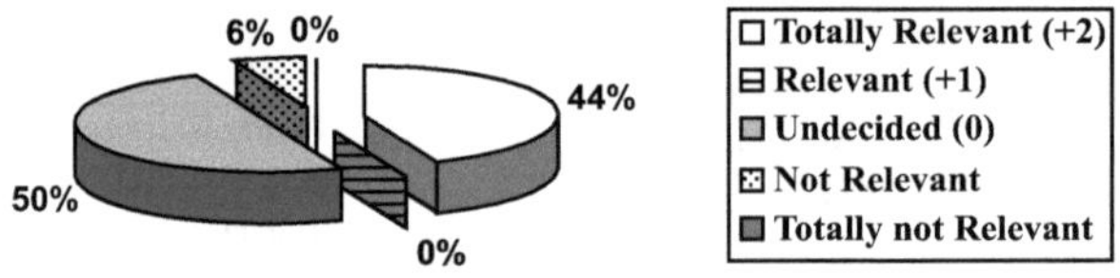

5.3.3.3 Virtues 1: (Cardinal Virtues): The Following items are desirable virtues in their own right:

5.3.3.3.1 Truth telling

QUALITATIVE ANALYSIS	
On this first cardinal virtue, our question elicited a very strong response of affirmation. 75% of the respondents were strongly agreed that this virtue is desirable in its own right. 13% simply agreed. 12% were undecided. We recorded no dissent on this point.	Strongly yes (+2) 75% Yes (+1) 13% Undecided (0) 12% No (-1) 0%

Virtues 1: Truth telling is desirable in its own right!

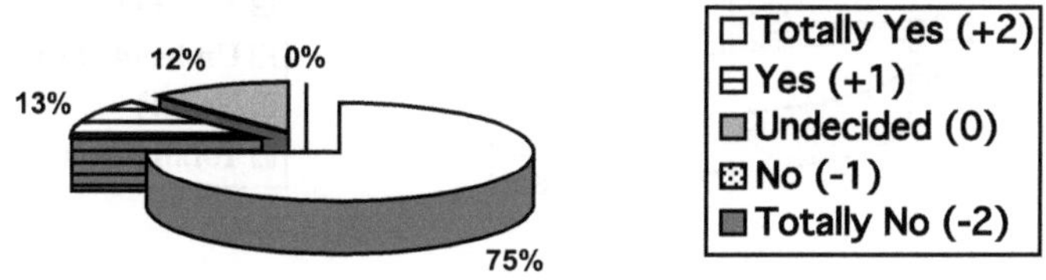

5.3.3.3.2 Justice

QUALITATIVE ANALYSIS	
On justice as a cardinal virtue, which is desirable on its own right, 80% of our respondents were strongly agreed to that. 15% simply agreed. 5% were undecided. Like in truth telling (Vide, Supra) we equally recorded no dissents on this virtue as desirable in its own right.	Strongly yes (+2) 80% Yes (+1) 15% Undecided (0) 5% No (-1) 0% Strongly No (-2) 0%

Virtues 2: Justice is desirable in its own right!

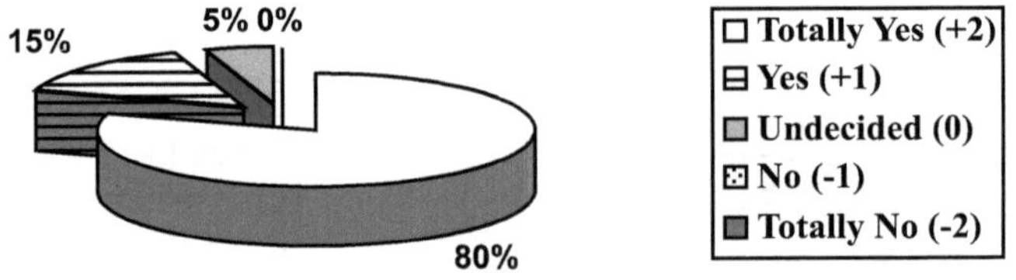

5.3.3.3.3 Prudence

QUALITATIVE ANALYSIS	
On prudence as a virtue desirable in its own right, we saw 69% of the respondents strongly agreeing with it. 20% simply agreed. 11% were undecided. And like in the two preceding virtues of cardinal import, we recorded equally no dissent here.	Strongly yes (+2) 69% Yes (+1) 20% Undecided (0) 11% No (-1) 0% Strongly No 0%

Virtues 3: Prudence is desirable in its own right!

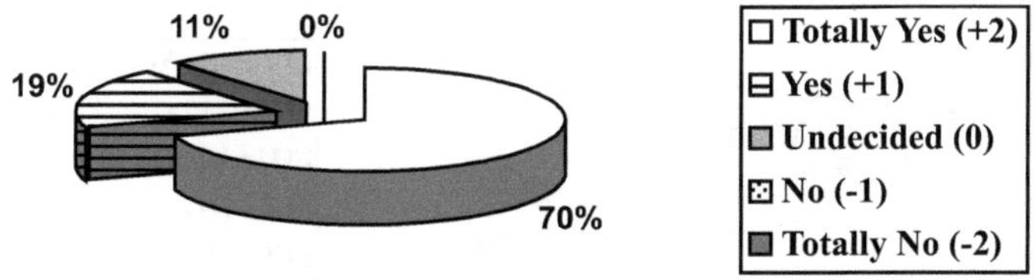

5.3.3.3.4 Courage in the sense of steadfastness

QUALITATIVE ANALYSIS	
On courage being desirable in its own right, our respondents followed a pattern which is almost becoming a trend fort he cardinal virtues. Here as in the others a high percentage 75% in this case were strongly agreed to it. 6% simply agreed while 19% remained undecided. Like in the three preceding ones we equally recorded no dissents here.	Strongly yes (+2) 75% Yes (+1) 6% Undecided (0) 19% No (-1) 0% Strongly No (-2) 0%

Virtues 4: Courage in the sense of steadfastness is desirable in its own right!

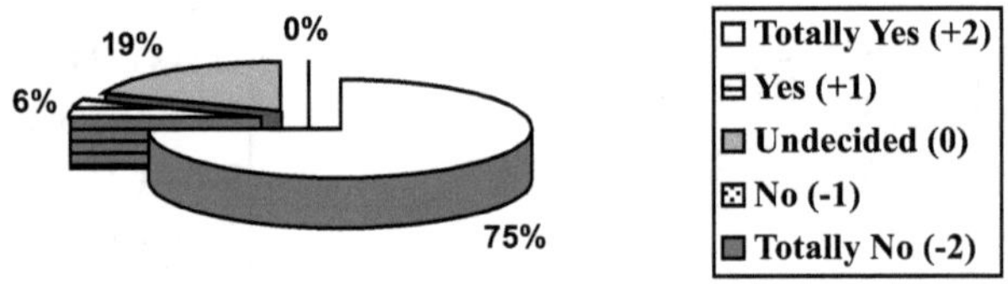

5.3.3.3.5 Peacefulness

QUALITATIVE ANALYSIS	
On peacefulness being a virtue that is desirable on its own, 68% of the respondents were strongly in agreement. 13% were simply in agreement. 19% were undecided. And like in the preceding ones, no dissent was recorded.	Strongly yes (+2) 68% Yes (+1) 13% Undecided (0) 19% No (-1) 0% Strongly No (-2) 0%

Virtues 5: Peacefulness is desirable in its own right!

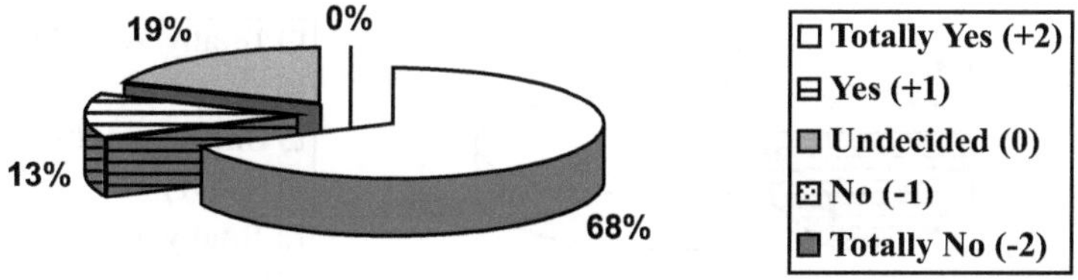

5.3.3.3.6 Sense of proportion and restraint

QUALITATIVE ANALYSIS	
On the sense of proportion and restraint as a virtue desirable in its own right, 55% were strongly in agreement. 20% were simply in agreement. 25% sat comfortably on the fence. And equally on this point, we recorded no disagreement as to the desirability of this virtue on its own terms.	Strongly yes (+2) 55% Yes (+1) 20% Undecided (0) 25% No (-1) 0% Strongly No (-2) 0%

Virtues 6: Sense of proportion and restraint is desirable in its own right!

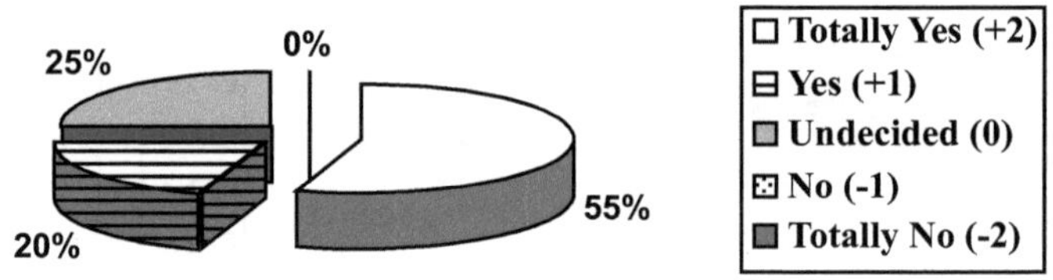

5.3.3.4 Virtues 2 (Secondary Virtues): The following items are desirable virtues to the extent that they are practised in the service of higher moral principles. To the extent they are placed in service of low moral principles, they stop being virtues!

5.3.3.4.1 Diligence

QUALITATIVE ANALYSIS	
On this first secondary virtue, and its desirability based on the extent to which it serves higher moral ideals and principles, 63% were strongly agreed to it. 6% simply agreed. 18% remained undecided while 13% strongly disagreed with it.	Strongly yes (+2) 63% Yes (+1) 6% Undecided (0) 18% No (-1) 0% Strongly No (-2) 13%

Secondary Virtues 1: DILIGENCE is desirable to the extent that it is practised in the service of higher moral principles. To the extent it is placed in the service of low moral principles, it stops being a virtue!

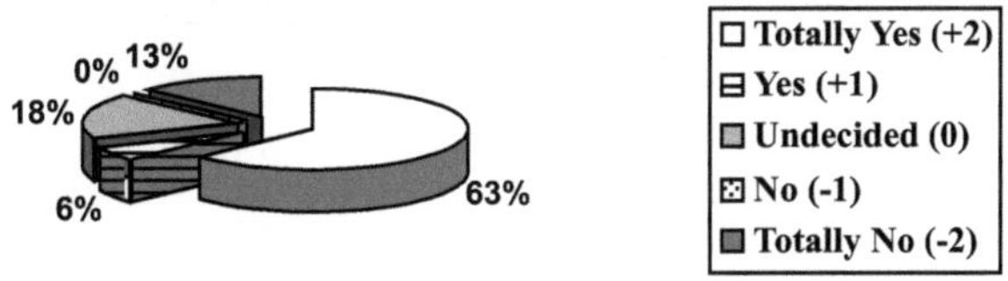

5.3.3.4.2 Punctuality

QUALITATIVE ANALYSIS	
On punctuality, 50% were strongly in agreement, construing it as desirable in so far as it serves higher moral principles and ideals. 18% simply agreed to that. 13% were undecided while another 13% strongly disagreed with it. They reasons offered were so various and could not establish a pattern.	Strongly yes (+2) 50% Yes (+1) 18% Undecided (0) 13% No (-1) 0% Strongly No (-2) 13%

Secondary Virtues 2: PUNCTUALITY is desirable to the extent that it is practised in the service of higher moral principles. To the extent it is placed in the service of low moral principles, it stops being a virtue!

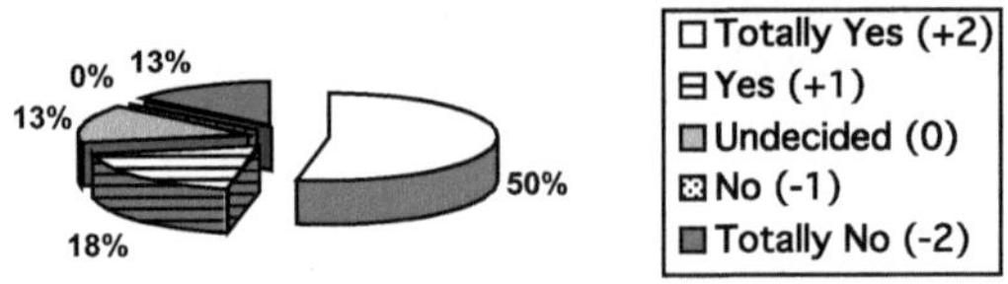

5.3.3.4.3 Cleanliness

QUALITATIVE ANALYSIS	
Cleanliness as a virtue desirable in so far as it serves higher moral principles and ideals attracted strong agreement with 50% of the respondents. 13% simply agreed with it. 25% were undecided. 6% lightly disagreed and another 6% strongly disagreed.	Strongly yes (+2) 50% Yes (+1) 13% Undecided (0) 25% No (-1) 6% Strongly No (-2) 6%

Secondary Virtues 3: CLEANLINESS is desirable to the extent that it is practised in the service of higher moral principles. To the extent it is placed in the service of low moral principles, it stops being a virtue!

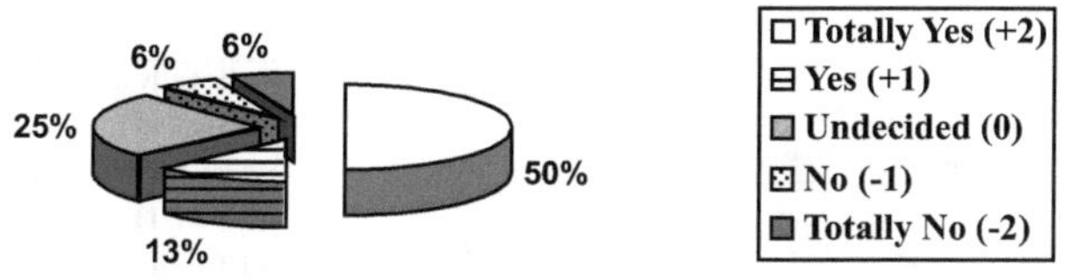

5.3.3.4.4 Orderliness

QUALITATIVE ANALYSIS	
On orderliness as a secondary virtue which is relevant in as much as it serves higher moral ideals, 61% were strongly in favour. 13% were simply in favour of it. Another 13% were undecided and we recorded another 13% that were strongly in disagreement with it.	Strongly yes (+2) 61% Yes (+1) 13% Undecided (0) 13% No (-1) 0% Strongly No (-2) 13%

Secondary Virtues 4: ORDERLINESS is desirable to the extent that it is practised in the service of higher moral principles. To the extent it is placed in the service of low moral principles, it stops being a virtue!

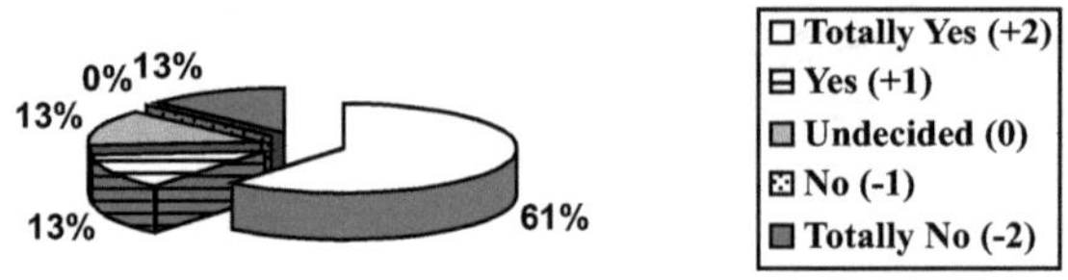

5.3.3.4.5 Obedience

QUALITATIVE ANALYSIS	
70% of the respondents were strongly agreed that obedience is a virtue which should serve higher moral principles in order to become a virtue. 8% were lightly in agreement.12% of the respondents were undecided. 6% disagreed and 4% disagreed totally with it.	Strongly yes (+2) 70% Yes (+1) 8% Undecided (0) 12% No (-1) 6% Strongly No (-2) 4%

Secondary Virtues 5: OBEDIENCE is desirable to the extent that it is practised in the service of higher moral principles. To the extent it is placed in the service of low moral principles, it stops being a virtue!

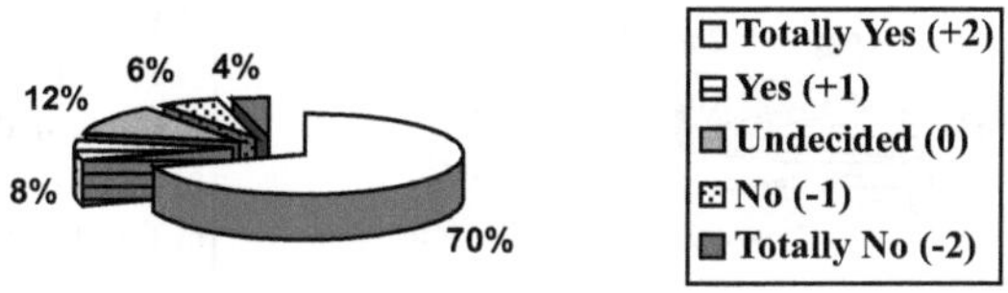

5.3.3.4.6 Flexibility

QUALITATIVE ANALYSIS	
On flexibility as a virtue which is a virtue in as much as it serves a higher moral principle, 68% of our respondents were strongly in agreement. 18% were lightly in agreement. 12% decided to sit on the fence, taking none of the sides. 2% lightly disagreed.	Strongly yes (+2) 68% Yes (+1) 18% Undecided (0) 12% No (-1) 2% Strongly No (-2) 0%

Secondary Virtues 6: FLEXIBILITY is desirable to the extent that it is practised in the service of higher moral principles. To the extent it is placed in the service of low moral principles, it stops being a virtue!

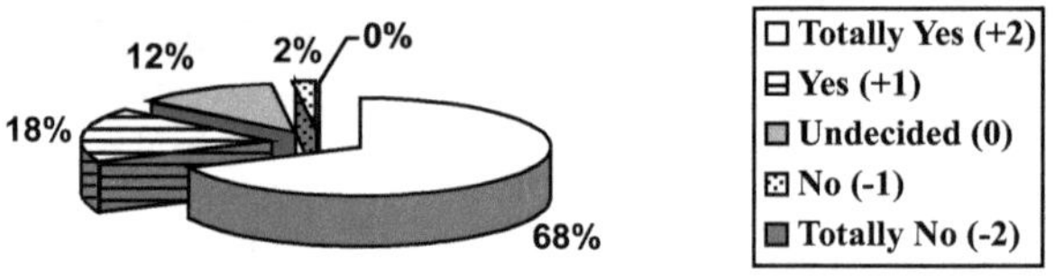

5.3.3.4.7 Mobility

QUALITATIVE ANALYSIS	
Mobility as a secondary virtue attracted the strong agreement of 69% of our respondents. 13% were lightly in agreement. 18% of the respondents were undecided. Here we recorded no dissents. No one disagreed.	Strongly yes (+2) 69% Yes (+1) 13% Undecided (0) 18% No (-1) 0% Strongly No (-2) 0%

Secondary Virtues 7: MOBILITY is desirable to the extent that it is practised in the service of higher moral principles. To the extent it is placed in the service of low moral principles, it stops being a virtue!

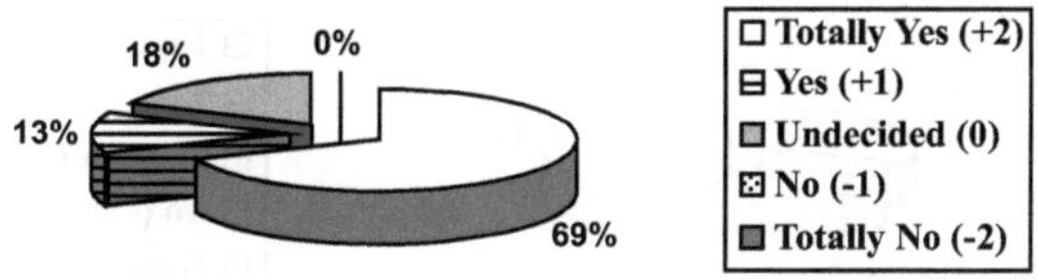

5.3.3.4.8 Empathy

QUALITATIVE ANALYSIS	
On this last secondary virtue; empathy, we recorded 44% strong agreement and 25% light agreement. 31% stayed undecided. Like the preceding one, we recorded equally here no disagreements.	Strongly yes (+2) 44% Yes (+1) 25% Undecided (0) 31% No (-1) 0%

Secondary Virtues 8: EMPATHY is desirable to the extent that it is practised in the service of higher moral principles. To the extent it is placed in the service of low moral principles, it stops being a virtue!

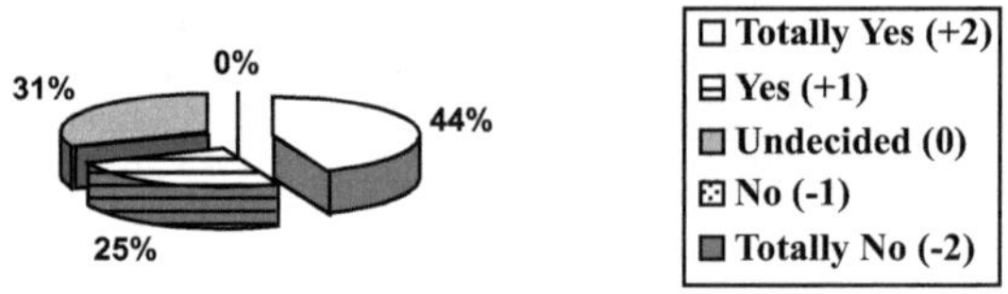

5.4 Summary and Conclusion

5.4.1 RESPONSES TO THE 10 GENERAL MORAL PRINCIPLES (%)

Principle	Strongly yes (+2)	yes (+1)	Undecided (0)	no (-1)	Strongly no (-2)
1	100	0	0	0	100
2	75	13	6	6	0
3	88	0	0	0	12
4	94	0	6	0	0
5	68	13	13	0	6
6	100	0	0	0	0
7	100	0	0	0	0
8	88	6	0	6	0
9	94	0	6	0	0
10	63	0	25	0	12
Totals	870	32	56	12	30
Averages	87	3.2	5.6	1.2	3

Strongly yes	87 %
yes	3.2 %
Undecided	5.6 %
no	1.2 %
Strongly no	3 %
Total	100 %

Total Average of the responses to the Relevance or otherwise of the 10 General Moral Principles of Frankfurt-Hohenheim Guidelines applied to the Nigerian Context

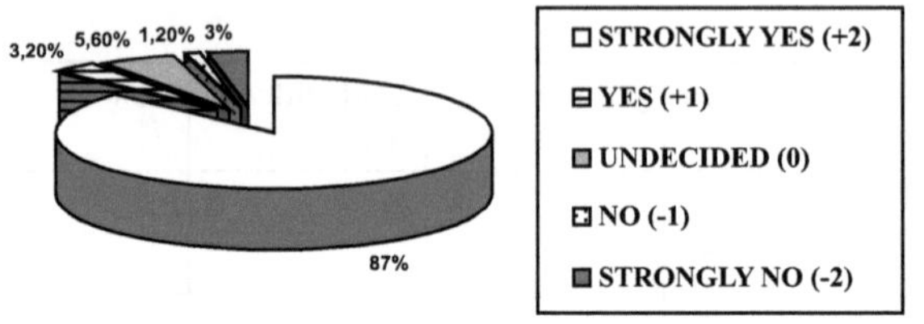

5.4.2 Responses to Questions Flowing from the General Moral Principles (%)

Question Number	Totally Relevant (+2)	Relevant (+1)	Undecided (0)	Not Relevant (-1)	Totally not Relevant (-2)
1.1	69	0	25	6	0
2.1	69	6	6	6	12
4.1	44	0	12	19	25
4.2	56	0	13	6	25
4.3	44	6	31	6	13
4.4	56	0	6	19	19
4.5	44	6	38	6	6
5.1	50	25	19	6	0
6.1	69	0	13	6	12
6.2	70	18	12	0	0
7.1	68	21	6	3	2
8.1	44	13	12	12	19
8.2	35	13	31	7	14
8.3	50	12	31	0	7
9.1	94	0	6	0	0
10.1	75	12	6	0	6
Totals	**937**	**132**	**267**	**102**	**160**
Simple Averages	**58.56**	**8.25**	**16.68**	**6.37**	**10**

Totally Relevant	59 %
Relevant	8 %
Undediced	17 %
Not Relevant	6 %
Totally not Relevant	10 %
Total	100 %

Total Average of the responses to the Relevance or otherwise of the 16 Questions flowing from the General Moral Principles of Frankfurt-Hohenheim Guidelines applied to the Nigerian Context

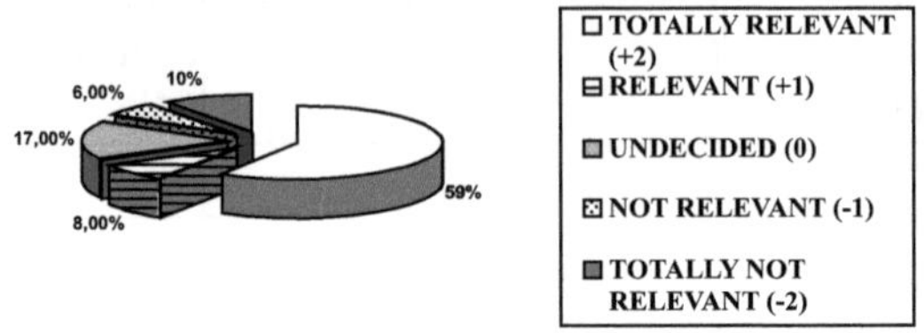

5.4.3 Responses to the Anthropologically Given Motivational Factors (%)

Motivation-al Factor	Strongly Yes (+2)	Yes (+1)	Undecided (0)	No (-1)	Strongly No (-2)
1.	56	0	25	6	13
2.	56	25	13	0	6
3.	44	19	19	6	12
4.	31	31	19	7	12
5.	25	19	31	6	19
Totals	**212**	**94**	**107**	**25**	**62**
Simple Averages	**42.4**	18.8	21.4	5	12.4

Strongly Yes	42.4 %
Yes	18.8 %
Undecided	21.4 %
No	5 %
Strongly No	12.4 %

Total Average of the responses to the Relevance or otherwise of the 5 Anthropologically Given Motivational Factors of the Frankfurt-Hohenheim Guidelines applied to the Nigerian Context

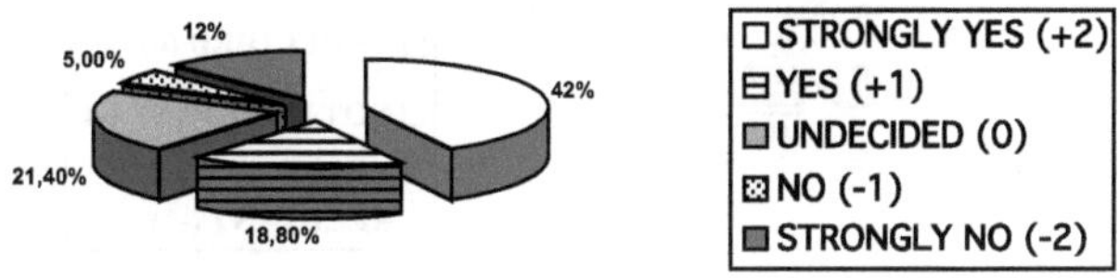

5.4.4 Virtues and Orientations

5.4.4.1 Responses to the Orientations

Orientations	Totally Relevant (+2)	Relevant (+1)	Undecided (0)	Not Relevant (-1)	Totally not Relevant (-2)
1.	50	13	18	6	13
2.	44	0	50	6	0
Total	**94**	**13**	**68**	**12**	**13**
Average	**47**	**6.5**	**34**	**6**	**6.5**

Totally Relevant	47 %
Relevant	6.5 %
Undecided	34 %
Not Relevant	6 %
Totally Not Relevant	6.5 %
Total	100%

Total Average of the responses to the Relevance or otherwise of the 2 Orientations of Cultural Compatibility of the Frankfurt-Hohenheim Guidelines applied to the Nigerian

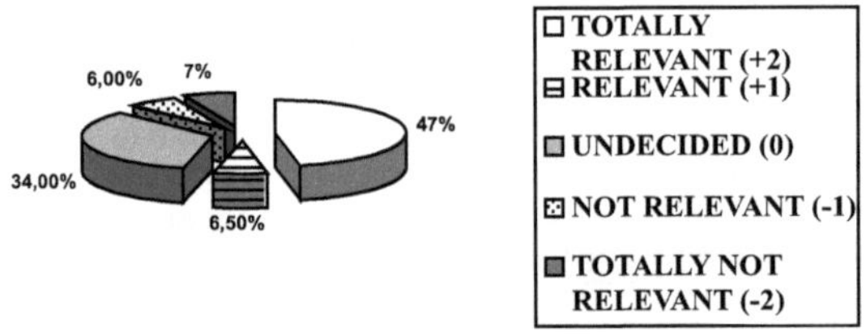

5.4.4.2 Response to the Cardinal Virtues

Cardinal Virtues	Strongly Yes (+2)	Yes (+1)	Undecided (0)	No (-1)	Strongly No (-2)
Truth-telling	75	13	12	0	0
Justice	80	15	5	0	0
Prudence	69	20	11	0	0
Courage in the sense of stead-fastness	75	6	19	0	0
Peacefulness	68	13	19	0	0
Sense of propor-tion	55	20	25	0	0
Totals	422	87	91	0	0
Simple Average	70.33	14.5	15.16	0	0

Strongly Yes	70 %
Yes	15 %
Undecided	15 %
No	0 %
Strongly No	0 %

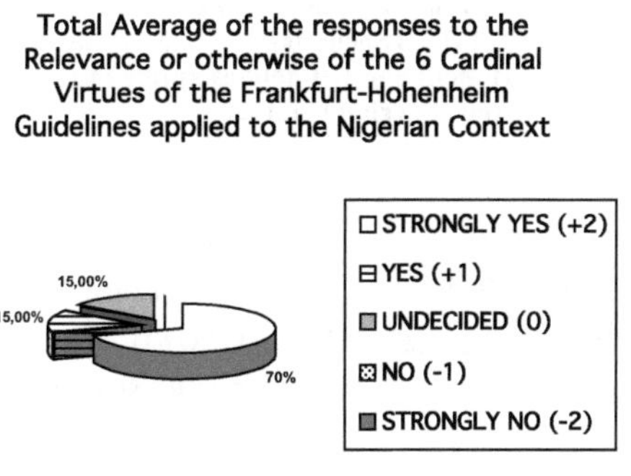

5.4.4.3 Response to the Secondary Virtues

Secondary Virtue	Strongly Yes (+2)	Yes (+1)	Undecided (0)	No (-1)	Strongly No (-2)
Diligence	63	6	18	0	13
Punctuality	50	18	13	0	13
Cleanliness	50	13	25	6	6
Orderliness	61	13	13	0	13
Obedience	70	8	12	6	4
Flexibility	68	18	12	2	0
Mobility	69	13	18	0	0
Empathy	44	25	31	0	0
Total	**475**	**114**	**142**	**14**	**49**
Simple Average	59.37	14.25	17.75	1.75	6.12

Strongly Yes 14 %
Undecided 18 %
No 2 %
Strongly No 6 %

Total Average of the responses to the Relevance or otherwise of the 8 Secondary Virtues of the Frankfurt-Hohenheim Guidelines applied to the Nigerian Context

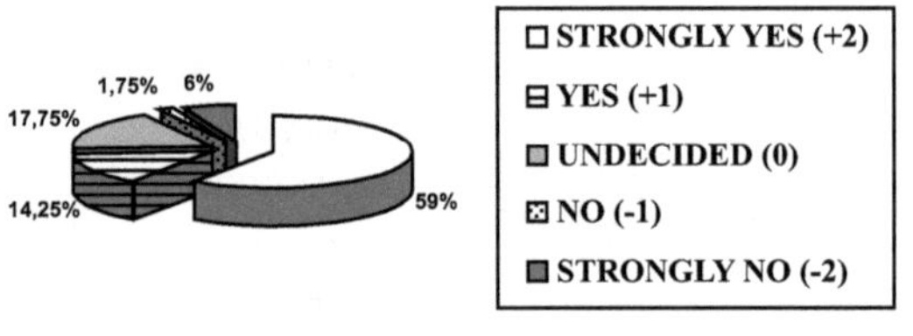

5.5 Test of Relevance

Our simple test of the relevance of a particular question rests on which value is greater than 50% of the whole values elicited. The same holds for all area sof cultural compatibility, as well as cultural compatibility as whole. This rests on the comparative summation of the total averages of two positives and the two negatives, and comparing them. Anyone of them that crosses the > 50% average becomes the result. When the positives trump the negatives by more than the average of 50%, then the particular area is deemed relevant, and vice versa. The responses that were undecided were naturally excluded from the computation.

This is mathematically represented thus:

Test of Relevance =
Relevant = (+2) + (+1) = > 50%
Not Relevant = (-2) + (-1) = > 50%
Undecided = (+2) + (+1) = (-2) + (-1)

Our research on Cultural compatibility in Nigeria, was along the 4 areas of cultural compatibility, namely, the anthropologically given motivational factors, the general moral principles, the value concepts or what we designated as orientations, and the virtues; both cardinal and secondary.

5.5.1 Comparative Summation ot the Two Givens

Summing the Positives (+1) +(+2) = Relevant	Undecideds Excluded (0)	Summing the Negatives (-1) +(-2) = Not Relevant
1.1 General Moral Principles **R= (+2) + (+1) = 87 + 3 = 90%** **1.2 Questions flowing from the General Moral Principles** **R= (+2) + (+1) 59 + 8 = 67%**		**NR= (-2)+ (-1)= 1 +3 = 4%** **NR= (-2)+ (-1)= 6 +10 = 16%**
2. Anthropologically Given Motivational Factors **R= (+2) + (+1) =42 + 19 = 61%**		**NR= (-2)+ (-1)= 5 +12 =17%**
3. Value Concepts (Orientations) **R= (+2) + (+1) =47 + 7 = 54%**		**NR= (-2)+ (-1)= 6 + 7 = 13**
4.1 Cardinal Virtues **R=(+2) + (+1) =70 + 15 = 85%** **4.2 Secondary Virtues** **R= (+2) + (+1) =59 + 14 = 73%**		**NR= (-2)+ (-1)= 0%** **NR= (-2)+ (-1)= 2 + 6 = 8**
Total Average= 71.6%		9.6%

CULTURAL COMPATIBILITY RELEVANCE IN THE NIGERIAN CONTEXT

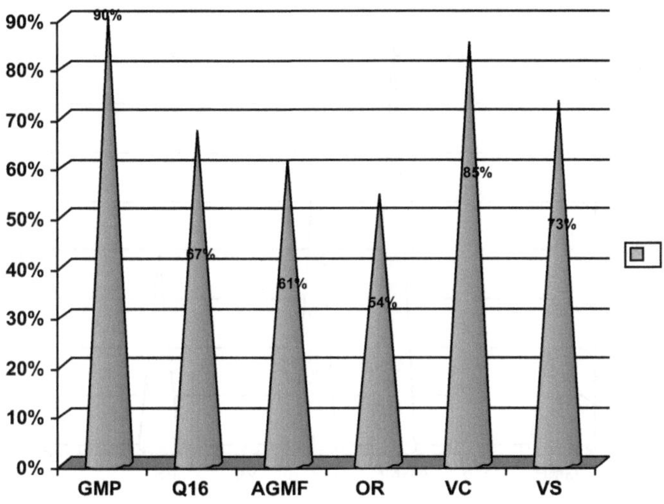

Key

1. GMP = General Moral Principles
2. Q16 = The 16 Questions flowing from the General Moral Principles
3. AGMF = Anthropological Given Motivational Factors
4. OR= Value concepts (What we designated here as Orientation, hence OR)
5. VC = Cardinal Virtues
6. VS = Secondary Virtues

CULTURAL COMPATIBILITY IRRELEVANCE IN THE NIGERIAN CONTEXT

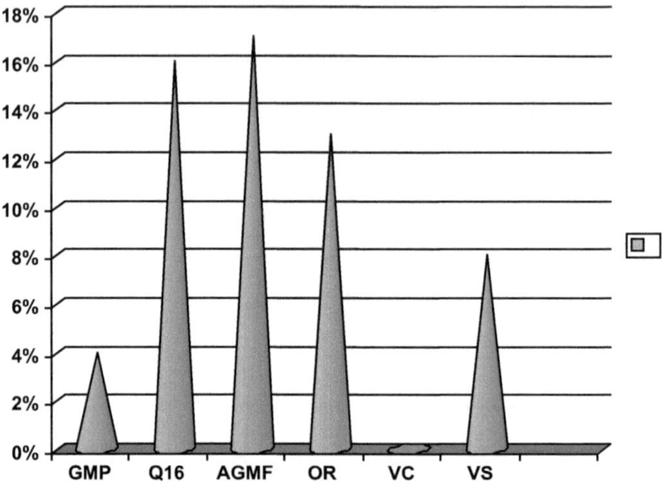

The analysis shows that with 71.6% average, the respondents are of the opinion that the FHG cultural compatibility criteria are relevant in the Nigerian context. This proves our hypothesis positive. An average of 9.6% of the responses deemed it not relevant in the Nigerian context. And 19.8% were undecided.

On the strength of this, we can say that our hypothesis, that over all, the Frankfurt-Hohenheim Guidelines Cultural Compatibility criteria has been proved positive; as relevant in the Nigerian context.

Proof of Hypothesis for Cultural Sustainability Criteria

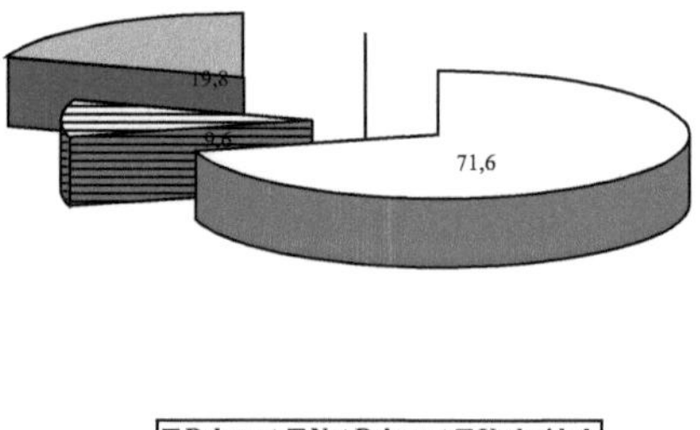

6. Examining the Relevance of the Social Compatibility Criteria in the Nigeria Context

6.1 Social Compatibility / Sustainability Survey

6.2 Hypothesis

Over all, the Social Compatibility/Sustainability of the Frankfurt–Hohenheim Guidelines is relevant to the Nigerian context!

6.3 Questionnaire Evaluation and Results

The questionnaire here was addressed and distributed to the CEOs and executive and top executive level officers of over 300 Microfinance Banks in Nigeria. These are the captains and doyens of this nascent industry. Our presumption is that they are in the know of what should validly apply to the industry under their watch.

6.3.1 Question 1: Commitment to Corporate Social Ethics

Is it relevant to ask whether companies in your specific industry have corporate policies covering social/ethical aspects (e.g. health and safety, non discrimination, freedom of association, suppliers, etc?)

QUALITATIVE ANALYSIS	
To this leading question, 65% of the respondents found it totally relevant to any ethical-ecological criteriology destined for the Nigerian context. 13% believe it is relevant. Another 13% were undecided. 4% found it not relevant and another 4% found it totally not relevant. Between those who found it totally relevant and relevant, some recurring reasons seemed to inform their choice. Most of the respondents in this category averred that such corporate policies covering the social/ethical aspects are relevant for the corporate existence and future of their various organizations, against the backdrop of the increasing sensitivity to ethical and ecological issues in various segments of the global audience. Some others equally in this category averred that such policies promote business growth and sustainability, while some others in this category equally opined that these issues are very relevant to the creation of good working environment. Between those who found it not relevant and totally not relevant, a host of answers informed their choice. Many in this category claimed that theirs is a new industry in the Nigerian formal business environment and to this end; their social/ethical corporate policies are not yet fully developed.	Totally Relevant (+2) 65% Relevant (+1) 13% Undecided (0) 13% Not relevant (-1) 4% Totally Not relevant (-2) 4%

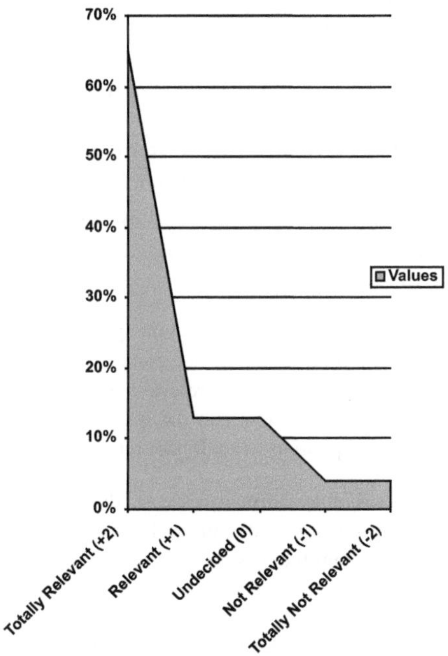

The reactions to this first question must be contextually situated to aid a fuller understanding. As earlier reiterated, formal Microfinance is a new experiment in the Nigerian business environment. The enabling law was promulgated in 2005, which allowed community banks to metamorphose into Microfinance banks. To this end, many of the respondents who viewed this question as not relevant were looking at the time picture or time constraints. They feared not having the requisite history or time to run a fully developed ethical/social corporate policy akin to that proposed by the Frankfurt-Hohenheim Guidelines. Some contend that the primary function of their industry is in the social arena since they cater for the community in all ways in relation to poverty eradication, which entails a lot of socio-ethical themes, as poverty and its alleviation cuts across a host of disciplines.

To this end, most of the companies are new in the sense that microfinance Banking is a new experiment in Nigeria. Many of them metamorphosed from co-operatives, and Non-governmental actors into full-fledged microfinance banks at the 2005 promulgation of the Central Banks Microfinance Regulatory and Supervisory Framework. But the responses show that this does not in any way detract from the enthusiasm and desire of the major actors in this sector, to see some ethical-ecological safeguards applied equally to their industry. To this first question, we can say that their responses, if it continues along these lines, will to a great extent validate our hypothesis that the Frankfurt-Hohenheim Guidelines of Social and Cultural Sustainability are equally relevant in the Nigerian context.

6.3.2 Question 2: The Relevance of Units dealing with Socio-ethical Issues

Is it relevant to ask whether companies in your specific industry have units apart from personnel administration dealing with social/ethical issues (responsibility for ethical policies, community projects, social advisors, etc.)

QUALITATIVE ANALYSIS	
30% of the respondents here were of the opinion that the question as a part of an ethical/ecological criteria fort he Nigerian context is totally relevant. 39% preferred to say that it is simply relevant. 17% sat on the fence; undecided. 4% were of the view that the question is not relevant, while 9% construed the question as totally not relevant. The question went on to ask, if they deem it relevant, they should name the unit and specify its function (vide: annex 1). Some of the units named, which were apart from the personnel administration are as follows: -***Internal Audit Department***, which checkmates the over all operation of the companies at all level -***Corporate Services***, which is identified as responsible for dealing with the public and identifying relevant social areas where the companies can contribute -***Corporate Social Responsibility Unit,*** which is designated as been there to identify the needs of the community and make proposals for possible assistance. It is equally identify as responsible for identifying grievances against the firm and how to mitigate them	Totally Relevant (+2) 30% Relevant (+1) 39% Undecided (0) 17% Not relevant (-1) 4% Totally Not relevant (-2) 9%

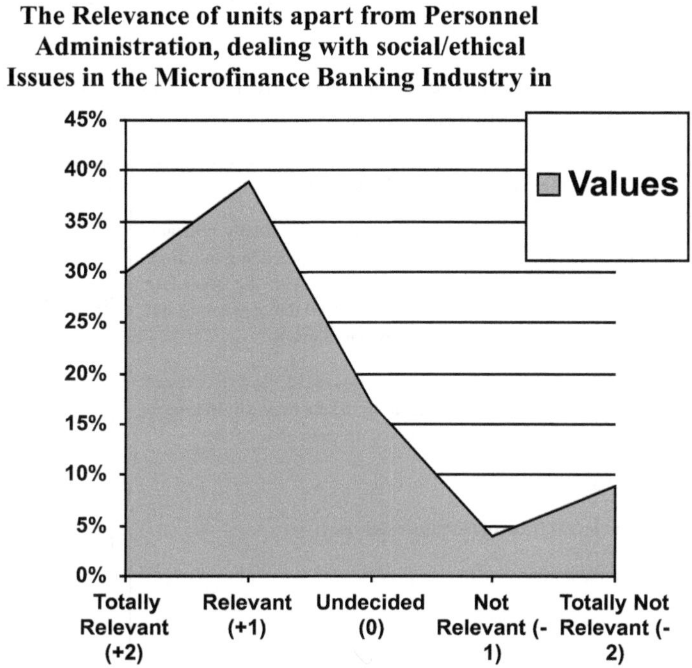

From the reasons advanced for the responses to Question 2: One could see a reactionary climate reminiscent of a sector still in its infancy. Here, ethical/Social issues are still in the thraldom of the over all contractarian model of business which is the hallmark of the Nigerian business environment. The companies and their management as was established in (chapter 2) still view social and ethical responsibility as philanthropy, which the company involves itself in as a matter of charity. To this end, we argue that the stakeholder model or communitarian model of business, which is the basis upon which the Frankfurt-Hohenheim Guidelines is established should be the default software for operation in the Nigerian business clime, if this reactionary bent is to give way to a holistic and all-inclusive consideration that business is not only about profit for the individual companies, but also should be about a win for all stakeholders, including our society and our environment in the long run.

6.3.3 Question 3: The Location of Social/Ethical Affairs in the Management Hierarchy

Is it relevant to ask, at which level of corporate hierarchy the full time head of Social/Ethical Affairs is located?

QUALITATIVE ANALYSIS	
To this question, 31% of the respondents deemed it totally relevant. This is in the neighbourhood of the answer to the preceding question. 39% deemed it relevant, which is on all fours with the preceding question. 9% decided to be undecided. 4% viewed the question as not relevant, while 17% construed it as totally not relevant. The question, gave a room to those who responded "yes" to expand more on the level of the corporate hierarchy where they would love to see this located. Some of the levels thrown up were as follows: -Middle level Management -Management level-(Head of Corporate Services) -Head of Administration -Board in charge of Management -Governing Board Level -Managing Director -Managerial Level	Totally Relevant (+2) 31% Relevant (+1) 39% Undecided (0) 17% Not relevant (-1) 4% Totally Not relevant (-2) 9%

The Relevance of asking at which level of the corporate hierarchy the full time Head of Social/Ethical Affairs is located

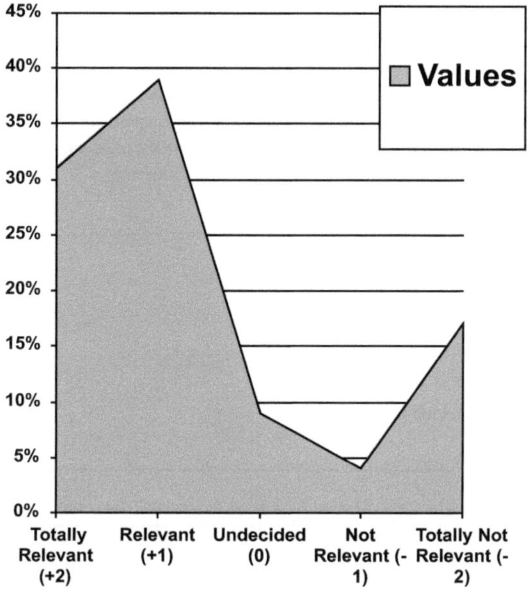

When one looks at the corporate hierarchy level where majority of the respondents who viewed the question as relevant desired that this head of social and ethical affairs should be located, the picture emerges that these administrators deem that the office or position is important as to merit a place in top level management of the company. None of the respondents advocated for a junior staff to man the position, or for the position to be located at the junior management level. Their suggestions could be seen to range from mid level, to the top level management. This as one could see is an encouraging signal that these executives are at home with the importance of ethical and social issues in their industry. This further consolidates the validity of our hypothesis that the Social Compatibility rating of the Frankfurt-Hohenheim Guidelines is relevant to the Nigerian context.

6.3.4 Question 4: Confidential Possibilities of Reporting Grievances related to Working conditions

Is it relevant to ask, whether companies in your specific industry offer possibilities, which allow employees to report grievances related to work place/working conditions in a confidential way?

QUALITATIVE ANALYSIS	
To this question, 66% of our respondents construed it as totally relevant, while 30% viewed it as relevant. Here we recorded no "undecideds" or anyone who deemed not relevant to the least degree. The question like the preceding ones tried to elicit the level of the corporate hierarchy where this should be located. The respondents' answers range is within the mid-level and top management officers. Some of the answers included, but not limited to the following -The Board of Directors -Chairman of the Board -The Management -The CEO -The Heads of the various Departments	Totally Relevant (+2) 66% Relevant (+1) 30% Undecided (0) 0 Not relevant (-1) 0 Totally Not relevant (-2) 0

Many respondents here submitted the fact that their companies are already using the ***Suggestion box*** to this end. Some others stated that ***ad hoc committees*** are empanelled as the cases arise to deal with grave cases or complaints emanating from the employees. Some others contended that they have an ***open door policy***, which gives an aggrieved employee the access to the top-management level executives to air his grievances and obtain redress or consideration of them.

The Relevance of asking whether Companies in the Nigerian Microfinance Banking Industr offer possibilities, which allow employees to report grievances related to workplace/working conditions in a confidential way

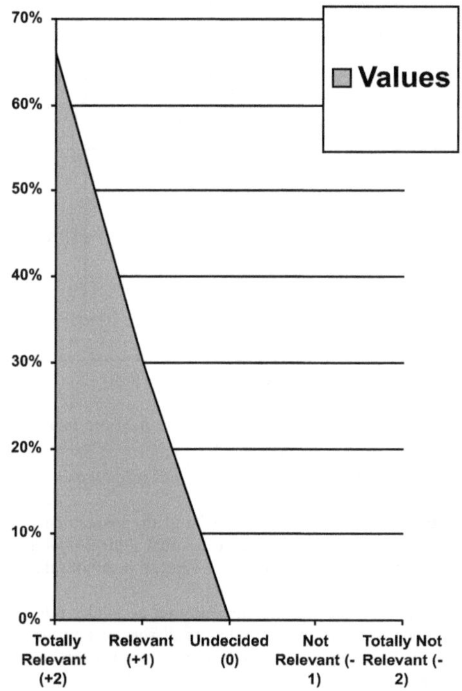

6.3.5 Question 5: Audit and Surveys in Employee Satisfaction, health and Safety, Non Discrimination, etc.

Is it relevant to ask whether companies in your specific industry conduct audits or surveys to monitor social/ethical aspects on the following areas, viz employee satisfaction, health and safety; non-discrimination, etc?

Area	Totally Relevant (+2)	Relevant (+1)	Undecided (0)	Not Relevant (-1)	Totally not Relevant (-2)
Employee Satisfaction	61%	17%	13%	4%	4%
Health and Safety	52%	21%	4%	0%	0%
Non Discrimination	35%	17%	13%	0%	0%
Other (Trading, Supplies and Contract awards)	17%	4%	0%	0%	0%

QUALITATIVE ANALYSIS

On whether it is relevant to ask whether firms in the Nigerian Microfinance banking industry conduct audits or survey to monitor social/ethical aspects, like employee satisfaction, health and safety of employees, non-discrimination and other issues of concern, our respondents reacted as follows:

1. **Employee Satisfaction**: Here, we recorded 61% of the respondents construing the question in relation to this item to be of total relevance to such ethical-ecological criteria. 17% deem it relevant. 13% were undecided while 4% apiece deemed it as not relevant and totally not relevant respectively.
2. **Health and Safety**: Here, 52% deemed the question as totally relevant and 21% deemed it as relevant. 4% were undecided and we recorded no dissensions on this score. The others chose to absent themselves from casting a vote in favour or against the relevance or otherwise of the question on this score.
3. **Non Discrimination**: Here 35% of the respondents deemed it totally relevant. 17% deemed it relevant. 13% were undecided and the rest absented themselves from venturing an opinion on this score, as we recorded no dissensions here as well.
4. **On other issues of concern**: So many respondents raised the issue that it relevant to ask whether companies in this sector conduct audits on their trade contract award policies or supplies whether it violates basic ethical codes or the laws of the land, or whether the contract award regime conduces to misappropriation, corruption and embezzlement of companies funds. Here we recorded 17% who deemed this issue to be totally relevant, and 4% who deemed it relevant.

Reviewing most of the reasons submitted for the above answers, most of the respondents' views transcended the framework we have for this point. Majority here were of the opinion that all aspects of the firms activities and operations should be subject to audit; and that there should be no sacred portfolios, offices, operations or policies which should be exempt from audit.

Another area that generated comments was on the relevance of conducting audit in the area of non-discrimination in the company. Many respondents here contended that discrimination should not be discouraged at all levels, especially where people are discriminated against based on their tribe or religion. We noticed that the perception of discrimination here in relation to this question revolves chiefly around tribal affinity and religious affiliation. This is a pointer that Nigerians may be more united on their common discountenance of tribalism or religious bigotry than their politics or the media suggest them to be. It is a very important point since tribalism has been the albatross and waterloo of development since Nigeria's independence.

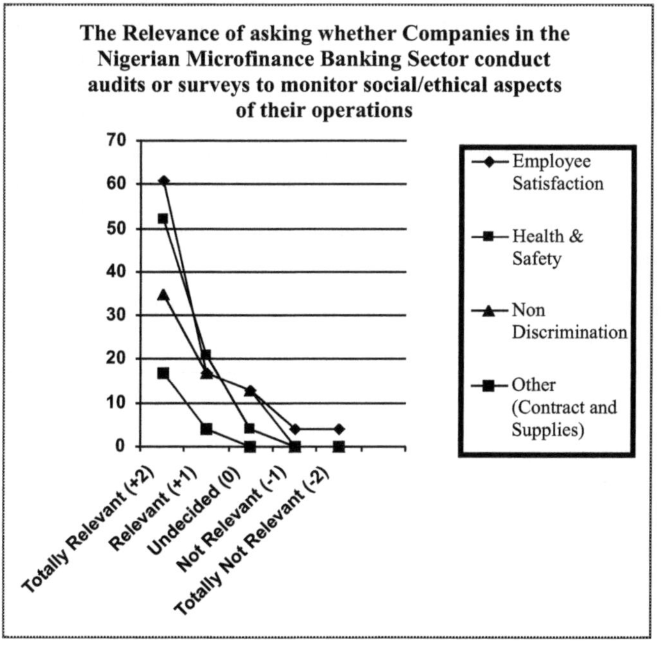

6.3.6 *Question 6a: Internal and External Reporting of Social/Ethical Performance*

Is it relevant to ask, how companies in your specific industry report internally/ externally on their social/ethical performance?

QUALITATIVE ANALYSIS	
On this score, 43% of the respondents were of the opinion that it is totally relevant that any ethical-ecology criteria for the Nigerian context should contain or rather ask how companies in the microfinance banking industry report on social/ethical performance. 17% believe that it is relevant. 4% remain undecided, while 9% of the respondents view the question as totally not relevant. In relation to the reasons for the answers, the major currents include: -The need for is a need for the employees and the public to be able to check the contributions and efforts of the related companies in this regard -Utmost transparency boost integrity, facilitates the participation of staff and other stakeholders -Report on the Social/ethical performance encourages the staff and increases customer confidence	Totally Relevant (+2) 43% Relevant (+1) 17% Undecided (0) 4% Not relevant (-1) 0 Totally Not relevant (-2) 9%

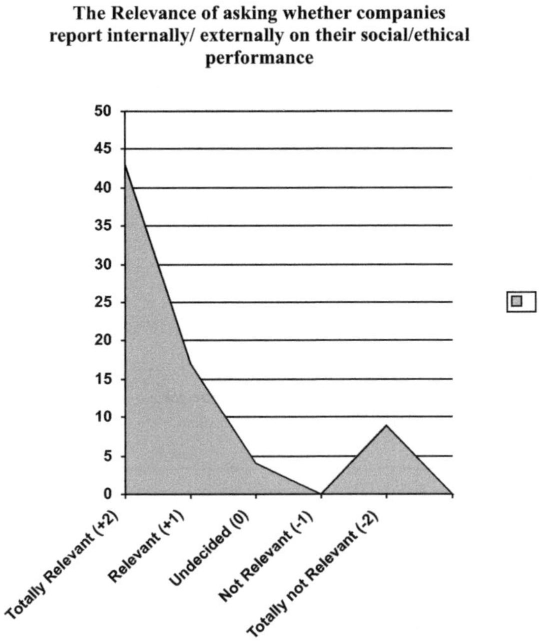

6.3.7 Question 6b: Relevant Media in Reporting Social/Ethical Performance

Are the following media relevant in reporting the social/ethical performance of the companies?

Medium of Reporting	Totally Relevant (+2)	Relevant (+1)	Undecided (0)	Not Relevant (-1)	Totally Not relevant (-2)
Social Report (Printed)	51%	28%	20	0	0
Social Report (via Homepage)	13%	13%	17%	4%	0
Staff Magazines	56%	18%	22%		

QUALITATIVE ANALYSIS

Social Report (Printed):

As can be seen from the table, those in who are of the opinion that the Printing the Social Report is totally relevant were 51% of the respondents. 28% felt that it is relevant. 20% stood undecided and we recorded no one who deemed it irrelevant.

Social Report (via the Homepage)

13% apiece viewed this way as totally relevant and relevant respectively. 17% were undecided and 4% deemed it as not relevant.

Staff Magazines

Here 56% of the respondents saw Staff Magazines as totally relevant. 18% viewed it as relevant. 22% were undecided. We recorded no dissensions.

One could see that the majority of our respondents favour the print medium as the most relevant way of publishing the Social report of companies. This may lie in the not so wide diffusion of other technologies in the Nigerian context.

Social Report (Printed)

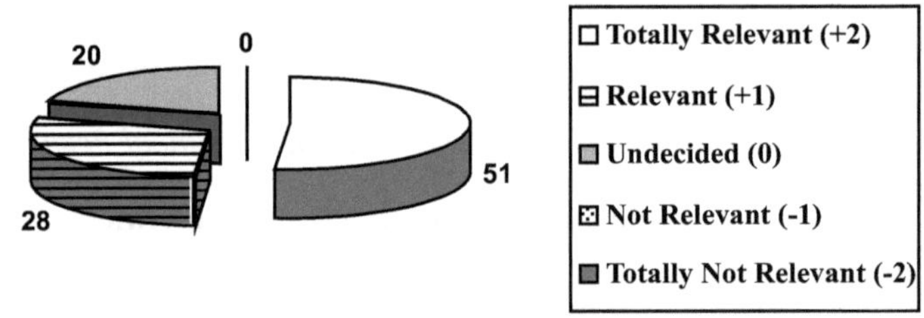

Social Report (via Homepage)

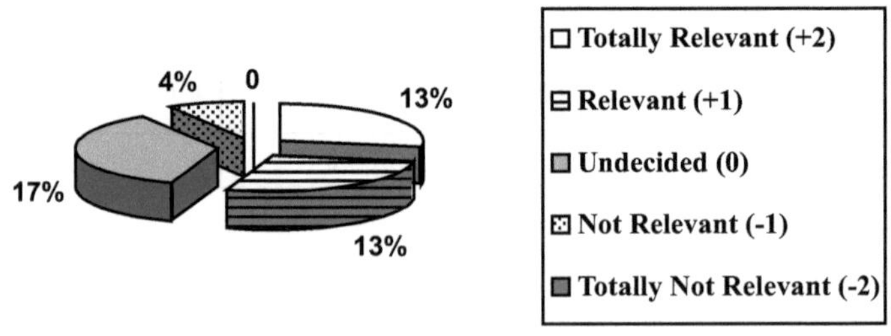

Publication of Social Report on Staff Magazines

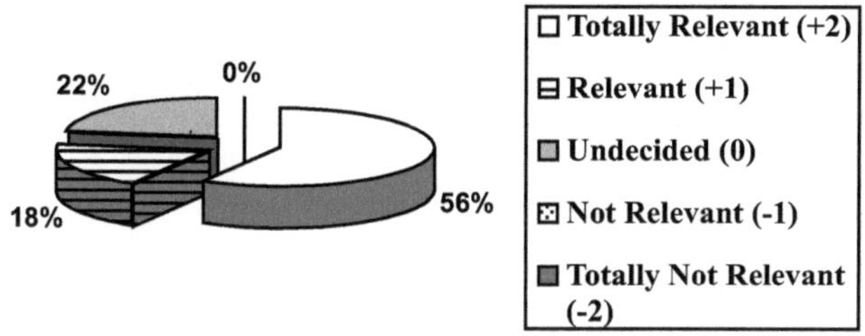

6.3.8 Question 7: Is it relevant to ask, how companies in your specific industry ensure freedom of association for all employees (e.g. through group policy, staff committees, etc.)

QUALITATIVE ANALYSIS	
On the relevance of querying how companies ensure freedom of association for all employees as a veritable part of an ethical-ecological criteriology for the Nigerian context, 78% of our respondent viewed it as totally relevant, while 17% construed it as relevant. We recorded 4% of our respondents contending that it is totally not relevant.	Totally Relevant (+2) 78%
Suffice it to note that some of those who disagreed contended that this is not relevant since the freedom of association is already provided for in the Nigerian constitutions and that Banks and every other corporate citizen are bound by it; and that making it a part of such a criteriology is equal to a duplication of what is already there.	Relevant (+1) 17% Undecided (0) 0%
The fact must be reiterated that the Nigerian constitution provides for the freedom of association. To this end, in every financial institution in Nigeria, especially in the banking sector, employees are allowed to form unions. And for many of our respondents, this is rightly so because unions seem to be the most unprejudiced way of representing the employees' aspiration and needs before the management. Many contend that the Human Resources Department of many firms are simply annexes or extensions of the management or board, or owners of the company, and hence subject to influences outside that of the employees.	Not Relevant (-1) 0% Totally Not Relevant (-2) 4%
Many of our respondents on the positive side contended that companies should extend incentives for their employees to unionize and not antagonize unions unnecessarily with threats of retrenchment.	

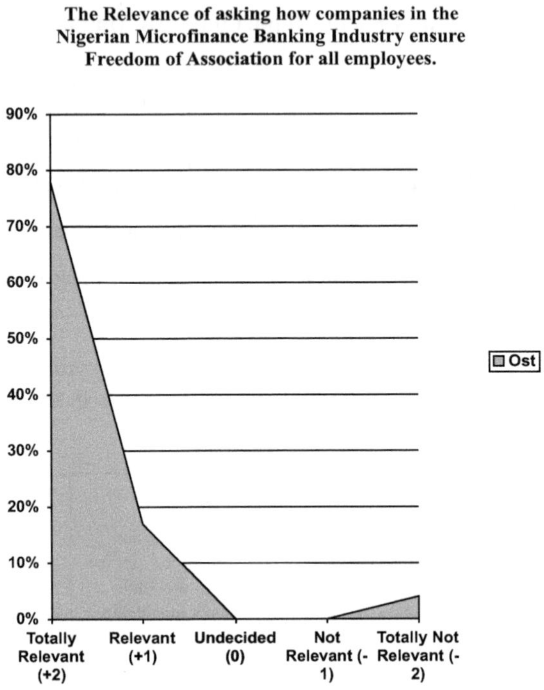

6.4 Staff Relations

6.4.1 Employee Participation

6.4.1.1 Question 1: Channels of Communication

Is it relevant to ask, which channels companies in your specific industry offer for employee participation or influence on decision making? If relevant, the following,

1. Incentives to promote employee proposals for what % of Staff?
2. Staff/employee committees with decision-making power for what % of Staff?

QUALITATIVE ANALYSIS	
On the relevance of asking about the channels companies use to facilitate employee participation or influence decision making, 48% of our respondents deemed it totally relevant. 4% construed it as relevant. 18% were undecided. The rest decided to absent themselves and their votes here. A major thread running through the reasons offered by those who deemed it as totally relevant include the following: ❖ Any company that wants to survive and progress in the tough competitive Nigerian environment must carry its employees along in all matters. ❖ Employees perform better when they are given a sense of responsibility in the direction in which the company goes ❖ When employees participate in decision making, their loyalty to their employer and to the company are enhanced. ❖ Involving employees in decision making secures their commitment to the implementation of company policies and programmes. Reacting to question (sub. 1), the respondents would love a situation where incentives to promote employee proposal is offered to 100% of Staff, both on the senior and the junior echelons of the company. And in reacting to question (sub.2) they would love to have staff/employee committees with decision making power for 60% of the staff.	Totally Relevant (+2) 48% Relevant (+1) 4% Undecided (0) 18% Not Relevant (-1) 0% Totally Not Relevant (-2) 0%

The Relevance of asking which channels companies in the Nigerian Microfinance Banking Industry offer for employee participation or influence on decision making.

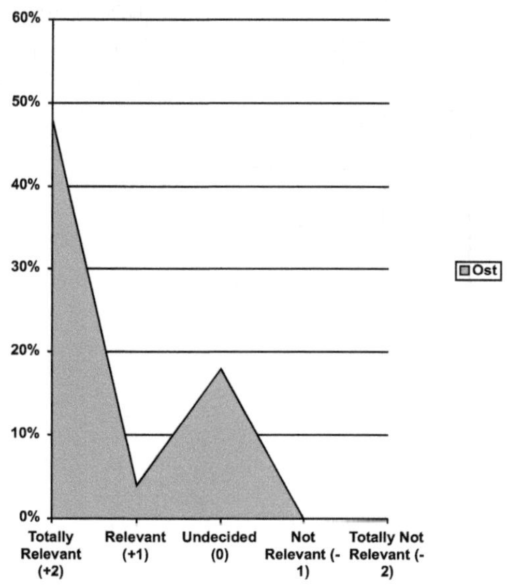

6.4.2 Working Time

The regular working time across the Banks, as supplied by our respondents are as follows:

Item	Maximum	Average
Working times per week	40 hours per week	40 hours per week
Daily Working time	8 hours per day	8 hours per day
Number of Vacations days per year	30 days	21 days

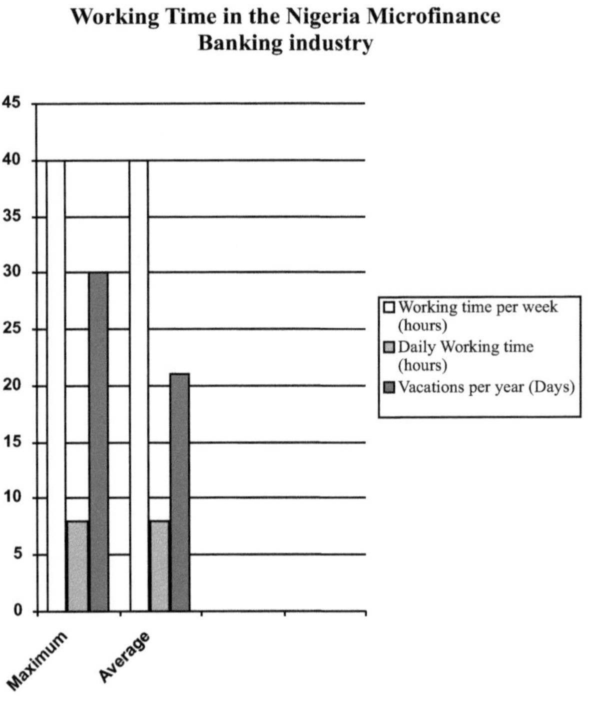

6.4.2.1 Question 2: Items Relevant for Compensation of Overtime

Which of the following items are relevant for the compensation of overtime in your company?

Item	Totally Relevant (+2)	Relevant (+1)	Undecided (0)	Not Relevant (-1)	Totally not Relevant (-2)
1. No Compensation					
2. Financial Compensation	100%	0	0	0	0
3. Compensation in the form of leisure time	2%	–	–	–	–
4. Other such as Promotion and awards	4%	8%		0	0

QUALITATIVE ANALYSIS

All our respondents, 100%, laid great emphasis on financial compensation as the most relevant item for the compensation of overtime in their various companies. This may not be unrelated to the fact that a section of the Nigerian labour law laid this down as the form of compensating for work done over the legal time limit of 8 hours a day. In 1974, the Nigeria military government changed by decree, the working hours from a 35 hour work week to a 40 hour work week, and stipulated payment for extra work done over the legal limit.

Over and above that, some of the reasons advanced by our respondents suggest that in a cash economy like Nigeria, which is in dire straits at the moment, that financial compensation is more motivational. They suggest that it encourages the staff to put in more; boosts their motivation in order to work hard for the progress of the institutions. Others suggests that financial compensation is more acceptable and determinable, while other suggests that in lieu of the low salary, which obtains across the industry, that financial compensation is more appreciated.

Another fact we encountered in the responses suggests that financial compensation is determined based on the level of those working overtime. This is to say, that everyone does not get the same thing.

2% of the respondents stated that compensation in the form of leisure time is a totally relevant item in consideration of compensation in their companies.

Another dimension was noticed equally from the responses. 4% stated that awards of prizes and promotions are relevant items in the consideration of compensation for overtime in their various companies. 8% thought it relevant.

The Relevant items for compensation of overtime in the Nigerian Microfinance Banking Sector

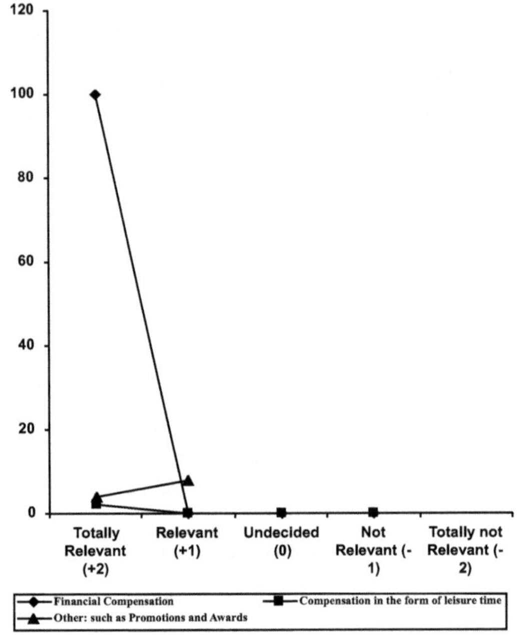

6.4.2.2 Question 3: Possibility of Flexible Working Time

Please specify the percentage of staff which is offered the possibility to use the following

Item	Totally Relevant	Relevant	Undecided	Not Relevant	Totally not Relevant
1. Part time jobs	0%	0%	0%	0%	0%
2. Flex time jobs	N/A	N/A			
Working time accounts					

Home based work	0%	0%	0%	0%	0%
Unpaid leave					
Other (Youth Corpers)	14%				

QUALITATIVE ANALYSIS

Many of the respondents feel that this question has no relevance in the Nigerian context. In an economy where unemployment is as high as 40% in urban areas, flex time jobs or part time jobs in an industry like the financial services sector seems to be a luxury. Some contend that since Nigeria is an economy with low technology and telecommunication density that most of the categories here do not apply. To this end, most staff of the banks works full time.

The only exception here is in the case of youth Corp members who are posted to serve on some of these institutions. They work full time except on the days they are billed for community service or any other activity bordering on their service.

6.4.3 Safeguarding Jobs

6.4.3.1 Question 4: Is it relevant to ask, whether companies in your industry offer limited appointments for their employees (What is the rate of limited appointments compared to appointments for an indefinite period?

QUALITATIVE ANALYSIS

Most of our respondents seemed not to be keen in answering this part of the questionnaire. This is understandably so, bordering on the same factors encountered in the immediately preceding question. In most cases in the MF industry, appointments are indefinite. Limited appointments are very rare. To this end, most of the MF banks offer full time employments.

We attribute this equally to the fact that microfinance banks are quite a very young experience in the Nigerian financial industry.

This situation holds and applies for questions 4 and 5 of our questionnaire

6.4.3.2 Question 6: Is it relevant to ask, whether in the last four years staff was laid off in your specific industry due to restructuring and economic reasons?

QUALITATIVE ANALYSIS	
21% of our respondents deemed this question totally relevant. 17% deemed it relevant. 34% were undecided. 9% construed it as not relevant, while 17% deemed it as totally not relevant. We noticed a trend where many are of the opinion that since microfinance banking is simply 3 years old in Nigeria, there has not be a major crisis in this sector to warrant laying off of workers. Some of the respondents recognized though that over and above the guidelines and regulations laid down by the Central Bank, that many individual companies operate within the terms of their corporate visions, which differ from one bank to another.	Totally Relevant (+2) 21% Relevant (+1) 17% Undecided (0) 34% Not Relevant (-1) 9% Totally Not Relevant (-2) 17%

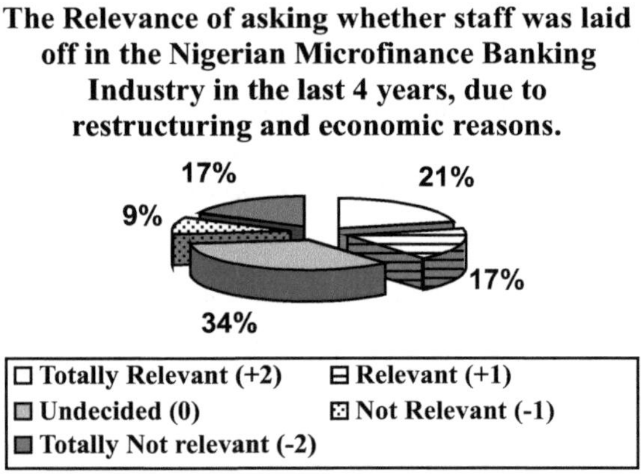

6.4.3.3 Question 7: Is it relevant to ask, what measures were implemented to help your former staff to find new employment and to reduce their economic hardship?

QUALITATIVE ANALYSIS	
At this juncture, it is important not to lose sight of who our respondents are. They are top level management of many microfinance banks in Nigeria. This is to say that they are the crème la crème of that nascent industry. This is what makes the responses to this question so very interesting. 43% view the question being a part of an ethical-ecological criteriology for the Nigerian context as totally relevant. 9% deemed it relevant. 26% remained undecided. Another 9% deemed it not relevant, while 13% deemed it totally not relevant. When asked to proffer or specify how the companies do promote this, many of our respondents suggested that companies could help their former staff find new employment by issuing testimonials, recommendations and reference letters to help them in their future job search. Others suggested simply paying them off as stipulated by the law.	Totally Relevant (+2) 43% Relevant (+1) 9% Undecided (0) 26% Not Relevant (-1) 9% Totally Not Relevant (-2) 13%

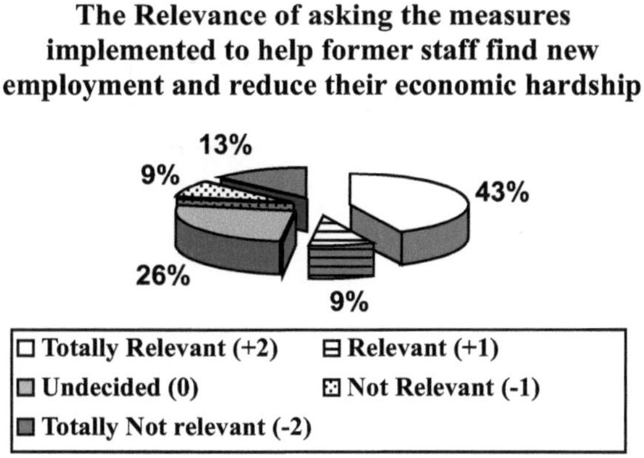

6.4.3.4 Question 8: Benefits Offered Workers

Is it relevant to ask, whether employees are offered the following benefits

	Totally Relevant (+2)	Relevant (+1)	Undecided (0)	Not Relevant (-1)	Totally not relevant (-2)
Share of Profit	42%	19%	–	4%	13%
Regular health insurance	64%	17%	–	6%	9%
Regular pay in case of illness	58%	35%	4%	–	–
Regular Pension Scheme	100%	–	–	–	–
Maternity Grants	72%	22%	6%		
Paid Parental Leave	43%	19%	29%		
Canteen/Subsi-dized lunch	68%	32%	–	–	–

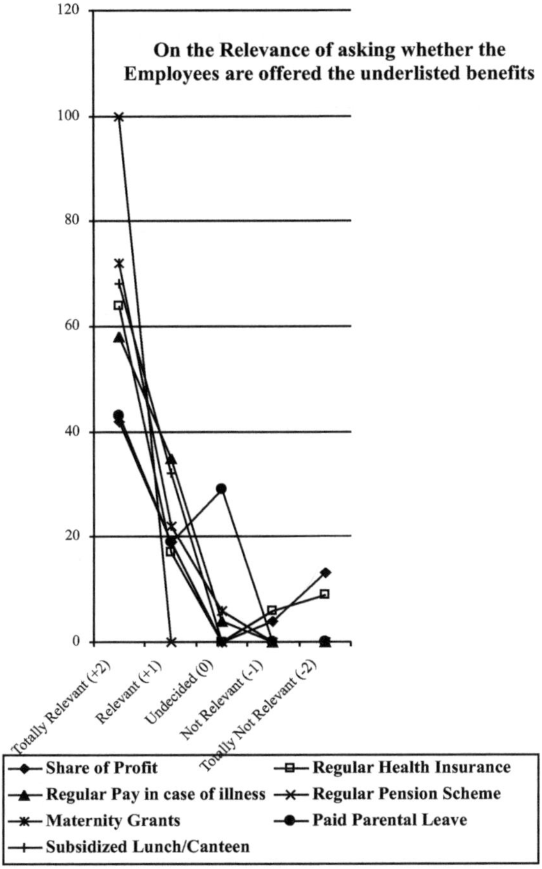
On the Relevance of asking whether the Employees are offered the underlisted benefits
120
100
80
60
40
20
0
Totally Relevant (+2)
Relevant (+1)
Undecided (0)
Not Relevant (-1)
Totally Not Relevant (-2)
Share of Profit
Regular Health Insurance
Regular Pay in case of illness
Regular Pension Scheme
Maternity Grants
Paid Parental Leave
Subsidized Lunch/Canteen

6.4.3.5 Question 9: Training Program for Staff

This question asked our respondents to provide data on the training program for their staff.

On this score, only 48% of the respondents were able to furnish us with this data. And from the collation of this data we were able to determine that the total average rate of the staff joining further training programmes here is 69% of the Staff. And the total average training hours is 80 hours per staff per year. This translates to some 3.3 days in a year.

6.5 Health & Safety

6.5.1 Question 10: Is it relevant to ask, whether companies in your industry offer a health and safety program?

<table>
<tr><th>QUALITATIVE ANALYSIS</th><th>Totally Relevant (+2)</th><th>65%</th></tr>
<tr><td rowspan="4">65% of our respondents view the question as totally relevant, while 4% viewed it as relevant. 13% were sitting on the fence of indecision. 9% apiece viewed as it not relevant and totally not relevant respectively.

Most of those who viewed it as relevant were of the view that this is and should be an essential part of the welfare package. Some contended that since health insurance schemes does not seem to be functional in Nigeria, that companies and banks should devise their own means of offering healthcare as apart of the welfare package, either in paying extra money as health benefits monthly to help the workers attend to their health needs.

Some of the safety programmes they listed as relevant are as follows: Minimal dust exposure, fire prevention programmes, electric shock prevention, humidity control</td><td>Relevant (+1)</td><td>4%</td></tr>
<tr><td>Undecided (0)</td><td>13%</td></tr>
<tr><td>Not Relevant (-1)</td><td>9%</td></tr>
<tr><td>Totally Not Relevant (-2)</td><td>9%</td></tr>
</table>

The Relevance of asking, whether companies in the Nigerian Microfinance Banking industry offer a health and safety program for its employees

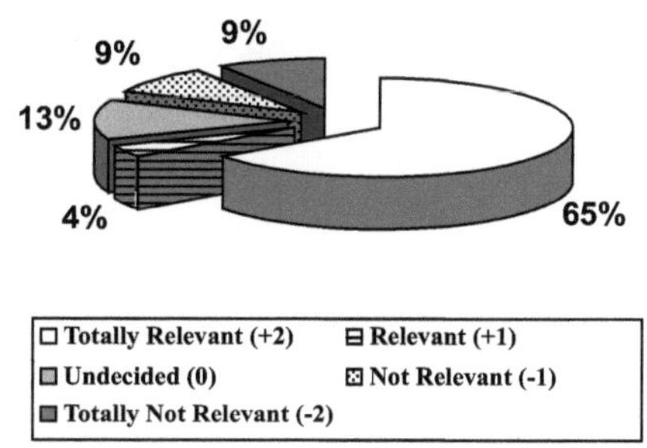

6.5.2 Question 11: Welfare Facilities for Employees

Please specify the % of staff with direct access to the following facilities

a. Medical care
b. Non-smoking offices

QUALITATIVE ANALYSIS

Medical care:

To this question, our respondents failed to come up with figures. Of all the respondents, none of them provided information which showed that any of their staff have direct access to medical care provided or paid for by the banks. Our conclusion is that either that these banks have no provisions for the medical care of their employees. This is understandable against the backdrop of the Nigerian context where health insurance is dysfunctional to say the least.

Non-Smoking Offices:

100% of our respondents opined that all their offices are non-smoking offices, as the employees who are smokers or who want to smoke must either do it outside or at any other place outside the office. Our conclusion here is that there seems to be a general discountenancing of smoking in the offices. This is equally understandable in the Nigerian context where the majority don't entertain a positive view of smoking.

6.5.3 Question 12: Health and Safety Standards for Employees

Is it relevant to ask, whether company's employees are protected by high minimum standards regarding health and safety standards are set either by law or through labour agreements?

QUALITATIVE ANALYSIS	
To this question, 52% of our respondents deemed it totally relevant. 4% deemed relevant and 22% were undecided. 13% deemed it not relevant and 9% went to the extreme of viewing as totally not relevant. The programme most of them specified is the National Health Insurance Scheme (NHIS). **The National Health Insurance Scheme** is a laudable attempt of the Nigerian government to redesign access to health care of the ordinary Nigerian along the lines of those standards obtained in the developed countries, where the costs of medical care is equitably shared and shoulder. The decree for this scheme was promulgated by the military government under General Abdulsalam Abubakar in 1999, but was eventually launched in 2003 under the civilian government of Olusegun Obasanjo. Under this scheme, participation is optional except for workers in public and private sectors, who will contribute 5% of their basic salary, while their employers pay 10% for each worker, which entitles a contributor, a spouse and four children to access healthcare from any approved service provider. But the implementation of this scheme seems not to have diffused into all sectors of the economy as can be seen in the preceding responses of our respondents, which indicates that this is not in place in their various organizations.	Totally Relevant (+2) 52% Relevant (+1) 4% Undecided (0) 22% Not Relevant (-1) 13% Totally Not Relevant (-2) 9%

The Relevance of asking, whether company's employees are protected by high minimum stadards regarding health and safety standards, which are either set by law or through labour agreements.

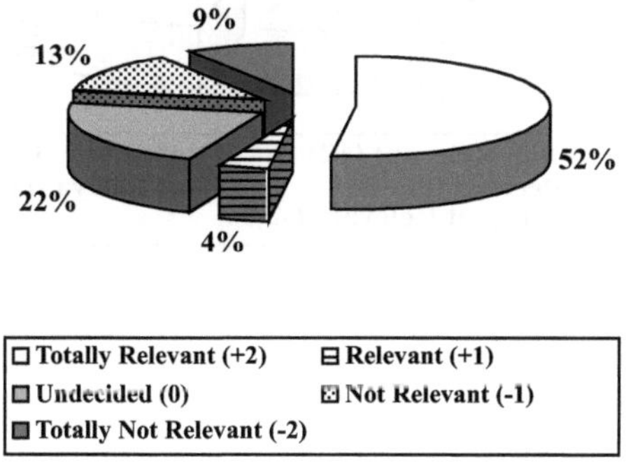

6.5.4 Question 13: Compliance of Company to Health and Safety Regulations

Is it relevant to ask, whether in recent years fines related to health and safety case were imposed on companies in your industry (job related fatal accidents)?

QUALITATIVE ANALYSIS		
On this score, 30% of our respondents deemed it totally relevant. But most of them cited the ambiguous nature of its realization and are doubtful of its application in the Nigerian context, where policy somersault from the government in promulgating the National Health Insurance scheme, leads the way in the lack of policy coherence and fluidity, which greatly mitigates against the application of such worthwhile aspirations to better the condition of workers and elevated motivation in the workplace. 4% deemed it relevant. Many of our respondents who deemed it totally relevant and relevant, in spite of their answers contended that this is relevant for a general criteriology but not so very relevant for their sector.	Totally Relevant (+2)	30%
	Relevant (+1)	4%
	Undecided (0)	13%
	Not Relevant (-1)	18%
On the other hand 13% were undecided as it relates to the relevance of the question. 18% deemed it not relevant, and 35% deemed it totally not relevant. Many of those here argued that production related or industrial accidents are minimal in the banking sector.	Totally Not Relevant (-2)	35%

The Relevance of asking whether in recent years fines related to health and safety cases were imposed on companies in your industry as it relates to the Microfinance Banking industry in Nigeria

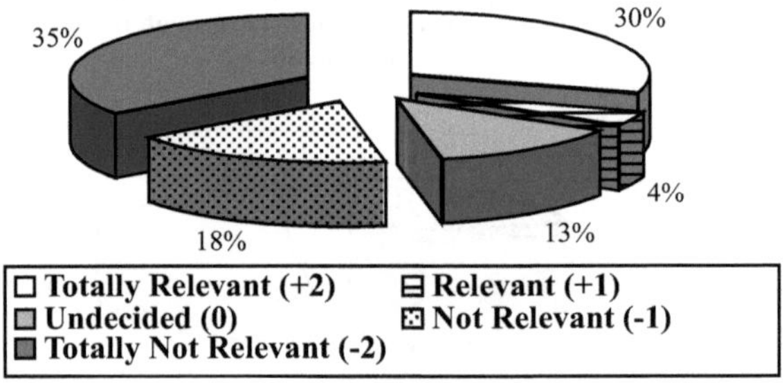

6.6 Equal Opportunities

6.6.1 Question 14: Application of Anti-discrimination Policies

Is it relevant to ask, whether companies in your industry apply policies to avoid discrimination on the basis of race, colour, sex, religion, political opinion, sexual preference or social origin?

QUALITATIVE ANALYSIS	
52% of the respondents viewed this question as totally relevant, while 12% viewed it as relevant. 13 were undecided and another 13% viewed it as not relevant. Only 9% saw it as totally not relevant. From the responses gathered, there does not seem to be any formal policy in relation to discrimination which the banks subscribe to. This is left to the provisions of the Nigerian constitution, which in Chapter 4 section 42, prohibits all forms of discrimination against any Nigerian based on circumstance of birth, sex or tribe and so on.	Totally Relevant (+2) 52% Relevant (+1) 12 % Undecided (0) 13 % Not Relevant (-1) 13 % Totally Not Relevant (-2) 9%

The Relevance of asking whether companies in the Microfinance Banking Industry in Nigeria apply policies to avoid discrimination on the basis of race, colour, sex, religion, political opinion, sexual preference or social origin

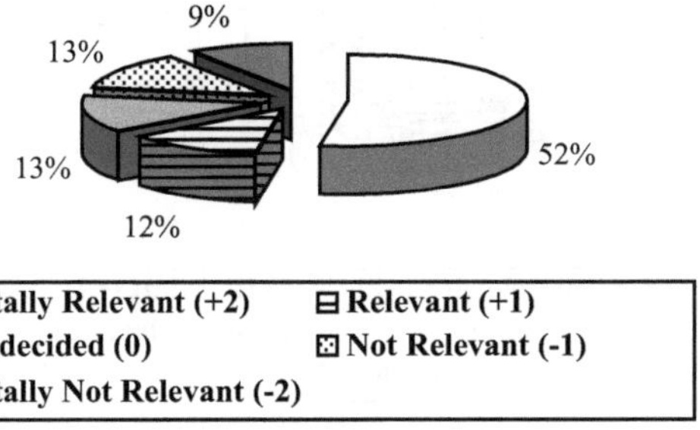

6.6.2 Question 15: Minimum Wage for Employees

Is it relevant to ask, whether companies in your industry apply legally required minimum wages for unskilled workers

QUALITATIVE ANALYSIS	
53% of our respondents agreed to the fact that the question is totally relevant. 9% saw it as relevant. 20% remained undecided and some 13% construed it as totally not relevant. The responses must be critically viewed against the backdrop that the legally required minimum wage in Nigeria as of 2000 according to the National minimum wage Amendment Act, 2000 makes it the duty of every employer in Nigeria to pay nothing less 5, 500 naira per month as minimum wage to every worker in his establishment. That translates to around $40 dollars a month. This is what the law says. But whether this is the case on the ground is another thing. Some of our respondents contend that the question is relevant although firms pay wages based on their size and earning. The fact as we discovered is that most companies don't follow government stipulations in this regard. On the reasons for their answers, some of those who viewed it as totally relevant contended that a minimum wage higher than the minimum wage rate motivates their employees to work better	Totally Relevant (+2) 53% Relevant (+1) 9% Undecided (0) 20% Not Relevant (-1) 0% Totally Not Relevant (-2) 13%

The Relevance of asking whether companies in the Microfinance Banking Industry in Nigeria apply legally required minimum wages for unskilled workers

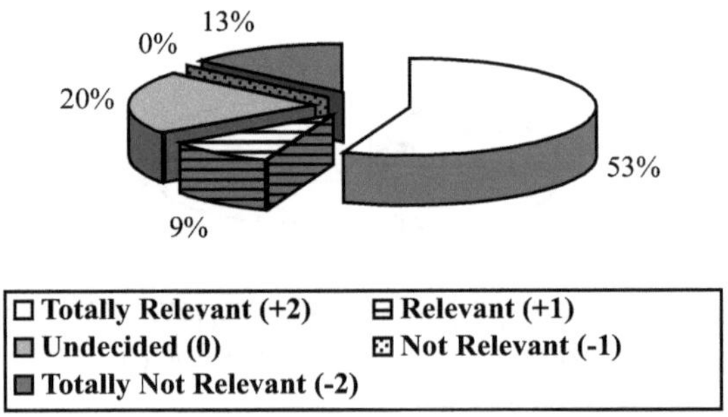

6.6.3 Question 16: Ensuring Safe Workplace and Adherence to Relevant Working condition-related Regulations

Is it relevant to ask, how companies in your industry ensure a safe workplace as well as adherence to relevant regulations for employees under 18 years of age (regarding dangerous work, night work) in your facilities?

QUALITATIVE ANALYSIS	
To this question, 45% of the respondents deemed it totally relevant. 20% remained undecided and 9% apiece viewed it not relevant and totally not relevant respectively. The rest did not respond to that. Those who deemed it totally relevant showed a marked intolerance for underage employment; some going as far as stating that it should never be tolerated. Some others anchored the relevance of the question on the fact that all safety appliances should be in place to save lives in cases like fire outbreaks and so on.	Totally Relevant (+2) 45% Relevant (+1) 0% Undecided (0) 20% Not Relevant (-1) 9% Totally Not Relevant (-2) 9%

The Relevance of asking whether companies in the Microfinance Banking Industry in Nigeria ensure a safe working place as well as adherence to relevant regulations for employees under 18% of age (regarding dangerous or night work)

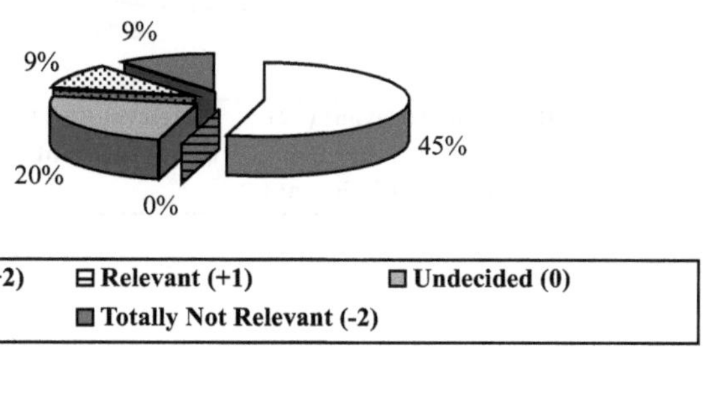

6.6.4 Question 17: Non Discriminatory Remuneration

Is it relevant to ask, whether companies in your industry ensure equal pay for men and women with equal qualification and experience?

QUALITATIVE ANALYSIS	
On the relevance of this question, 86% of our respondents were of the opinion that it is totally relevant to any ethical/ecological criteria for assessing firms in the microfinance banking sector in Nigeria. 4% followed suit concurring that it is relevant. 9% stood undecided. Here we recorded no dissensions. Many of our respondents transcended constitutional provisions to favour a non discriminatory and empowerment policy for women.	Totally Relevant (+2) 87% Relevant (+1) 4% Undecided (0) 9% Not Relevant (-1) 0% Totally Not Relevant (-2) 0%

The relevance of asking whether companies in the Nigerian Microfinance Banking Industry ensure equal pay for men and women with equal qualification and experience

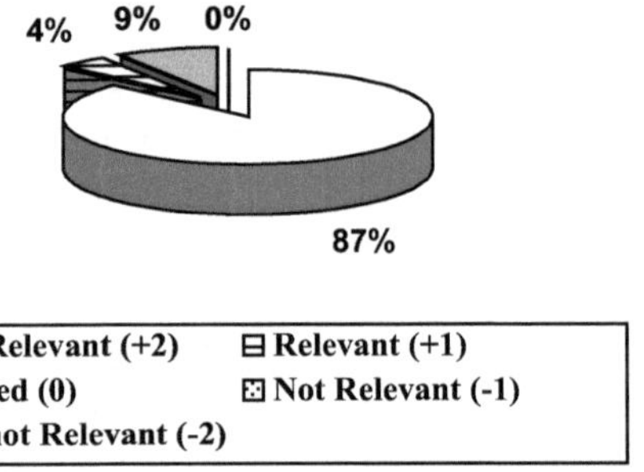

6.6.5 Question 18: Gender Distribution of Management Positions

The data concerning gender distribution at the top executive and management levels of the Nigerian Microfinance Banking industry

Position	Male	Female
Executive Board	66%	34%
Management Positions	55%	36%

The average rate of women working in the industry is 30%

18c: **On the efforts of the firms to avoid**

1. Many of the executive respondents did not answer the questions on their efforts to avoid sexual harassment and mobbing of female employees. Many claimed never to have any cases of sexual harassment. Others claimed that it is not an issue of immediate concern, but they are dealt with whenever such situations arise. Some others claimed that the board constitutes a disciplinary committee to investigate each case as it arises on an ad hoc basis. Punishments for defaulters range from the possibility of facing a disciplinary committee and dismissal. Another form of punishment listed by our respondents is that any case of sexual harassment is subject to investigation after which the guilty part is handed over to the Police for prosecution.
2. The inference could be drawn that either that the executives are uncomfortable discussing such issues, as this attitude cannot be divorced from what obtain from the general population. In Nigeria, the issues of sex and sexual harassment are to an extent still clothed in corrugated layers of taboo. Open discussion of sex is considered in bad taste. Women, who are sexually harassed or sometimes raped, are not forthcoming with their plight. The ventilation of their trauma shows them off as damaged goods, which jeopardises their chances of marriage or good odour in the society.
3. On the efforts to curb mobbing, we could not get a clear line of action proposed by the respondents in relation to this question. Many claimed that it does not exist in their working environment.

Gender Distribution of those employed in the Nigerian Microfinance Banking Industry

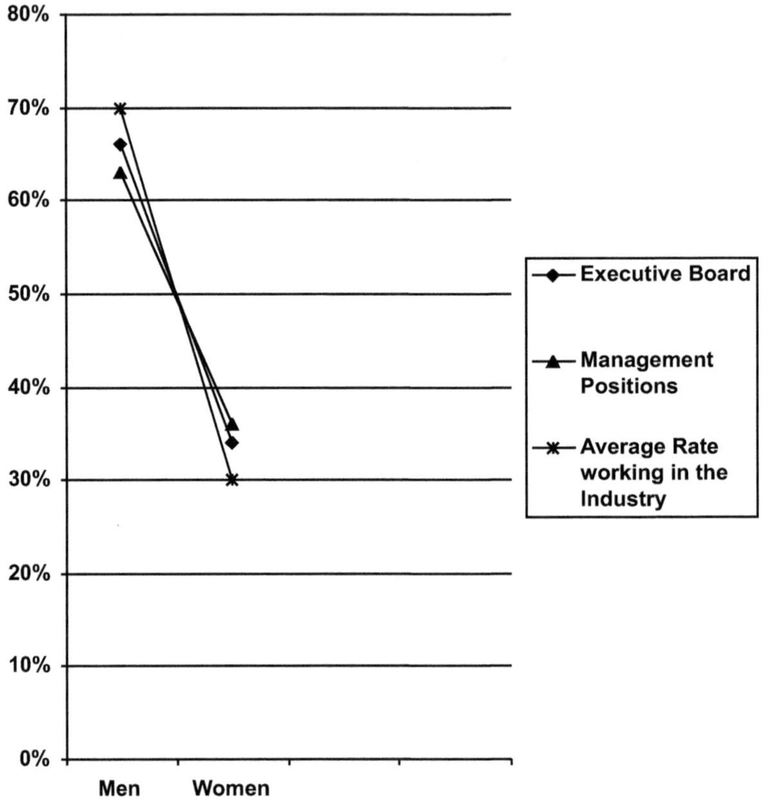

6.7 Relations with External Stakeholders

6.7.1 Customer and Product Responsibility

6.7.1.1 Question 1: Responsible Marketing and Data Protection

Is it relevant to ask, whether companies in your industry have policies regarding responsible marketing and data protection?

QUALITATIVE ANALYSIS	
48% of our respondent deemed the question totally relevant although they stated that no such policies exist in the microfinance industry in Nigeria. 4% deemed it relevant. 17% were undecided. 4% deemed it not relevant. The remainder did not venture an opinion here. As reiterated earlier, many of the respondents contended that no such policy exists independently outside the Central Bank of Nigeria's regulations on Microfinance banks, which stipulates the rules and regulation guiding the conducts of microfinance banks. But some of our respondents remarked that this question is relevant for the larger banking industry in Nigeria, where young girls are used in a sexually exploitative way to secure customers for the banks. They deemed this practice a form of irresponsible marketing. And that no banks can pass any ethical test without passing this question.	Totally Relevant (+2) 48% Relevant (+1) 4% Undecided (0) 17% Not Relevant (-1) 4% Totally Not Relevant (-2) 0%

The relevance of asking whether companies in the Nigerian Microfinance Banking Industry have policies regarding responsible marketing and data protection

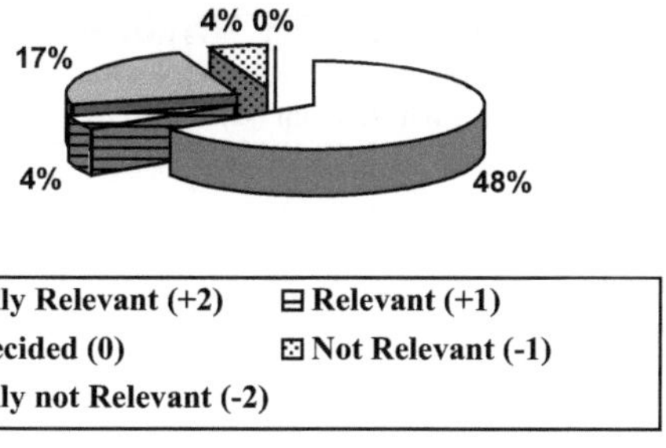

6.7.1.2 Question 2: Non Discriminatory Access to Financial Services

Is it relevant to ask, whether companies in your industry have policies/measures on granting access to financial services without discrimination (Social financial inclusion for low income groups)

QUALITATIVE ANALYSIS	
This question goes to the heart of this industry. The industry as reiterated in the opening pages is all about granting the poor access to finance without collateral, in order to finance their enterprise and escape from poverty. To this question, 61% deemed it totally relevant, while 9% deemed it relevant. 13% of the respondents were undecided while 17% deemed it totally not relevant. Majority of those who deemed it totally not relevant were of the opinion that since the raison d'être of the industry is to provide loans to the poor without discrimination, that the question has to that end being relegated to irrelevance.	Totally Relevant (+2) 61% Relevant (+1) 9% Undecided (0) 13% Not Relevant (-1) 0% Totally Not Relevant (-2) 17%

The relevance of asking whether companies in the Nigerian Microfinance Banking Industry have policies/measures on granting access to financial services without discrimination (social/financial inclusion for low income groups)

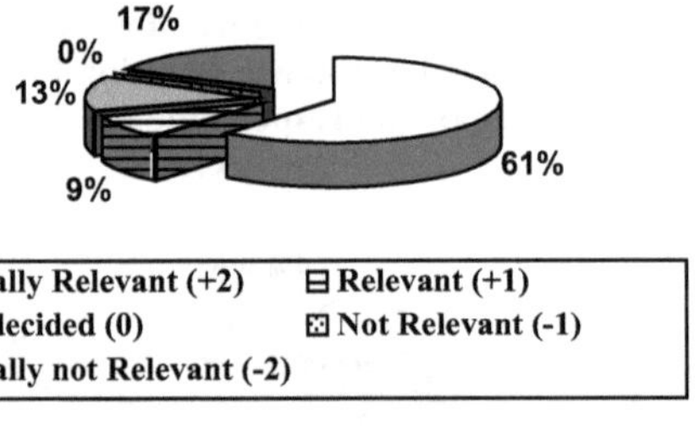

6.7.1.3 Question 3: Options Open to Customers with Debt Repayment Problems

Is it relevant to ask, whether companies in your industry have policies/measures regarding customers with debt repayment problems (e.g. Debt counselling, ombudsman, co-operation with customer protection organizations)

QUALITATIVE ANALYSIS	
On this score 59% of our respondents contended that it asking about such measures and policies is totally relevant, while 18% deemed it relevant. 12% were undecided and 10% deemed it totally irrelevant.	Totally Relevant (+2) 59% Relevant (+1) 18% Undecided (0) 12% Not Relevant (-1) 0% Totally Not Relevant (-2) 10%

The relevance of asking whether companies in the Nigerian Microfinance Banking Industry have policies/measures regarding customers with Debt Repayment Problems

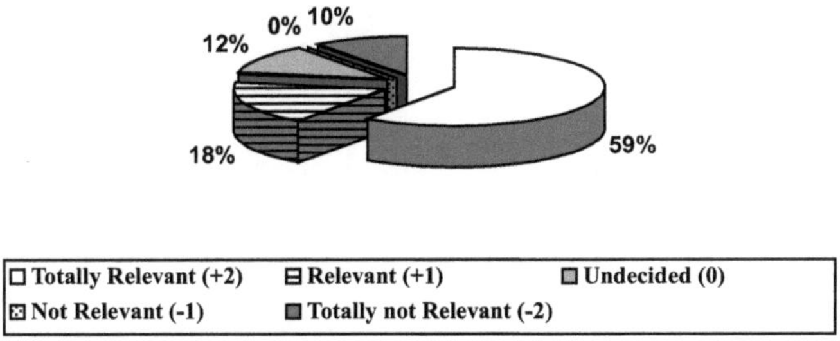

6.7.1.4 Question 4: Companies' Social Engagement

Is it relevant to, ask whether companies in your industry lend to companies / projects with high social benefits (e.g. microcredit programmes, community lending/investments, special conditions for SMEs)

On this question, we scarcely got a response, but a variety of remarks, which when summarized states that this question is not relevant to the industry since the essence of the industry is to lend to projects with high social benefits; to SMEs, and to individuals to help snatch them from the jaws of poverty.

6.7.1.5 Question 5: Disclosure of Mutual Funds voting Behaviour

Is it relevant to ask, whether mutual funds managed by the company disclose their voting behaviour in annual general meetings to the fund owners.

To this question as well, majority of our respondents voted out rightly that it is not relevant because it does not apply in this case. This inheres in the fact that microfinance banks in Nigeria do not manage mutual funds.

6.8 Corporate Governance

6.8.1 Independene and Effectiveness of Board

6.8.1.1 Question 6: Separations of Powers at the Top Management Level

Is it relevant to ask, whether companies in your industry separate the power between the CEO and Chairman of the Board?

QUALITATIVE ANALYSIS	
68% of our respondents were agreed that this is totally relevant while 11% deemed it as relevant.16% were undecided and 5% viewed the question as totally not relevant. Most of the respondents indicated that in their outfit, the CEOs are answerable not only to the board chairman, but to the entire board of directors. To ensure delineation of duty areas and to forestall undue overlapping or interference of the Board Chairman in the day to day working of the company; to define the powers of the CEOs, the board is placed over him are some of the reasons tendered by our respondents who deemed it totally relevant.	Totally Relevant (+2) 68% Relevant (+1) 11% Undecided (0) 16% Not Relevant (-1) 0% Totally Not Relevant (-2) 5%

The relevance of asking whether companies in the Nigerian Microfinance Banking Sector separate the power between the CEO and the Chairman of the Board

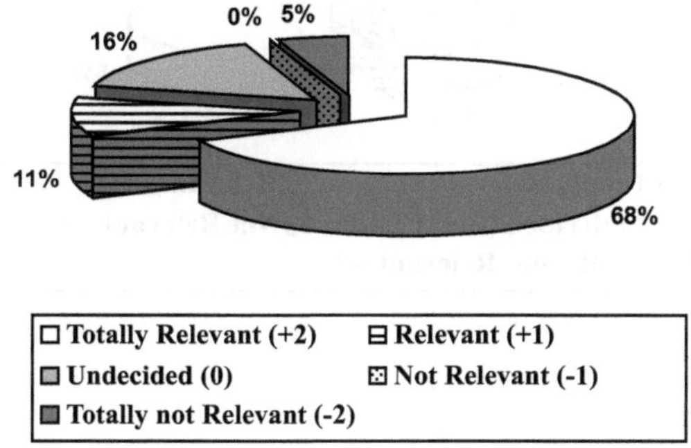

6.8.1.2 Question 7: Independence of Board from Executive Managers

Is it relevant to ask, whether companies in your industry maintain different board committees which are independent of executive managers (e.g. remuneration committee, audit committee, nomination committee, etc.)

QUALITATIVE ANALYSIS	
On this score, 56% of our respondents were of the opinion that the question is totally relevant, while 6% deemed it relevant. 17% of our respondents were undecided and 11% deemed it not relevant. Only some 9% construed it as totally not relevant.	Totally Relevant (+2) 56% Relevant (+1) 6% Undecided (0) 17% Not Relevant (-1) 11% Totally Not Relevant (-2) 9%

The relevance of asking whether companies in the Nigerian Microfinance Banking Sector maintain different boardd committees which are independent of executive managers

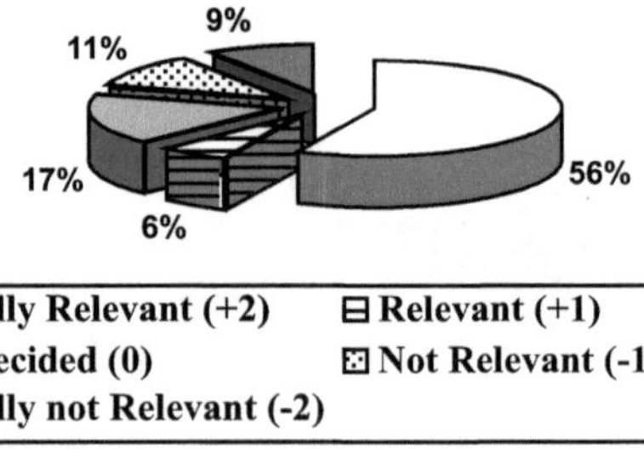

6.9 Shareholder Democracy

6.9.1 Question 8: Restrictions on Voting Rights

Is it relevant to ask, whether companies in your industry maintain any restrictions on voting rights (e.g. one share entitles the owner to one vote)?

QUALITATIVE ANALYSIS	
On this score, we have 41% attesting to its total relevance while 12% considered it relevant. 18% of the respondents were undecided. 12% and 16% of the respondents viewed it as not relevant and as totally not relevant respectively.	Totally Relevant (+2) 41% Relevant (+1) 12% Undecided (0) 18% Not Relevant (-1) 12%

The relevance of asking whether companies in the Nigerian Microfinance maintain any restrictions on voting rights (e.g. one share entitles the owner to one vote)

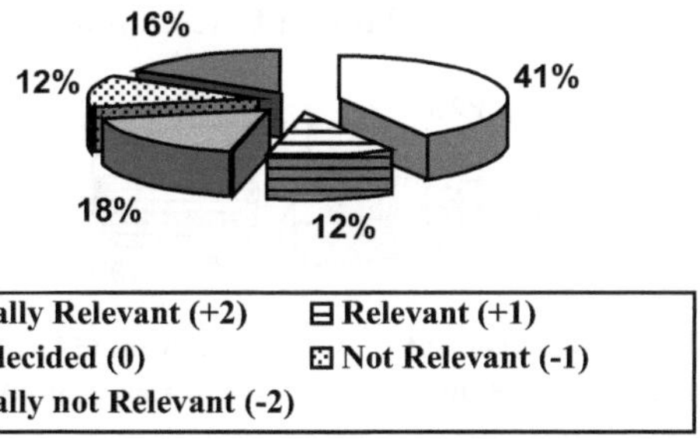

6.9.2 Question 9: Shareholding Size as Precondition for Submitting Resolution at the AGM

Is it relevant to ask, whether companies in your industry consider the size of the shareholding as a pre-condition on submitting a resolution at the annual general meeting.

QUALITATIVE ANALYSIS	
On this score, 29% of our respondents viewed it as totally relevant. 18% viewed it as relevant while 24% were undecided. 6% and 22% respectively construed it as not relevant and totally not relevant respectively. Some of our respondents considered the question and the point very relevant but opined that in most cases, this is not being considered due to the size of most companies in this sector. Others contend that in their own companies, shares determine the number of votes, but not the submission of resolutions.	Totally Relevant (+2) 29% Relevant (+1) 18% Undecided (0) 24% Not Relevant (-1) 6% Totally Not Relevant (-2) 22%

The relevance of asking whether companies in the Nigerian Microfinance sector consider the size of shareholding as a precondition on submitting a resolution at the annual general

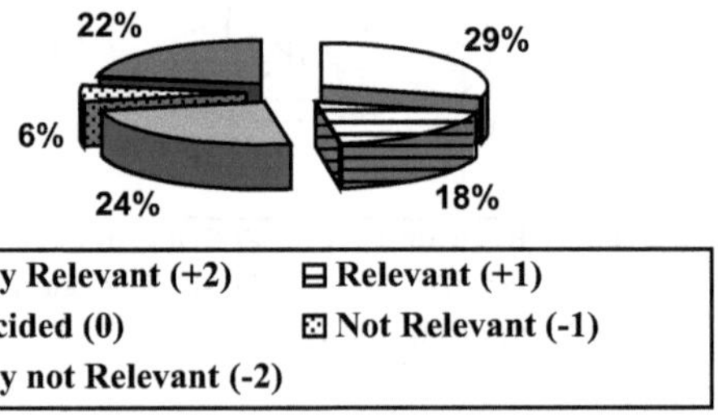

6.9.3 Question 10: Facilitating Shareholder Participation

Is it relevant to ask, whether companies in your industry facilitate shareholder participation by broadcasting the annual general meeting and giving the shareholders the opportunities to vote on proxy resolution via the internet

QUALITATIVE ANALYSIS	
Here 56% of our respondents deemed the question totally relevant and 6% deemed it relevant. 28% were standing in the middle; casting their votes neither way. 5% apiece deemed the question not relevant and totally not relevant respectively. Most of our respondents who were on the positive side deem the question relevant with a caveat. This caveat is that votes per internet are almost impossible in the Nigerian context where limited access to internet is the order of the day coupled with the literacy and computer literacy level of the shareholders. Lack of electricity is equally fingered as a factor which makes the internet option, an impossibility in the Nigerian context.	Totally Relevant (+2) 56% Relevant (+1) 6% Undecided (0) 28% Not Relevant (-1) 5% Totally Not Relevant (-2) 5%

The relevance of asking whether companies in the Nigerian Microfinance sector facilitate shareholder participation by broadcasting the annual general meeting and giving shareholders the opportunities to vote on proxy resolutions

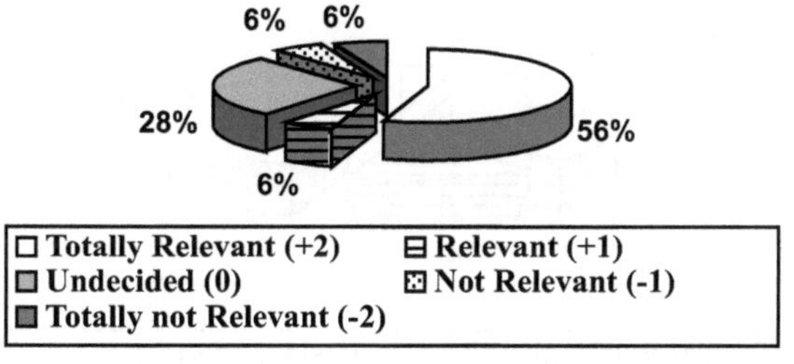

6.9.4 Question 11: Disclosure of Compensation Scheme for Executive Board members

Is it relevant to ask, whether companies in your industry disclose the compensations schemes for executive board members?

QUALITATIVE ANALYSIS	
On this score 44% of our respondents deemed the question totally relevant and 17% deemed it relevant. Another 17% were undecided. 15% of the respondents deemed the question as not relevant, while a 6% deemed it totally not relevant. Those who disagreed cited the security situation in Nigeria; for instance, the rampant case of armed robbery, assassinations, and kidnapping of people in Nigeria and the huge ransom sums being demanded by the kidnappers, as a reason why it is not desirable to publicize such an information. Some contended that this would expose their board members to unnecessary security risks.	Totally Relevant (+2) 44 % Relevant (+1) 17% Undecided (0) 17 % Not Relevant (-1) 15 % Totally Not Relevant (-2) 5%

The relevance of asking whether companies in the Nigerian Microfinance sector disclose the compensation schemes for executive board members

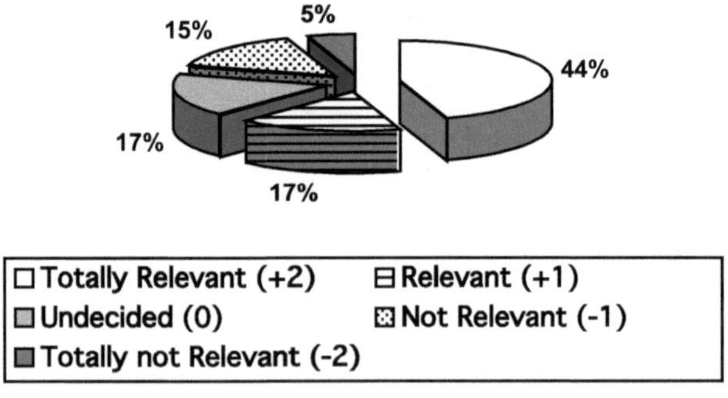

6.10 Community Involvement

6.10.1 Question 12: Responsibility for Community projects

Is it relevant to ask, whether companies in your industry take responsibility for community projects? If yes, the following

Project	Totally Relevant (+2)	Relevant (+1)	Undecided (0)	Not Relevant (-1)	Totally Not Relevant (-2)
1. Social Projects	54%	6%	17%	11%	6%
2. Cultural Projects	28%	0%	22%	6%	0%
3. Environmental Projects	33%	20%	4%	4%	0%

QUALITATIVE ANALYSIS

Social Projects

On this score, we see the majority of the respondents, 54% submit that asking whether companies in their sector take responsibility for social projects is totally relevant. 6% stated that it is relevant, and 17% were undecided. 11% of the respondents deemed it not relevant, while 6% deemed it totally not relevant.

Cultural Projects

Here, 28% deemed it totally relevant and 22% were undecided. 6% submitted that it is not relevant and the rest abstained.

Environmental projects

33% views the question on this score as totally relevant, while 20% viewed it as relevant. 4% were undecided and 4% deemed it as totally not relevant.

On the social project, we saw a deluge of diverse opinion as regards the reasons for their various answers. The majority of those who deemed the question as totally not relevant contended that this question is dangerous in a country like Nigeria. This they contended lies in the fact that if companies are expected or made to shoulder the responsibility for social and environmental projects, that will hand the government a blank check to shirk and evade its responsibilities, which Nigerian governments have been so good at doing since independence. They contended that this is not the province of companies; that companies should like everyone else behave itself like good corporate citizens; obeying the laws and following on the cues laid down by the law and the policies laid down by the government; and not usurping the role of governments for their subjects.

The trend noticed among those who concurred that on the relevance of the question is their belief that it is a part of their social and corporate responsibilities as parts of the society; as well as a way the companies burnish their images and creates rapport between the company and their clients or local communities in their surroundings.

We did not get answers on the percentage of their profits they dedicate or would dedicate to community projects.

The Relevance of asking, whether companies in the Nigerian Microfinance Banking sector take responsibility for community projects

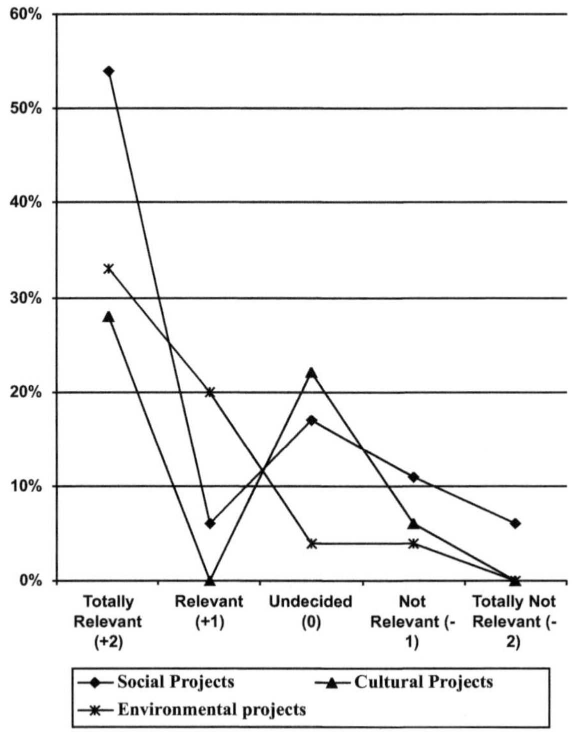

6.10.2 Question 13: On Making Political Contributions

Is it relevant to ask, whether companies in your industry make political contributions?

QUALITATIVE ANALYSIS	
On this score, 26% deemed it as totally relevant to ask whether companies in the industry make political contributions, while 13% remained undecided. 17% deemed it as not relevant, while 43% deemed it as totally not relevant. Most of the respondents contended that, although this question is relevant for a criteriology that it does not apply to the microfinance industry since it is a very young experience in the Nigerian formal business sector.	Totally Relevant (+2) 26% Relevant (+1) 0% Undecided (0) 13% Not Relevant (-1) 17% Totally Not Relevant (-2) 43%

The Relevance of asking, whether companies in the Nigerian Microfinance sector make political contributions.

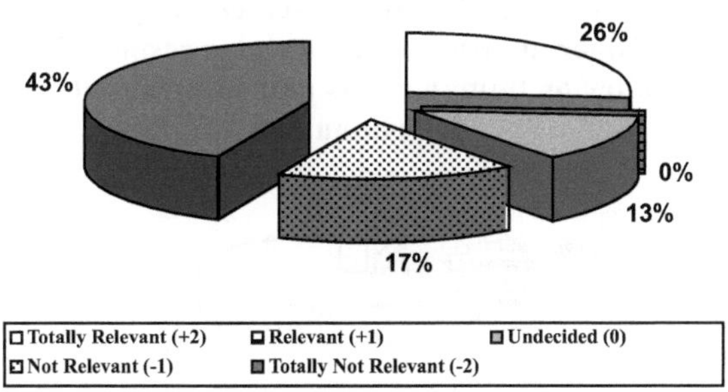

6.11 Society

6.11.1 Question 14: Respect for Human Rights

Is it relevant to ask, whether companies in your industry respect the policy on human rights and cultural self determination?

QUALITATIVE ANALYSIS	
On this question, 72% deemed it totally relevant and 11% deemed it relevant. Another 11% were undecided and 6% deemed it not relevant. The overwhelming majority are of the opinion that human rights must be respected by business as well as the state. But they did not offer us concrete applications of how their industry is doing this, outside the pervading belief that could be gleaned from their reasons, that poverty alleviation, which is their fort is a way of elevating human dignity, which they believe is equally a very important component of human rights.	Totally Relevant (+2) 72% Relevant (+1) 11% Undecided (0) 11% Not Relevant (-1) 6% Totally Not Relevant (-2) 0%

The Relevance of asking, whether companies in the Nigerian Microfinance sector respect the policy on human rights and cultural self-determination

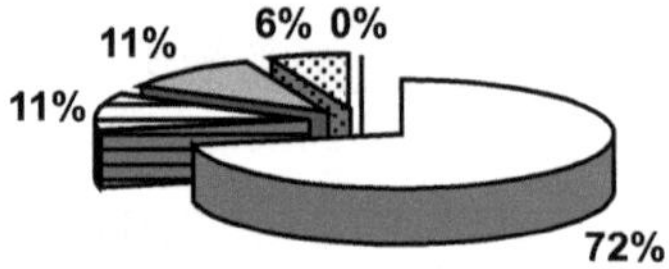

Totally Relevant (+2)	Relevant (+1)
Undecided (0)	Not Relevant (-1)
Totally Not Relevant (-2)	

6.11.2 Question 15: Fair treatment of peoples affected by Companies' activities

Is it relevant to ask, whether companies in your industry have policies on how to deal fairly with peoples affected by companies' activities?

QUALITATIVE ANALYSIS	
Here 37% construe the question as totally relevant and 21% view it as relevant. 10% remained undecided. On the other end of the spectrum, 16% apiece deemed the question as not relevant and totally not relevant respectively. Many of the respondents here on either side of the divided submitted no reasons for their choices, but they made their choices anyway.	Totally Relevant (+2) 37% Relevant (+1) 21% Undecided (0) 10% Not Relevant (-1) 16% Totally Not Relevant (2) 16%

The Relevance of asking, whether companies in the Nigerian Microfinance sector have policies on how to deal fairly with peoples affected by companies' activities

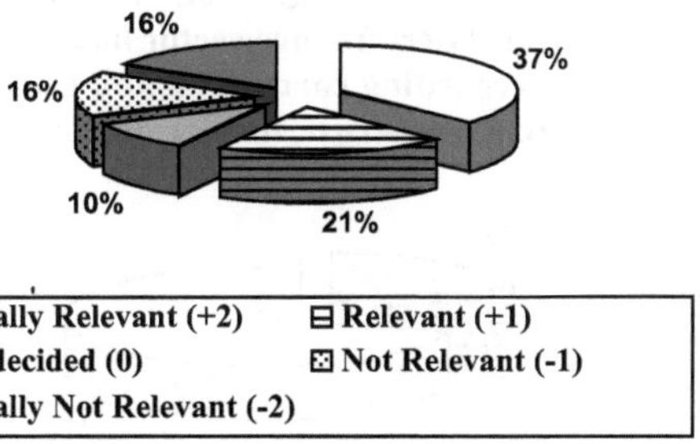

6.12 Fair Business Practices

6.12.1 Question 16: Code of Conduct regarding corruption and economic fraud

Is it relevant to ask, whether companies in your industry have a code of conduct regarding corruption and economic fraud (e.g. antitrust, insider dealing)

QUALITATIVE ANALYSIS	
On this score 70% of our respondents were of the opinion that the question is totally relevant and 10% deemed it relevant. 20% of the respondents were undecided. The trend inferred from the reasons submitted by the respondents include that the question is relevant because corruption and economic fraud erodes customer confidence of any bank or finance house that tolerates it. And that is really risky for business in this competitive sector. Over and above that, Nigeria instituted an Economic and Financial Crimes commission, which seems to be tightening the controls and sensitizing the public on the dangers and risks of economic fraud.	Totally Relevant (+2) 70% Relevant (+1) 10% Undecided (0) 20% Not Relevant (-1) 0% Totally Not Relevant (2) 0%

The Relevance of asking, whether companies in the Nigerian Microfinance sector have a code of conduct regarding corruption and economic fraud (e.g. anti-trust, insider dealing, etc.)

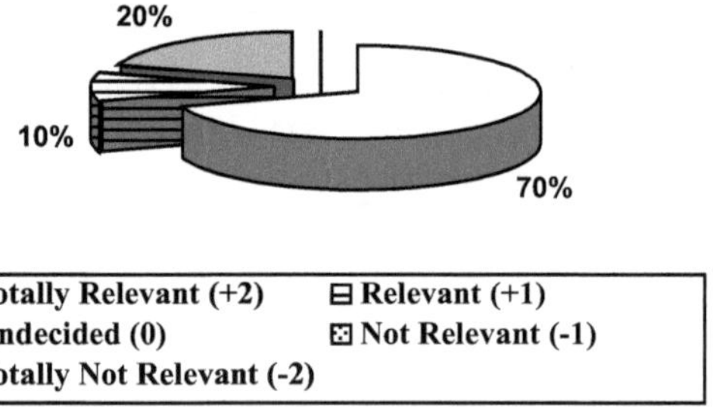

6.12.2 Question 17: Measures to ensure fair business practices

Is it relevant to ask, whether these measures are taken up by the companies in your industry to ensure fair business practices (e.g. against corruption, antitrust, insider dealing, etc.

Measure	Totally Relevant (+2)	Relevant (+1)	Undecided (0)	Not Relevant (-1)	Totally Not Relevant (-2)
1. Training	70	10	20	0	0
2. Audits	90	10	0	0	0
3. Compliance Officers	48	25	7	20	0
4. Hotlines	62	18	20		

QUALITATIVE ANALYSIS

On training, as the table shows, 70% of the respondents deemed it totally relevant, while 10% deemed it relevant. 20% of the respondents were undecided. Here we recorded no dissents. We witness an equally high score on the positive side for AUDITS. Here 90% deemed it totally relevant and 10% deemed it relevant. Here like in training, we witnessed no dissents. The pictures changed a bit as we came to COMPLIANCE OFFICERS. Here 48% deemed it totally relevant, while 25% deemed it relevant. 7% stood undecided and 20% deemed it not relevant. On HOTLINES, 62% deemed it totally relevant and 18% deemed it relevant. 20% stood undecided. Here we equally had no dissents.

The Relevance of asking whether these measures are taken up by companies in the Nigerian Microfinance Banking sector to ensure fair business practices

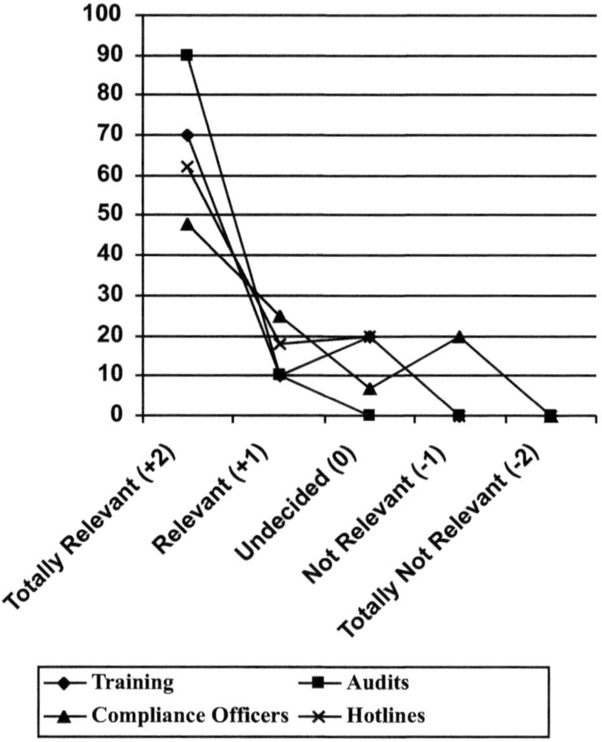

6.13 Summary and Conclusion

6.13.1 Total Average of the Responses to the Social/Cultural Management (A.1)

Question Number	Totally Relevant (+2)	Relevant (+1)	Undecided (0)	Not Relevant (-1)	Totally Not Relevant (-2)
1.	65	13	13	4	4
2.	30	39	17	4	9
3.	31	39	17	4	9
4.	66	30	0	0	0
5a.	61	17	13	4	4
5b.	52	21	4	0	0
5c.	35	17	13	0	0
5d.	17	4	0	0	0
6a.	43	17	4	0	9
6b.	51	28	20	0	0
6c.	13	13	17	4	0
6d.	56	18	22	0	0
7.	78	17	0	0	4
Totals	598	273	140	20	39
Averages	46	21	10.76	1.5	3

Totally Relevant	46 %
Relevant	21 %
Undecided	11 %
Not Relevant	2 %
Totally Not Relevant	3 %
Total absent on this section	17 %

6.13.2 Text of Relevance for A.1

Test of Relevance =

Relevant = (+2) + (+1) = > 50%

Not Relevant = (-2) + (-1) = > 50%

Undecided = (+2) + (+1) = (-2) + (-1)

Relevant = (+2) + (+1) = 46 + 21 = 67%

Not Relevant = (-2) + (-1) = 2 + 3 = 5%

A 1 = Relevant in the Nigerian context: Q.E.D

Total Average responses to the Social/Cultural Management (A.1)

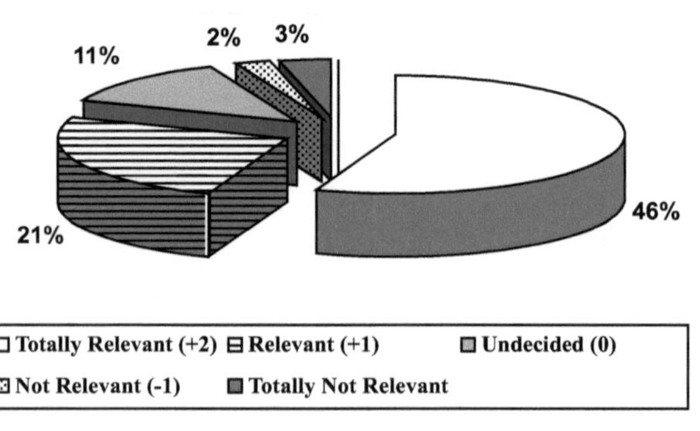

6.13.3 Total Average of the Responses to Staff Relations (A.2)

Question Number	Totally Relevant (+2)	Relevant (+1)	Undecided (0)	Not Relevant (-1)	Totally Not Relevant (-2)
1.	48	4	18	0	0
2a.	100				
b.	2	0	0		0
c.	4	8	0	0	0
6	21	17	34	9	17
7.	43	9	26	9	13
8a.	42	19	0	4	13
b.	64	17	0	6	9
c.	58	35	4	0	0
d.	72	22	6	0	0
e.	43	19	29	0	0
f.	68	32	0	0	0
g.	100	0	0	0	0
10.	65	4	13	9	9
12.	52	4	22	13	9
13	30	4	13	18	35
14.	52	12	13	13	9
15.	53	9	20	0	13
16.	45	0	20	9	9
17.	87	4	9	0	0
Totals	**1049**	**219**	**227**	**90**	**136**
Averages	**52. 45**	**10.95**	**11.35**	**4.5**	**6.8**

Totally Relevant	52 %
Relevant	11 %
Undecided	11 %
Not Relevant	5 %
Totally Not Relevant	7 %
Total absent on this section	14 %

Total Average responses to the Staff Relations (A.2)

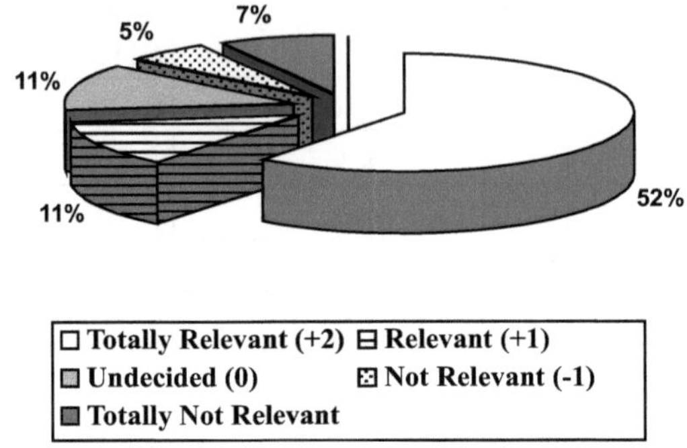

6.13.4 Text of Relevance for A.2

Test of Relevance =

Relevant = (+2) + (+1) = > 50%

Not Relevant = (-2) + (-1) = > 50%

Undecided = (+2) + (+1) = (-2) + (-1)

Relevant = (+2) + (+1) = 52 + 10 = 62%

Not Relevant = (-2) + (-1) = 5+ 7 = 12%

A 2 = Relevant in the Nigerian context: Q.E.D

6.13.5 Total Average of the Responses to Relations with External Stakeholders (A. 3)

Question Number	Totally Relevant (+2)	Relevant (+1)	Undecided (0)	Not Relevant (-1)	Totally Not Relevant (-2)
1.	48	4	17	4	0
2.	61	9	13	0	17
3.	59	18	12	0	10
6.	68	11	16	0	5
7.	56	6	17	11	9
8.	41	12	18	12	16
9.	29	18	24	6	22
10.	56	6	28	5	5
11.	44	17	17	15	5
12a	54	6	17	11	6
b.	28	0	22	6	0
c.	33	20	4	4	0
13	26	0	13	17	43
14.	72	11	11	6	0
15	37	21	10	16	16
16.	70	10	20	0	0
17.a	70	10	20	0	0
B	90	10	0	0	0
C	48	25	7	20	0
D	62	18	20	0	0
Totals	**1052**	**232**	**306**	**133**	**154**
Averages	**52.6**	**11.6**	**15.3**	**6.65**	**7.7**

Totally Relevant	53 %
Relevant	12 %
Undecided	15 %
Not Relevant	7 %
Totally Not Relevant	8 %
Total absent on this section	14 %

Total Average responses to Relations with External Stakeholders

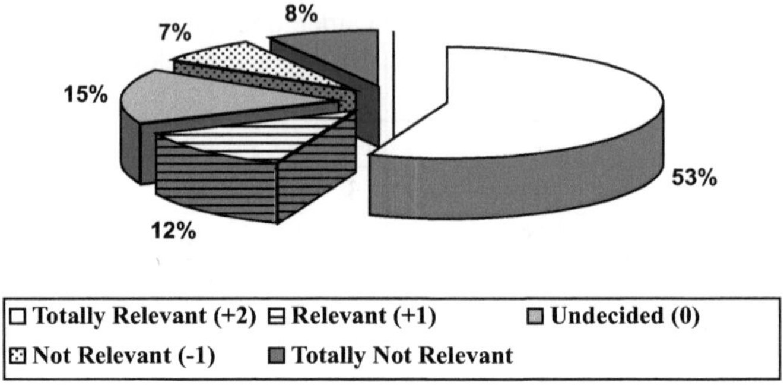

6.13.6 Test of Relevance for A.3

Test of Relevance =

Relevant = (+2) + (+1) = > 50%

Not Relevant = (-2) + (-1) = > 50%

Undecided = (+2) + (+1) = (-2) + (-1)

Relevant = (+2) + (+1) = 53 + 12 = 65%

Not Relevant = (-2) + (-1) = 7+ 8 = 15%

A 2 = > 50%, there fore Relevant in the Nigerian context: Q.E.D

6.14 Overall Relevance of the Social Compatibility of the Frankfurt-Hoheheim Guidelines in the Nigerian Context

= Average Sum total of

A.1 + A.2 + A.3 = > 50%

That is 67 + 62 + 65 / 3 = > 50%

= 194 / 3 = >50%

= 65%

Therefore, the Social Compatibility of the FHG is relevant to the Nigerian context

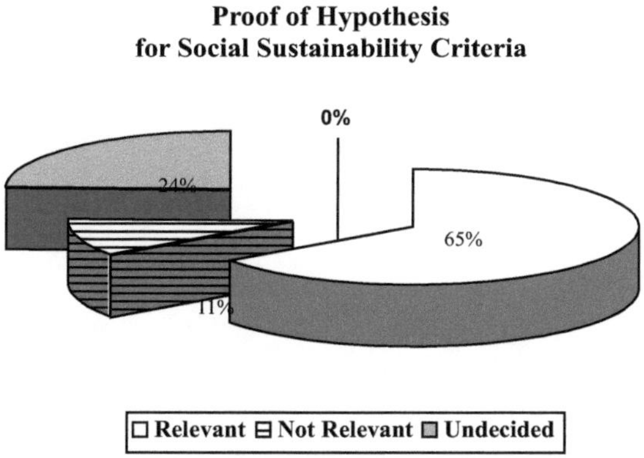

14 Overall Relevance of the Social Compatibility

7. Recapitulation and Synopsis

7.1 Major Moments of the Work

7.1.1 Theoretical Basis of the Investigation

In recapitulating and summarizing our enterprise in this work, we found and submitted as follows:

A few years ago, ecological or ethical investments were dismissed as idealistic combination of finance and ethics, which had a negative effect on yields. Although there had been an increasing realization across all spectrums of socio-economic and developmental discourse, that the need is there for a new ethical manifesto to dethrone the imperialism of economics over ethics; which decades of unbridled accent on capitalism has led the human race, the October, 2008 Stock market crash and the ripples it sent across the world, from which the global economy is yet to recover brought it back forcefully to the table of discourse. If the role of ethics in business and relevance of an ethical-ecological criteria for evaluating companies have been troubling those at the periphery of the discourse on the trajectory of human economic activities, and its portents on human desire not to self-destruct, the 2008 global financial crisis is their answer. Today, ethical assessment of companies has come to increasingly colour the way we invest our resources, and the way companies operate. It is increasingly becoming clear that companies, who fail to adapt or adjust to this trend, are heading towards extinction.

This realization is, among other factors also nourished by the conceptual shift in the traditional conception of a company, which is the basic unit of the economic system. This is the realization that "modern societies are not market economies, but organizational economies in which companies are the chief actors in creating value and advancing economic progress; and that the growth of firms, and therefore economies is primarily dependent on the quality of their management; and that the foundation of a firm's activity is a new 'moral contract' with employees and society replacing paternalistic exploitation and value appropriation with employability and value creation in a relationship of shared destiny."[289]

289 Sumantra, G. Bartlett, C.A., & Moran, P. A New Manifesto for Management, in Cusumano, M.A, and Markides, C.C. (eds.) Strategic Thinking for the Next Economy, San Francisco, MIT-Sloan Management Review, 2001, p.10

Prior to this realisation, a cannibalistic conceptual scheme, which has not fully exhausted itself even till today, held sway over much of modern business. In this scheme, companies strive to carve out, 'seize and keep for themselves as much as they can the values embodied in the products and services they deal with, while allowing as little of this value as possible to fall into the hands of others'. But the ethical bankruptcy of this scheme lies in the fact that it nourished and sustained the fundamentally defective conception that the interests of the company are incompatible with those of society and must be divorced therefrom.[290] This is one of the things that actually made ethical investment and consequently, ethical assessment of companies an inevitable necessity, as could be seen in the rise of the clamour for sustainable development and ecological justice.[291] And ethical investment is a strand of this movement.

Ethical criteria or rating for assessing companies are like their counterparts-the financial or credit rating, instruments geared towards evaluating companies on the basis of their social, environmental, ethical and cultural sustainability. Its goal is to make investments, businesses or companies to behave responsibly and ethically in their actions. In this area, subscription to ethical compatibility in business practices transcends the legal imposition of regulations. Companies and investors are informed to make decisions and choices based on ethical principles. And ethical investments are investments, which explicitly seek to take environmental, social and ethical issues into account.

In this way investors are given the opportunity of aligning the power of their money with the direction of values, which are socially credible, environmentally sustainable and ethically sound.

The origins of ethical investment date back to the 19th century, with religious movements like the Methodists and the Quakers, who were concerned with issues such as fair employment conditions and temperance. It has grown into a flourishing global market today in Europe and America and Asia. The same could be said of ethical rating agencies or companies. Most of the agencies or organizations which apply ethical or ecological criteria in rating companies which were born in the 1970s equally had origins traceable to the desire of religious institutions to have their ethics reflect in their investments. In for instance America, the first rating agencies arose to meet the needs of institutional investors like church-based or charity organizations and pension funds. They arose to provide these with the

290 Ibid., p.14

291 See the following: (1) World Commission On Environment and Development, Our Common Future, Oxford University Press, Oxford1987. (2) Meadows, Donella and Co. The Limits of Growth: A Report for the Club of Rome's Project on the Predicament of Mankind, Massachusetts Institute of Technology, 1972. (3) Sachs, Wolgang & Santarius, Tilman (eds.) Fair Future: Resource conflicts, Security and Global Justice, London, ZED Books, 2005

information that facilitated their exercise of their voting rights in a socially responsible manner. In the 1980s the landscape witnessed some changes. Consumer-oriented systems among consumer and human rights organizations emerged to assess companies according to ethical, social and environmental criteria. This time saw to the emergence of agencies like EIRIS in the United Kingdom in 1985. The formation of EIRIS laid the foundation for the systematic ethical, environmental and social evaluation of companies for British investors. And these movements in Britain like the one witnessed in the United States were set in motion by religious institutions.[292]

Ethical investment and ethical criteria for assessing companies all have a deeper source in ethics. Ethics has been a guide to human relationships with one another and with his environment. To this end, ethical criteria for assessing companies rose to contend that it is not nonsense to speak about fairness and virtue in today's capitalist economy.[293] This is philosophically based on the fact that fairness, construed as equality of opportunity (Chancengleichheit), remains the ethical index in a competitive society, in spite of the legitimate controversy, which sees fairness and competition as antagonistic and mutually exclusive.

This is the theoretical backdrop upon which we undertook to examine and test the relevance and functionality of an ethical criteriology in the Nigerian context, where such a criteriology for evaluating companies is lacking.

7.1.2 Ethical Rating in Nigeria

We discovered that there were no ethical rating agencies in Nigeria. And that in fact, Nigeria has no history of ethical investments or ethical-ecological criteria for assessing companies or investments. This absence could be attributed to a mixture of factors like Nigeria's history, the corporate governance framework which evolved on the basis of this history; as well as the geopolitical and socio-economic trajectory taken by the country, which all came together to make the Nigerian business context and public life what it is at the point of this study.

The country for instance never generated the industrial climate, manufacturing base, or industrial relationship that created the kind of evolutionary conflict, which really redefined the concept of profit; swung or refocused the accent of the economic process equally on the ethical behaviour of companies, like was the case in industrial societies of Europe and America.

292 See: Schäfer, et al: Who is Who in Corporate Social Responsibility Rating. Op. cit.

293 Kondo, Yoshiki. Fairness in Capitalist Competition: In Reisch, Lucia (ed.) Ethical-ecological Investment: Towards Global Sustainable Development. Frankfurt am Main, IKO Verlag,2001, p.39

In spite of the increasing realisation worldwide that the current global economic structure is no longer sustainable and does not conduce anymore to human welfare, local motivations in the Nigerian context, for the germination or emergence of an ethical-ecological consciousness in the public and business life are grossly retarded on so many fronts. Even in the face of grinding poverty, scandalous environmental destruction and ethical bankruptcy and corruption in many business quarters, the awareness or urge to stand against the factors causing the situation has not really taken hold in the Nigerian public space.

There could scarcely be any motivations for companies to be ethical in their relationship with their stakeholders in a country where unemployment rate is 40%, and 70% of the 150 million citizens are classified as poor; living on 1$ dollar a day. It is even worse when the situation is compounded by a history of bad, dysfunctional government, and pervasive corruption, derelict institutions and infrastructures. It is even worsened where the government is the greatest employer of labour as well as the most dysfunctional institution one can imagine.[294] In such a situation, many companies would not have a lot of motivation to be ethical in their relationships. Add this to the fact that no Nigerian company is a global player in the real sense of the word. To this end, international conventions and sanctions are not directly of consequence to their operations and profits. Throw a company law that supports a contractarian viewpoint, which sets its accent on the profit for shareholders as narrowly defined by the company; then the ground for ethical behaviour in business is not fertile and ethical criteria in business stands no chance of survival.

This absence of criteria for ethically evaluating companies in Nigeria has not augured well for the country. This could be seen in ecological damage engendered by oil companies in the Niger Delta and the impoverishment and hazards consequent on that. It could equally be seen in the failure of many banks and financial institutions, predicated on fraud and other sharp practices by the bank officials. It could equally be seen in the unethical practices of some companies in almost all sectors of the Nigerian economy, whose investments, activities and

294 According to the arguments of Robert Reich (cf: Supercapitalism, London, Icon Books, 2009, op .cit); only the governance structure or institutions and systems which real democracy creates and provides, can stand between the ontological inclination of capital to seek its survival and profitability over and above every other factor. Where democracy fails, or where the system is weakened, the forces of capital help themselves to laws that will make them more competitive even if that posture destroys the environment, sacks the culture of the people within its business area, or replicates impoverishment. In Nigeria where the government is so very dysfunctional, one witnesses bank chief executives defrauding their depositors, as well as Multinationals like Shell BP remorselessly destroying the Niger Delta ecology or pharmaceutical companies like Pfizer using Nigerians as guinea pigs to effect clinical trials of drugs that were not approved for human consumption.

operations destroy the Nigeria environment, degrade the dignity of their employees and endanger the life and wellbeing of the consumers across the country. In Nigeria, for instance, the relationship between employers and their employees are in certain cases akin to that between a house slave and his master. In some companies, strikes are construed as the exclusive province of those in public service or government employ; never for those who work for companies. This situation could be explained by the fact that since companies hold the lifeline over the livelihood of these people; against the backdrop of the fact that unemployment rate is 40% and that graduates are coming out of the university annually; joining the already swollen and bursting unemployment market, companies most times feel that if a worker joins a strike, he risks losing his job, which a million others are ready and waiting to snap for half the salary.

The fact that there are no ethical-ecological criteria for evaluating companies in Nigeria does not mean that the basis for such does not exist. Research[295] has shown that some local cultures across Nigeria, like the Omenala principle; a very ancient body of laws of the Igbos of Southern Nigeria, dating back to much more than 450BC, is in agreement with the basis of an ethical criteriology like the FHG, which was built upon the core principles of the Catholic Social Teaching. This is one of the cultural soils, upon which such criteriologies could be engrafted into the Nigeria business consciousness.

A historical instance lends credence to the possibility of a co-operation between these two pedestals. For instance, due to the fact ethics has forever been a living, breathing part of the Igbo cultural fabric, there were pre-colonial agitations in relation to the behaviour of the colonial government and its parastatals. The 1929 Aba women riots, which was embarked upon to protest the injustice of arbitrary taxation is construed by many historians, more as a political agitation, than as the action of workers protesting better conditions of service. But the 1949 coal miners strike in Enugu and the consequent massacre of the coal miners by the colonial authorities was more of the search for better conditions of service by the workers. It directed the searchlight on the colonial machine's treatment of its workers. The colonial administration reacted with the kind of brutality that we still witness sometimes in subdued tones in the relationship between the Nigerian government, which is the largest employer of labour in the country, and workers. Many labour leaders have done time in government jails, because they protested the bad conditions of service; the hunger wage they have been paid in the course of Nigerian history and the non-payment of their salaries and arrears. These two agitations could happen in Igbo country due to the principles harboured in their Omenala, which discountenances injustice. This could explain why the Igbo country constituted one of the major hubs of the anti-colonial agitations and fight for Nigerian independence.

295 See: Nnoli-Edozien, Ndidi; op. Cit.

Nigeria held interest for our exploration not only because it is our heritage, but equally because it is a new, expanding and important investment market in Africa. After years of political instability and military tyranny, this country of over 150 million people, was welcomed into the committee of democratic nations in 1999. To this end, many foreign companies are already locked and struggling for the market share in the oil sector. The banking industry is stabilizing after the consolidation exercise of the CBN in 2005. The telecommunication sector is showing great promise. Many foreign investors especially the Chinese are showing greater interest in Nigeria. And this landscape provides a fertile opportunity for the meeting of foreign business interests with the local realities available in the Nigerian context. In the past, the local context has never been prepared for this encounter, which has left it with a heritage of disadvantages. Nigeria needs development and she cannot isolate herself from the rest of the world. It is against this backdrop that an ethical-ecological consciousness as well as criteria for evaluating companies and institutions becomes imperative.

In the face of all these, the question which faced us then became: how does one go about trying to redress this scandalous lacuna? Pioneering into any field is never the rosiest of journeys. There exist no local frameworks in this direction upon which to build. The choice was either to abandon the enterprise and mourn its absence in Nigeria, or to extend the search for a framework to other business and cultural environments, where that exists to see what could be taken. Importing an alien framework to lead this paradigm shift is not without its cultural, hermeneutic and epistemic implications. Ethical criteriologies in this regard in other to be functional are essentially culture-specific. What obtains across Nigeria are cultural and epistemological basis that could act as authentic scaffolds for the introduction of an ethical criteriology from another cultural environment into the local Nigerian context, but no criteriology. So our search for a framework concentrated on one that could align with cultural pedestals available in Nigerian. This will present as little risk of rejection as possible.

The FHG which has its basis on the rich traditions of the Catholic Social Teaching possesses some core similarities with some cultures in Nigeria, which could act as a pedestal for its download into our sociocultural milieu, and prevent its being rejected. 'Omenala', which is the corpus of Igbo traditional laws and norms, has been in existence for almost 2000 years. The excavations of Thurstan Shaw in Igbo land attests to the fact that the Igbo civilization has been around as early as 450 BC. And this culture as was shown by the studies of Ndidi Nnoli Edozien has some core principles which align perfectly and are similar to the Catholic Social Teaching principles. The premium placed on human life and its sustenance in both traditions is for instance, a point of agreement that could scaffold any introduction of one into the other. A common tread in both traditions that have implications for the ethical criteria is the Igbo communal philosophy of life, extended kinship and concern for the less privileged, which in the Catholic Social teaching is alive and well in the principles of solidarity and subsidiarity. The Igbo concepts of 'Egbe belu Ugo belu'-'Live and let live'; 'Agbatobi onye bu nwanne ya'-one's neighbour is his brother' are all basis shared by the two tradition that have implications for our work. Ndidi Edozien showed for instance that the Omenala principles pervade and influence the conceptual landscape of many Igbo businesses; and that in establishing a company, the founder represents not only the founder but also his family. To this end, in his business decisions, the founder balances the demands of his business with his responsibility to his extended family, which could be the whole community sometimes.[296]

These are some of the important points that informed and facilitated our preference and choice of the FHG. These are the factors which informed our hypothesis that the FHG could be a basis for the development of an ethical criteriology for the assessment and evaluation of companies in the Nigerian context. And the results of the research have borne out the hypothesis.

7.1.3 The Frankfurt-Hohenheim Guidelines as the Framework of the Study

The framework for our investigation was the Frankfurt-Hohenheim Guidelines. The Frankfurt-Hohenheim Guidelines (FHG) as we clarified is an ethical-ecological criteriology for assessing and evaluating companies developed in the German cultural context. It is the product of the project Ecological Group led by Prof. Dr. Johannes Hoffman, Dr. Ott and Prof. Dr. Gerhard Scherhon. Building on a comprehensive and integral approach to the concept of sustainable development, the group developed a scientifically-based criteriology for the ethical assessment of companies. It was among others designed to bring the influence of moral reasoning to bear on the movements of capital in order to focus normative moral understanding, such as reflected in the ecological movement, and make it fruitful for the structuring of socio-economic life and for cultural development. This is in lieu of the belief that greater significance must accrue to moral communication within the context of the economic system.[297]

These FHG guidelines gave rise to the CRR, which was developed in conjunction with the Oekom Research AG and deployed in assessing companies' responsibility towards the natural environment (Environmental Sustainability); persons affected by corporate activities of the companies (Social Sustainability);

296 Amaeshi et. al, op. cit. p.18

297 Project group Ethical-Ecological Rating, op. cit. p.18

and society and Culture (Cultural Sustainability). This practical dimension has shown strong relevance in the assessment of companies and investments world wide across major economic sectors, as well as in other cultural contexts like India and some parts of Asia with surprising results. To that end, we decided to import the FHG into the Nigerian context and examine how relevant it would be in the development of a culture specific ethical criteriology for assessing companies, investments and even institutions in the Nigerian context.

7.1.4 Methodological Issues

The question then swung to how we are to accomplish this task of examining the relevance of the FHG in the Nigerian context. To resolve this question, we chose two of the arms of the FHG namely the Social compatibility and the Cultural Compatibility criteria. This choice was informed by the fact that environmental compatibility which is the third arm is more standardized and can apply without many problems across a broad spectrum of environments, cultures and countries.

Methodologically it was a logical and logistical impossibility to gather and analyse the opinion of all Nigerians across all sectors of the economic; and across the length and breadth of the country. Mindful of the fact that poverty remained one of the central, and grinding challenges facing Nigeria, where over 70% of the population are living in poverty; and coupled with the fact that microfinance, which is to an extent proving to be a new global sustainable investment vehicle seems to be catching on and making serious inroads in Nigeria since the 2005 promulgation of the Microfinance Supervisory and Regulatory Framework for Nigeria; we decided to use this young industry that is gaining popular interest both in terms of patronage and outreach, to test whether the FHG will survive a relevant test in Nigeria.

To conduct this relevance test, we readapted for the Nigerian context, questionnaires derived from the FHG by oekom research, AG and first deployed in such a study by Dr. James Agi Makil in the Indian context. Our hypothesis was that the Frankfurt-Hohenheim Guidelines (FHG) criteria of Social and Cultural Compatibility/Sustainability are relevant in the Nigerian context.

The questionnaires were two different questionnaires; one for each; namely social compatibility and cultural compatibility. The questionnaires both have 35 questions apiece, with each criterion in the FHG's Social and Cultural compatibility being converted to one question and posed to the respondents to determine their relevance in the Nigerian context, in which they are intimate participants.

The respondents were required to mark any of the following to indicate that which best captures their opinion of each question: namely;

a. Totally Relevant (+2)
b. Relevant (+1)
c. Undecided (0)
d. Not Relevant (-1)
e. Totally Not Relevant (-2)

600 participants took part in the study, 300 apiece for both criteria. For the study we choose the two extremes of the social ladder so to say; those a little higher the social ladder; bank managers, and those relegated to the periphery; namely the poor, who are in need of access to finance. For the social compatibility test, we choose 300 top managers of 300 different microfinance banks in the three regions of Nigeria that we selected; while for the cultural criteria, we choose the clients of these banks, or those who have had business with the banks.

The information from both questionnaires were collated, analysed and subjected to a simple relevant test. Our relevance test was a simple one. If a criterion garners relevant affirmation greater than 50%, then it is positive and relevant to the Nigerian context; if not, then the obverse obtains. At a > 50% affirmation, then our hypothesis is positive. At the end, we gathered the positives and the negatives together and did a comparative analysis of them for each of the questionnaires. And the trend that garners more than 50% becomes the answer to our hypothesis.

Our test in order to make the work a representative reflection of Nigeria, we divided Nigeria into three zones; namely North, West and South. We chose a State from each of these three zones to represent the tripodal geopolitical arrangement in Nigeria. We chose the states, Kano in the North, Lagos in the West and Enugu in the Southeast for the study. These as reiterated earlier where socio-cultural and business hubs of those three regions, around which the major currents of socio-economic, political and cultural trends in Nigeria revolve.

7.1.5 Summary of Findings

7.1.5.1 Cultural Sustainability/Compatibility Criteria

Our analysis and findings indicate that on the relevance or otherwise of the Frankfurt-Hohenheim Guidelines Cultural Compatibility criteria, that with 71.6% average, the respondents are of the opinion that the FHG cultural compatibility criteria are relevant in the Nigerian context. This proves our hypothesis positive. An average of 9.6% of the responses deemed it not relevant in the Nigerian context. And 19.8% were undecided.

The General moral principles, which is a major component of the Cultural compatibility criteria, polled an over all average of 90% relevant and 4% not relevant with 6% undecideds to posit its relevance for the Nigeria context. This result either transcended the religious constructs obtainable; were in agreement with them, or did not inform the responses. The smallness of dissent here could not be logically attributed to a single factor like religion because no trend was established in this regard.

The general moral principles are as follows:

3.2.1 You shall observe the fundamental bio-cultural norm in all spheres of activity
3.2.2 You shall not cause or inflict pain
3.2.3 You shall not render anyone incapable
3.2.4 You shall not deprive anyone of their freedom or opportunities
3.2.5 You shall deprive no one of their pleasure in something
3.2.6 You shall not deceive or defraud
3.2.7 You shall keep your promises
3.2.8 You shall respect the property of others
3.2.9 You shall obey the law
3.2.10 You shall subject no one to moral obligations beyond their ability to fulfil them

Each of the 10 commandments or general moral principles was given a number and the concrete applications derived there from, which were formulated as questions were the sub-numbers.

For the general principles, the respondents were expected to answer "Strongly yes" to show the highest affirmation to strongly No to show the highest rejection of that particular principle. In between we have merely Yes, undecided and Merely No. In the concrete applications, the respondents were required to answer "Totally Relevant" to show strongest support or affirmation, and "Totally No" to register their strongest dissent. In between we had "relevant" to show mere support and "not relevant" to register a mere rejection. In between we have undecided to show neither support nor rejection of the particular concrete application in question.

One notices that under the general moral principles, the majority of our respondents saw them as totally relevant. But the dial began to shift as the case may be, when one comes to the specifics or concrete applications. Our respondents were overwhelmingly positive on the general principles, but had more guarded or diversified responses when it came to the concrete applications.

The above Decalogue with 16 questions flowing from them; together with 5 Anthropologically given motivational factors, 2 orientations, 6 cardinal virtues and 8 secondary virtues are the components or constituents of the cultural compatibility criteria.

Other components of the Cultural criteria equally polled strongly in Nigeria (vide: 4.5 Test of relevance), to stake claims of relevance to the Nigerian context. On the cardinal virtues, for instance, one notices that we recorded no dissents as to whether they are desirable in their own rights. That they are cardinal could be glimpsed from the responses to our questionnaire in that regard. We recorded Zero percent all through on their undesirability and recorded high averages as to their desirability.

7.1.5.2 Social Sustainability/Compatibility Criteria

On the Social Compatibility Criteria, our analysis and findings indicate that with a 65% average, the respondents were of the opinion that the FHG criteria of Social compatibility are relevant in the Nigerian context. This is to say that our hypothesis in this direction has equally been proved positive. On the strength of both results we can state that the FHG is relevant in the Nigeria context for the ethical evaluation and assessment of companies.

These findings are what informed our recommendations as we embarked upon our systematic reflection.

7.2 Reflection on the Findings

This study opened our eyes to the problematic of interface when a foreign cultural dynamic makes a landfall in another cultural ambient. One of the major features of culture is its dynamic nature. It is capable of changing itself and assimilating change from external influences. But be that as it may, cultures that were forced to change to the onslaught of greedy profit, huddled at the brink of extinction.[298] The Incas of Peru and the Amerindians of the American continent were examples in this regard.

Nigeria presented an interesting backdrop for our considerations and investigation. Granted that we are intimate participants in this country, which houses our heritage and most intimate acquaintances; it provided us endless opportunities to really deepen our knowledge of the conceptual currents underlying the Nigerian economic system. Many of the naïve prejudices we held in this regard were equally exploded. Without any intention of hoisting grand theories of illusory

298 See: Diamond, Guns, Gems and Steel.

provenance, our investigation and findings leads us to the following conclusions, which we gladly offer as a baseline for further study in this regard.

7.2.1 The FHG as an Innovative Instrument in Ethical-ecological Rating

The Frankfurt-Hohenheimer Guidelines would have been like every other ethical criteria for evaluating companies out there, if not for a very novel criteria, which it introduced into its criteriology; namely: the cultural sustainability criteria.

Measuring the cultural compatibility of enterprises over and above been one of the great innovations of the FHG is no doubt of paramount importance in any ethical evaluative criteriology for companies and investments. This inheres in the historical and contemporary observations that are there for all to see.

Like we have constantly re-echoed in this work, as mankind invented new production processes; new systems, structures, and economic vehicles, with which to deploy capital; capitalism on the heels of sociotechnological advancements, primed itself to construct and take along its own sociologies; introducing new synergies and relationships into any environment that it enters. To this end, we have seen big business coagulate into a supranational 'corporatocracy,' which for most part of the 20th century constituted itself into the new empire colonizing peoples and nations. Right from the monumental indiscretions of the robber barons, to the reckless impunity of contemporary investment bankers, the imperialism was totalizing. And like every empire this corporatocracy was in many instances, equally savage in its decimation of cultural, ethical, social and ecological realities that have been the furniture of peoples' life, and dignity in many parts of the world. And the results of this imperialism are there for to see. 'Executives at respected companies hire people at near-slave wages to toil under inhuman conditions in sweatshops. Oil companies wantonly pump toxins into rain forest Rivers, consciously killing people, animals, and plants, and committing genocide among ancient cultures. The pharmaceutical industry denies life-saving medicines to millions of HIV-infected Africans; and so on.[299]

History bears witness to the fact that this ogre most times casts off irreplaceable cultural heritages and values as hangovers of human evolutionary infancy, in its bid to create and market new products, new needs, new utilities and values. And since capitalism has never been a guarantee for social, cultural, ecological, or political justice, such constructs always created problems. Most of these problems arise because markets and the market system do not always meet the ethical and aesthetic criteria of society.[300]

299 John Perkins, The Confessions of an Economic Hit Man, op. cit. p.xii
300 Heilbroner and Thurow, op. cit. p.30

In Nigeria context and much of Africa for instance, colonialism introduced a fluid dynamic that wiped away so many cultural values and heritages, labelling what it could not understand as primitive or savage, even in those areas where these values summarized millenniums of life of the people inhabiting those regions. Nigeria lost a lot to this dynamic, which as it were, introduced new values and sociologies, some of which has continued to dog Nigeria's attempt at unity and progress. The country was equally plunged into a conceptual crossroad. The education and pedagogy, which many Nigerians got from the fall outs of this dynamic was savage in its relationship to autochthonous cultural realities and values. And the crisis of identity arising therefrom has really been at the root of most of the socio-cultural, political and economic problems bedevilling the country since its birth.

To this end, reason supports the conclusion that if we are not to further destroy the cultural heritages, which have underwritten and shouldered the social evolution and survival of peoples for ages, we must appraise carefully the way economic processes impact on the human culture, human society, human future and human ecology. This is important although 'many of today's social systems, at the cultural level, have their own problems as levers of change.

Over and above bringing culture back to the centre of economic consideration, the value of FHG's cultural compatibility criteria can equally be seen in the historical experiences which are shaping our contemporary situation. Our contemporary situation circa 2008 was defined by the raging conflict between two great forces, which really shaped the dawns of this century. These are the forces articulated by Benjamin Barber in his work of the same title as Jihad vs. McWorld (1995), or what Samuel Huntington captured as the Clash of civilizations. These forces seemingly collided with a cataclysmal impact as the planes hijacked by terrorists, pierced the twin-towers on the morn of September 11, 2001.

The blurred lines between the two forces as the encountered each other, and the reactions and reaction formations which arose as a result of this collision impacted immensely and have far reaching consequences on socio-cultural relations, geopolitics, economics, security and mutual existence as we know it today on the global level. These two forces created and have continued to generate very hot contentions and tensions.

On one side of the divide is the view characterized as McWorld. McWorld according to Benjamin Barber denotes the thrust of international capital, from its chief strongholds in Western Europe, North America and East Asia, to transform the whole world into a single marketplace (Global supermarket) with a single ideology and way of life.[301]

301 See: Barber, Benjamin. R; McWorld: How Globalism and Tribalism Are Reshaping the World, New York, Times Book, 1995: cited in W. Warren Wagar, "Tribe, Empire, or Global Commonwealth", in Didsbury, H.F. et al (eds.) Thinking Creatively in Turbulent Times, Maryland, World Future Society, 2004, p.248

The defenders of this march of capital' contend that Mcworld is a disparaging term for a 'noble' enterprise, in which capitalism marches to remake our world and bring progress, development and peace to all and sundry. They see those who oppose this march as reactionaries and pseudo-religious fanatics, who are bent on pulling the world back to medieval primitivity.

Those on the receiving end contend that this totalitarianism of capital destroys their culture, religion and way of life, and is an evil that must be fought. They hold the view that 'Jihad' may be actually just an ill-humoured trope for the legitimate aspirations of peoples to lead their own lives as they choose, free from imperialism political, economic and cultural.[302]

While rejecting this Manichean division raging in the cultural discourse of our times, which impact is equally felt in the socio-economic life of societies in our day, we are of the view that Cultural compatibility, as a part of the FHG ethical criteriology for evaluating enterprises, while not blind to these ideological currents, was not designed to take sides in this dichotomy. The FHG never envisioned its cultural compatibility criteria to scaffold or be the foundation for 'a balkanized world of thousands of sovereign tribes, each jealously guarding its sacred patrimony. Neither was it designed to support on the other hand a new world order, which is a vast global shopping mall, managed by a consortium of profiteering corporate giants under the protective shield of one or more capitalist superpowers. [303]

This non-partisan mediation of FHG on issues of ideological import is what ethics would recommend any day. This is because the two great forces listed above, and every other such ultra-parochial ideologies, are narrow in their vision of the world. Their insularity is their weakness. Jihad for instance, seeks the greatest possible advantage for one's own tribe. And as Wagar rightly argues, what is good for one tribe may be bad or even intolerable for its neighbours. McWorld on the other hand is helpless to save us because its engine is the relentless search for profit through maximizing production and sales and minimizing costs of both, above all the costs of labour. And many are rightly of the view that none of these two forces dominating contemporary history will be in charge of human destiny. Both of them will continue their malevolent competition for decades or even years to come, but with time, they will exhaust their relevance, as both are excellent recipes for planetary disaster.[304]

We must concede that although there have been many suggestions as to what would go for a sane alternative to these two conflicting conceptual schemes or movements. We have never been favourably disposed to the construction of a

302 Loc. cit

303 Wagar, loc. Cit. p.249

304 Wagar, op. Cit. p.249

democratically regulated system of global governance in which all tribes yield their sovereignty and all multinationals surrender their capital to overarching common authorities.[305] In an interdependent world rife with disparities and asymmetries, no tribe acting unilaterally can or should determine its own fate. In an interdependent world of finite resources and masses yearning for social justice, globalization on market principles is neither sustainable nor fair.[306]

The unwieldy impracticality of a globally regulated system of global governance is an insurmountable obstacle to it being considered. While we may spend eternity waiting for the realisation of this vision, we may have gone a long way in placing humanity in the orbit of self-destructive cannibalization. Instead of waiting for the emergence of a supranational Leviathan to operationalize these visions, the FHG's cultural compatibility offers itself as veritable alternative; which in time will create the kind of sociocultural pressures necessary in changing social attitudes and processes in human society.[307]

7.2.2 The Transferability of the FHG Social and Cultural Criteria

There are other many works and reflections that have dealt with the transferability of the FHG into other cultural contexts. Fuad Kandil found that inappropriate socio-cultural, socio-political, and socio-economic conditions make the feasibility of the CRR concept within contexts like the Arab-Islamic society very difficult, in spite of the positive components of the FHG.[308] One of the reasons, which he submitted for this difficulty, was what he identified as the 'latent suspicion' against all Western institutions prevalent in the Arab-Islamic world.[309] To that end, most people in the Arab-Islamic world according to this contention cannot understand that Western agencies should judge the compatibility of certain economic activities with their own Islamic culture.

In our studies, we found that if evaluation of companies is deemed as foreign, there are chances that it will be rejected as an unrealistic imposition from without, which is ignorant of local realities. But if this evaluation is the product of co-operative interaction or as originating from that cultural ambient, the chances

305 Ibid.

306 Ibid.

307 In system theory, we have political, economic, social and technological levers of change. And ours here will operate on the social and economic levels and can possibly evolve to the political level. (See: John Smart, The Political-Economic Pendulum, op. cit. p.65)

308 Kandil Fuad, Applicability of the CRR concepts to Arab-Islamic Societies: In Reisch, L. (ed.),op. cit. p.105-109

309 Ibid., p.109

are high that it will not suffer rejection or other prejudicial stances that potentially await such innovations. This stance identified by Fuad is important to a great extent in many other cultural environments. His may have echoes in the Arab-Islamic world, but could equally obtain in other places. In Nigeria, we framed and presented the guidelines in a way that called for local inputs. The questionnaires gave the respondents the opportunity of writing out what their views are whenever they agree or disagree or feel that something in the guidelines need modification. And it is our contention that once the stakeholders come to view the product as emanating from an effort in which they were consulted, or collaborated in making, it will be difficult to reject it.

For instance, Nigeria that has over 45% of its citizens as Muslims. But the opinions gathered from our research in Kano, which is an Islamic hub in Northern Nigeria showed no particular construction of the criteria as a Western invention. There was no specific singling out of any of the criteria as not applicable because it is Western. This some may contend may be thanks to the absence in Nigeria, of the kind of relationship and the reaction formations, which hardened Islamic sensibilities against western patterns in the Arab-Islamic world. But the method of presenting it to our respondents may have played a role there too. In fact, there was a very strong agreement with the 10 General moral principles of the Cultural sustainability criteria in Nigeria irrespective of the cultural and religious diversities of the respondents.

7.2.3 The Necessity of Ethical-ecological Criteria for Rating Companies in Nigeria

We must concede the fact that Corporate Social Responsibility (CSR) is making a gradual headway in Nigeria. But a criteriology for measuring companies' compliance with these hallowed principles that grace most of their company documents and websites is still lacking. To this end, the functional definition and praxis of CSR principles in Nigeria differ from company to company, and is most times at the good pleasures of the PR departments of these companies. And since CSR still wears the garbs of philanthropy in the Nigerian context, many companies practice it in a way that leaves one no other option than to identify it as a 'social bribe', which does not go far enough, but is there to keep dissents and discontents to the company's operation to the barest minimum. This is what could be seen in the Nigerian oil sector, where the big MNCs enjoy a field day polluting the environment, collapsing the ecology upon which the livelihood of many in the Niger Delta depend, and building paltry schools or doling out paltry sums to town unions led by corrupt profiteers to shush discontent to their reckless modus operandi in those areas.

To redress this absence as well as create a functional bridge between socio-ethical values and themes deeply embedded in the Nigerian psyche; which undergirded life in pre-colonial Nigeria, and gave meaning and significance to the lives of the people, and which baggage followed Nigerians even to the present time; but which failed to cross the Rubicon of colonial dynamic into modern business life in Nigeria; there is a need to find ways of making a culture-specific criteriology fit for the Nigerian context come alive in Nigeria. This attempt to be valid for our context must be a collaborative effort between Nigerian cultural pedestals and modern socio-economic thinking, which are increasingly going back to its ethical roots today.

Over and above every other criteriology for rating companies, the ethical criteriology for doing same, over and above the advantage of bringing a neutrality conducive to gaining public trust in its ratings, brings ethics into focus as the long term perspective of economic processes. Ethical criteriologies transcend short term profits to embosom the overall interest of all stakeholders. It expands the narrow definitions of profitability, and neutralizes the toxic amorality of capital; forcing it to take a stand for human survival and the dignity of the human person in his society and workplace. It is only in the ethical purview that profit means profit for capital, labour, nature and society. Ethical-ecological rating therefore repositions the discourse, placing the accent not on profit maximization for some narrow 'cabal of shareholders', but also on social, ethical and ecological questions arising from the deployment of capital and production processes. It contends and shows that it is not nonsense to speak about fairness and virtue in a capitalist economy.[310] It contends that fairness, which in Rawlsian terms means the equality of opportunity remains the ethical index in a competitive society, even when the contention is still out there that fairness and struggle are antagonistic and mutually exclusive.

A few years ago, ecological or even ethical investment was dismissed in many quarters as an idealistic combination of finance and ethics, which has a negative effect on profits and yields.[311] But today, it is increasingly being realised that companies that fail to embrace and sail with this wind, will find themselves out of business in the no distant future.

And the Nigerian business space is in dire need of this awareness, if it is not to compound the rot that bad governance has engendered and supports in the Nigerian society.

---

310 Cf. Kondo, Yoshiki. Fairness in Capitalistic Competition. In Reisch, Lucia (ed.) Op. cit. p.39

311 Robert Hassler. Corporate Responsibility Rating: An Innovative tool for Promoting Sustainable Development among Companies and on the Financial Market-A Rating Agency's Practical Experience. In Reisch, Lucia (ed.) Op. cit, p.55

7.2.4 The Potentials of FHG in the Nigerian Context

Our work was severely limited by the vastness and the multi-dimensional nature of the country Nigeria. To that end, the work cannot lay claim to being exhaustive of the various dimensions and sectors of the Nigerian economy, which need to be further studied in this regard to see how receptive these sectors would be to the possibilities of subscribing to ethical-ecological criteria for their evaluation and assessment. To this end, we submit that our work has pioneered into the Nigerian market, but has not exhausted the dimensions and possibilities, which this great socio-economic embrace holds for both investors and companies. We therefore deem it right that this is simply the starting point. And could and should be a basis for further exploration of Nigeria in relation to ethical investments, by future generations of scholars and scientists.

It is our educated conclusion based on our findings that an ethical-ecological criteriology for rating companies and that a rating agency, that rates or evaluates companies based on ethical criteriology is long overdue in Nigeria. We were not able to find any rating agency dealing with ethical criteriology in its rating.

This is not like it is a government's responsibility. Based on this, we submit that there is a market for ethical rating in Nigeria, and that any investor bent on establishing a rating agency in Nigeria will be pioneering into a market, where there are no competitors, outside the challenging business environment. But since every challenge is a reservoir of opportunities, the indicators are showing a positive trend in this regard.

7.2.5 The FHG with modifications can be downloaded in the Nigerian context

Every business finds itself in a cultural context. Sustainability is basically culture-specific. The assumption that firms and businesses are products of their contexts and socio-economic milieus is well founded. Firms are socio-economic creatures. They are entities created in specific contexts to fulfil specific needs; by producing and trading on goods and services pursuant to making profits, creating utility and satisfying human wants. The social environment sires and influences the way firms relate to their environment and conduct business. It exerts considerable influence on the ways, in which the firms view their socio-ethical responsibilities; manufacture and package their products. It also shapes the way in which the firms in turn contribute their own quota in creating, sustaining and responding to the chains of relationships, interactions, and heritage of influences, which the society is susceptible and amenable to.

To that end, any attempt to transfer a paradigmatic idea manufactured or developed in one cultural context into another is really an uphill task. It like transplanting a plant could be done. But whether it succeeds is another matter, which is dependent on some many factors like sensitivity to the demands and constituents of both cultures and one seeking points of contact which is a condition-sine-quanon, if the assimilation of the idea is what was intended. The non-examination of African cultural pedestals remains one of the tragic mistakes of colonialism. The international financial institutions, development agencies and NGOs working all over Africa today are following in the footsteps of the same mistake.[312] And this accounts for the failures of decades of development aid to effect any positive change in the lives and situation of many African economies.[313]

As our studies have shown, there are points of contact for downloading the FHG into the Nigerian context. To this end, our study found that Nigerians would be happy to have this in their context, but some pedestals of the FHG must be carefully modified to suit the situation without compromising the ethical and methodological validity of the FHG.

The Omenala principle as we have shown is one of these pedestals. Gerhard Scherhon argued that the present attitude to capital is amoral. And this amoral attitude towards money could be traced to the amorality of foreign trade as opposed to domestic business. To that end, as long as tradesmen dealt with fellow countrymen or women, they obeyed the law and followed the rules. But once the pendulum swings to people abroad, whom they regarded as strangers-possibly as savage people with barbarian and pagan customs and traditions, the urge or commitment to respect their views and norms, and treat them as men with equal rights evaporates. They most times regarded these peoples as potential enemies, which converts them into objects to be cheated and exploited.[314] The FHG criteriology is built on a basis which counters this amoral stance of capital. To that end, it shares something that is ontologically present in the Omenala principle. In the Omenala, there exists a pedestal which goes thus: ***"Agbatobi onye bu nwanne ya"***-One's neighbour is his brother"; and a similar one ***"O biara be onye abiagbuna ya"***-One should never do his host in, and his host should not invoke ill on him as he goes"-

These Omenala principles are affirmations of the universal brotherhood of man. And that one should never bear anyone ill, even if he is a stranger. This is one of the things that made capital respectful of man. There were capital in-

312 Cf. Manji, Firoze. The Missionary Position: NGOs and Development in Africa. In: International Affairs 78 3 (2002) 567-83, http://www.fahamu.org/downloads/missionaryposition.pdf

313 Cf. William Easterly, The Whiteman's Burden: Why the West's Effort to Aid the Rest have Done So Much Ill and So Little Good New York, Oxford University Press, 2006

314 Scherhon, G. Will Globalization Contribute to a World Culture: In: Reisch, Lucia (ed.) Ethical-ecological Investment: Towards Global Sustainable Development, Frankfurt am Main, IKO Verlag, 2001,p.6

vestments in the traditional sense in Igbo society. One could keep his She-goat as a capital with his neighbour. The neighbour contributes labour in caring for the goat. And the proceeds from the goat; which in this case are the offsprings, are divided between both parties according to an already agreed equation. Similar instances abound in Igbo worldview and tradition. But only a few of them made their way into the formal Nigerian business environment. But one could see people falling back to these pedestals when the formal system seems to have failed them. A perfect example of this could be seen in the fact of 'Isusu'. This is traditional revolving credit scheme mostly practiced by women in Igbo country. When many Nigerian banks were failing during the military government of Sanni Abacha, many women working in the banks in Enugu resorted to Isusu instead of saving their money in the bank, they chose saving it in one another. The contributed these monies and gave to one of them at a given time, who receives a bulk capital for her business, and it revolves till all the members have gotten their monies back. This was an eye opener in the sense that these educated women who worked in the formal financial sector had to fall back on a very ancient way of savings and capital accumulation, when the formal system, which they are intimate participants in failed them.

8. Closing Submissions

Our studies have been able to show that in spite of the absence of ethical criteria for assessing companies in Nigeria, that Frankfurt Hohenheim Guidelines of cultural and social compatibility are relevant and have a potential in the evaluation of companies in the microfinance banking sector of the Nigerian economy.

We have been able to see that there are cultural pedestals upon which the FHG can be downloaded into the Nigerian cultural context without fear of rejection as an alien conceptual criteriology. This could be seen for example in the Omenala principles, which shares ontological similarities with the core values of the Catholic social teaching upon which the Frankfurt-Hohenheim Guidelines were based. We argue that if anchored on cultural principles available in the Nigerian cultural environment, it will create an acceptable framework for culture-specific company evaluation in Nigeria.

We equally saw that CSR is making gradual inroads into Nigeria although the conceptual scheme which supports it leans heavily on the notoriously inadequate philanthropic direction. That offers no motivation for the functional assimilation of those principles into corporate life. In this purview, the principles are then subject to being treated as peripheral ad hoc concerns, which are to be taken up when the situation calls for it; to shore up their image or market their reputation even when their actions are at variance with the noble missions they profess.

Apart from introducing the noble values of the FHG to the Nigerian audience, it is hoped that this work will join the debate in refocusing attention on the role of ethics in business in the Nigerian context, which is a part of the process in mobilizing social and cultural forces within the Nigerian society to facilitate the diffusion and appreciation of corporate ethical responsibility by companies operating within our shores. It will contribute to the movement towards the creation of a moral or rather ethical-ecological counterweight to the power of economic relationships[315], in order to bring the destructive potentials of the economic system under control.

315 Schneider, Hans-Albert. Ethisches Rating, Op. Cit. p.19

Annex 1

Social Compatibility Questionnaire

GOETHE
UNIVERSITÄT
FRANKFURT AM MAIN

Emmanuel Franklyne Ogbunwezeh
Department of Social and Economic Ethics
Frankfurt Graduate School of Social Sciences and Humanities
Johann Wolfgang Goethe University,
Frankfurt am Main

To whom it may concern

Dear Sir/Madam,

We crave your help in this academic research designed to assess what Nigerians in the Finance sector would loved to see in the formulation of rating or assessment criteria for companies.

This questionnaire is designed to find out, what you would love to see as major components of any workable criteria directed at the ethical and ecological rating and/or assessment of companies in Nigeria, especially in your sector of the economy.

We would be most glad if you would cross an X in the relevant box as you deem fit, in answer to the questions.

All information obtained in this research are strictly for academic purposes and is not open or accessible to third parties for marketing purposes except as a part of a doctoral dissertation in fulfilment of the academic requirements for the award of a PhD in Social and Economic Ethics of the above-named university.

Your diligent completion of the questionnaire would be highly appreciated.

Yours very sincerely,

Emmanuel Franklyne Ogbunwezeh

A. Social Cultural Rating — Banks/Finance

A.1. Social / Cultural Management

1		Yes			No		
		+2	+1	0	-1	-2	
	Is it relevant to ask whether companies in your specific industry have corporate policies covering social / ethical aspects (e. g. health & safety, non discrimination, freedom of association, suppliers) (+2 = Totally relevant, -2 = Totally not relevant)?						
Please give reasons for your answer:							

2		Relevant			Not relevant		
		+2	+1	0	-1	-2	
	Is it relevant to ask whether companies in your specific industry have units apart from personal administration dealing with social / ethical issues (responsibility for ethical policies, community projects, social advisors etc.) (+2 = Totally relevant, -2 = Totally not relevant)?						
If yes, please name the unit and specify its function: CSR - Corporate Social Responsibility							

3			Yes			Not		
			+2	+1	0	-1	-2	
		Is it relevant to ask, at which level of corporate hierarchy the full time Head of Social / Ethical Affairs is located (+2 = Totally relevant, -2 = Totally not relevant)?						
If yes, please name the level of corporate hierarchy:								

4			Yes			Not		
			+2	+1	0	-1	-2	
		Is it relevant to ask, whether companies in your specific industry offer possibilities, which allow employees to report grievances related to the work place /working conditions in a confidential way (+2 = Totally relevant, -2 = Totally not relevant)?						
If yes, please name the level of corporate hierarchy: Yes there are CEO listening posts and Whistle Blower policies all of which aid in the same.								

5			Relevant			Not relevant		
			+2	+1	0	-1	-2	
		Is it relevant to ask, whether companies in your specific industry conduct audits or surveys to monitor social / ethical aspects (+2 = Totally relevant, -2 = Totally not relevant)? If relevant, the following:						
	1	Employee satisfaction						
	2	Health & Safety						
	3	Non-discrimination						
	4	Other (please describe)						
Please give reasons for your answers:								

5			Relevant		Not relevant			
			+2	+1	0	-1	-2	
		Is it relevant to ask, how companies in your specific industry report internally / externally on their social / ethical performance (+2 = Totally relevant, -2 = Totally not relevant)? If relevant, the following:						
	1	Social report (printed)						
	2	Social report (via homepage)						
	3	Other social / ethical information on Homepage						
	4	Staff magazines						
	5	Intranet						
	6	Dialog with NGOs						
	7	Other						
Please give reasons for your answers:								

6			Relevant		Not relevant			
			+2	+1	0	-1	-2	
		Is it relevant to ask, how companies in your specific industry ensure freedom of association for all employees (e. g. through group policy, staff committees) (+2 = Totally relevant, -2 = Totally not relevant)?						
Please specify how companies promote this: Though Unions are seen as a less preferred route to represent employee needs. The HR function is seen as a proactive grouping who takes the interest of the employee into consideration in all of its action. The competitive market dynamics ensure that								

A.2 Staff Relations

A.2.1 Employee participation

1			Relevant			Not relevant		
			+2	+1	0	-1	-2	
		Is it relevant to ask, which channels companies in your specific industry offer for employee participation or influence on decision making (+2 = Totally relevant, -2 = Totally not relevant)? If relevant, the following:						
	1	Incentives to promote employee proposals for ___% of staff						
	2	Staff / employee committees with decision-making power for ___% of staff						
Please give reasons for your answers:								

A.2.2 Working time

2. Please provide the following aspects regarding regular working time in your company (excluding management):

Working time per week (hours/week)	____max,	____ average
Daily working time	____max,	____ average
Number of vacation days per year	____max,	____ average

3			Relevant			Not relevant		
			+2	+1	0	-1	-2	
		Which of the following items are relevant for the compensation of overtime in your company (+2 = Totally relevant, -2 = Totally not relevant)?						
	1	No compensation						
	2	Financial compensation						
	3	Compensation in the form of leisure time						
	4	Other, such as:						
Please give reasons for your answers: Recognition awards								

4			Relevant			Not relevant		
			+2	+1	0	-1	-2	
		Please specify the % of staff which is offered the possibility to use the following (+2 = Totally relevant, -2 = Totally not relevant)?:						
	1	Part time jobs, (___% of staff groupwide)						
	2	Flex time jobs, (___% of staff groupwide)						
	3	Working time accounts, (___% of staff groupwide)						
	4	Home based work						
	5	Unpaid leave (___ months)						
	6	Other						
Please give reasons for your answers: While we have flexibility the percentage is statistically insignificant.								

A.2.3 Safeguarding of jobs

5.		Relevant			Not relevant		
		+2	+1	0	-1	-2	
	Is it relevant to ask, whether companies in your industry offer limited appointments for their employees (+2 = Totally relevant, -2 = Totally not relevant)? What is the rate of limited appointments compared to appointments for an indefinite period: ___%						
Please specify how companies promote this: Contractual employment is offered for specific periods when the situation demands. As a practice we offer full time employment							

6. Please provide the following data:
a) Average period of notice: _4___ days/weeks/months
b) Staff fluctuations _____% (employees leaving the company compare to total number of staff per year)

7		Relevant			Not relevant		
		+2	+1	0	-1	-2	
	Is it relevant to ask, whether in the last four years staff was laid of in your specific industry due to restructuring and economic reasons (+2 = Totally relevant, -2 = Totally not relevant)?						
Please specify how companies promote this:In the current economic environment that is not a very necessary question							

8		Relevant			Not relevant		
		+2	+1	0	-1	-2	
	Is it relevant to ask, what measures were implemented to help your former staff to find new employment and to reduce their economic hardship (+2 = Totally relevant, -2 = Totally not relevant)?						
Please specify how companies promote this: Yes though we don't do it within our organisation							

9			Relevant			Not relevant		
			+2	+1	0	-1	-2	
		Is it relevant to ask, whether employees are offered the following benefits (+2 = Totally relevant, -2 = Totally not relevant)?						
	1	Share of profit, ____% of staff (groupwide)						
	2	Regular health insurance, ____% of staff (groupwide)						
	3	Regular pay in case of illnes, ____% of staff (groupwide)						
	4	Regular pension scheme, ____% of staff (groupwide)						
	5	Maternity grants, ____% of staff (groupwide)						
	6	Paid parental leave, ____% of staff (groupwide)						
	7	Canteen/subsidized lunch, ____% of staff (groupwide)						
Please give reasons for your answers: All the above are part of typical benefits offered in many companies of standing. Its good to know what happens when local companies and small companies consider these benefits								

10. Please provide the following data for training programs for staff:
a) Rate of staff joining further training programs: ____%
b) Average hours of further training per employee/year: ____ hours

A.2.4 Health & Safety

11		**Relevant**			**Not relevant**		
		+2	+1	0	-1	-2	
	Is it relevant to ask, whether companies in your industry offer a health & safety programm (+2 = Totally relevant, -2 = Totally not relevant)?						
Please specify the program:							

12. Please specify the % of staff with direct access to the following facilities:
a) Medical care, _100___% of staff (groupwide)
b) Non-smoking offices, _100___% of staff (groupwide)

13		**Relevant**			**Not relevant**		
		+2	+1	0	-1	-2	
	Is it relevant to ask, whether company's employees are protected by high mimimum standards regarding health and safety standards which are set either by law or through labor agreements (+2 = Totally relevant, -2 = Totally not relevant)?						
Please specify the program:							

14		Relevant			Not relevant		
		+2	+1	0	-1	-2	
	Is it relevant to ask, whether in recent years fines related to health and safety cases were imposed on companies in your industry (job related fatal accidents) (+2 = Totally relevant, -2 = Totally not relevant)?						
Please specify the program:							

A.2.5 Equal opportunities

15		Relevant			Not relevant		
		+2	+1	0	-1	-2	
	Is it relevant to ask, whether companies in your industry apply policies to avoid any discrimination on the basis of race, color, sex, religion, political opinion, sexual preference or social origin (+2 = Totally relevant, -2 = Totally not relevant)?						
If yes, please specify the policy:							

16			**Relevant**			**Not relevant**		
			+2	+1	0	-1	-2	
		Is it relevant to ask, whether companies in your industry apply legally required minimum wages for unskilled workers (+2 = Totally relevant, -2 = Totally not relevant)?						
	1	Wages are based on legally required locial minimum wages						
	2	Our minimum wages are generally ___% higher than local min.wages						
	3	We refer to living wages						

Please give reasons for your answers:Our wages are many times the minimum wage so the question is more relevant in the case of companies bordering on the unorganised

17			**Relevant**			**Not relevant**		
			+2	+1	0	-1	-2	
		Is it relevant to ask, how companies in your industry ensure a safe work place as well as adherence to relevant regulations for employees under 18 years of age (regarding dangerous work, night work) in your facilities (+2 = Totally relevant, -2 = Totally not relevant)?						

Please give reasons for your answers:

18		Relevant			Not relevant		
		+2	+1	0	-1	-2	
	Is it relevant to ask, whether companies in your industry ensure equal pay for men and women with equal qualification and experience (+2 = Totally relevant, -2 = Totally not relevant)?						
If yes, please specify the policy:							

19. Please specify the following data concerning gender distribution:
a) Executive Board: ____% female ____% male
b) Management positions: ____% female ____% male
b) Rate of women working in the company: ____% female
c) Please describe your efforts to avoid
- Sexual harassment:
- Mobbing:

A.3 Relations with external stakeholders

A.3.1 Customer and product responsibility

1		Relevant			Not relevant		
		+2	+1	0	-1	-2	
	Is it relevant to ask, whether companies in your industry have policies regarding responsible marketing and data protection (+2 = Totally relevant, -2 = Totally not relevant)?						
If yes, please specify the policy:Especially in BPO industry where this is a crucial concern							

2		Relevant			Not relevant		
		+2	+1	0	-1	-2	
	Is it relevant to ask, whether companies in your industry have policies / measures on granting access to financial services without discrimination (social / financial inclusion for low income groups) (+2 = Totally relevant, -2 = Totally not relevant)?						
If yes, please specify the policy:							

3		Relevant			Not relevant		
		+2	+1	0	-1	-2	
	Is it relevant to ask, whether companies in your industry have policies / measures regarding customers with debt repayment problems (e.g. Debt councelling, ombudsman, cooperation with consumer protection organizations) (+2 = Totally relevant, -2 = Totally not relevant)?						
If yes, please specify the policy: Personally not aware of details							

4		Relevant			Not relevant		
		+2	+1	0	-1	-2	
	Is it relevant to ask, whether companies in your industry lend to companie / projects with high social benefits (e. g. microcredit programs, community lending/investment, Special conditions for SMEs) (+2 = Totally relevant, -2 = Totally not relevant)?						
If yes, please specify the policy: We have a huge effort in the areas of sustainability and specifically in Microfinance							

5		Relevant			Not relevant		
		+2	+1	0	-1	-2	
	Is it relevant to ask, whether mutual funds managed by the company disclose their voting behavior in annual general meetings to the fund owners (+2 = Totally relevant, -2 = Totally not relevant)?						
If yes, please specify the policy:							

A.3.2 Corporate Governance

A.3.2.1 Independence and effectiveness of the Board

6			Relevant			Not relevant		
			+2	+1	0	-1	-2	
		Is it relevant to ask, whether companies in your industry separate the power between CEO and chairman of the Board (+2 = Totally relevant, -2 = Totally not relevant)?						
If yes, please specify the policy:								

7			Relevant			Not relevant		
			+2	+1	0	-1	-2	
		Is it relevant to ask, whether companies in your industry maintain different board committees which are independent of executive managers (remunaration committee, audit committee, nomination committee) (+2 = Totally relevant, -2 = Totally not relevant)?						
If yes, please specify the policy:								

A.3.2.2. Shareholder democracy

8		Relevant			Not relevant		
		+2	+1	0	-1	-2	
	Is it relevant to ask, whether companies in your industry maintain any restrictions on voting rights (e. g. one share entitlesthe owner to one vote) (+2 = Totally relevant, -2 = Totally not relevant)?						
If yes, please specify the policy: Not relevant except in the case of Financial Services Industry specifically where there are restrictions on Voting rights. Limited to 10%.							

9		Relevant			Not relevant		
		+2	+1	0	-1	-2	
	Is it relevant to ask, whether companies in your industry consider the size of the shareholding as a precondition on submitting a resolution at the annual general meeting (+2 = Totally relevant, -2 = Totally not relevant)?						
If yes, please specify the policy: Not able to understand relevance							

10			Relevant			Not relevant		
			+2	+1	0	-1	-2	
		Is it relevant to ask, whether companies in your industry facilitate shareholder participation by broadcasting the annual general meeting and giving shareholders the opportunities to vote on proxy resolutions via the internet (+2 = Totally relevant, -2 = Totally not relevant)?						

If yes, please specify the policy: In I ndia we are a branch presence so some of these questions are not strictly relevant But it is done internationally

11			Relevant			Not relevant		
			+2	+1	0	-1	-2	
		Is it relevant to ask, whether companies in your industry disclose the compensation schemes for executive board members (+2 = Totally relevant, -2 = Totally not relevant)?						

If yes, please specify the policy:

A.3.3 Community involvement

12			Relevant			Not relevant		
			+2	+1	0	-1	-2	
		Is it relevant to ask, whether companies in your industry take responsibility for community projects (+2 = Totally relevant, -2 = Totally not relevant)? If yes, the following						
	1	Social projects						
	2	Cultural projects						
	3	Environmental projects						
Please give reasons for your answers: We do a lot with environment and Children and women								

Portion of profit: __?__%

13			Relevant			Not relevant		
			+2	+1	0	-1	-2	
		Is it relevant to ask, whether companies in your industry make political contributions (+2 = Totally relevant, -2 = Totally not relevant)?						
If yes, please specify the policy: We don't and companies genrally don't atleast officially								

A.3.4 Society

14			Relevant			Not relevant		
			+2	+1	0	-1	-2	.
		Is it relevant to ask, whether companies in your industry respect the policy on human rights and cultural self-determination (+2 = Totally relevant, -2 = Totally not relevant)?						
If yes, please specify the policy:								

15			Relevant			Not relevant		
			+2	+1	0	-1	-2	.
		Is it relevant to ask, whether companies in your industry have policies on how to deal fairly with peoples affected by companies activities (+2 = Totally relevant, -2 = Totally not relevant)?						
If yes, please specify the policy: Pls clarify more								

A.3.5 Fair business practices

16			**Relevant**			**Not relevant**		
			+2	+1	0	-1	-2	
		Is it relevant to ask, whether companies in your industry have a code of conduct regarding corruption and economic fraud (e. g. antitrust, insider dealing) (+2 = Totally relevant, -2 = Totally not relevant)?						
If yes, please specify the policy: This is relevant								

17			**Relevant**			**Not relevant**		
			+2	+1	0	-1	-2	
		Is it relevant to ask, whether measures are taken up by the companies in your industry to ensure fair business practices (e. g. against corruption, antitrust, insider dealing) (+2 = Totally relevant, -2 = Totally not relevant)?						
	1	Training						
	2	Audits						
	3	Compliance officers						
	4	Hotlines						
	5	Others						
Please give reasons for your answers: We have a detailed modular program which most staff have to complete mandatorily								

Name: ………………………………………………………………………………..
Company/Sectorofoperation:…………………………………………………………
Department: ……………………………………………………
Size of company (sales/employees): ………………………………..

Annex 2

The Cultural Compatibility Questionnaire

GOETHE
UNIVERSITÄT
FRANKFURT AM MAIN

Emmanuel Franklyne Ogbunwezeh
Department of Social and Economic Ethics
Frankfurt Graduate School of Social Sciences and Humanities
Johann Wolfgang Goethe University,
Frankfurt am Main

To whom it may concern

Dear Sir/Madam,

We crave your help in this academic research designed to assess what Nigerians in the Finance sector would loved to see in the formulation of rating or assessment criteria for companies.

This questionnaire is designed to find out, what you would love to see as major components of any workable criteria directed at the ethical and ecological rating and/or assessment of companies in Nigeria.

We would be most glad if you would cross an X in the relevant box as you deem fit, in answer to the questions.

All information obtained in this research are strictly for academic purposes and is not open or accessible to third parties for marketing purposes except as a part of a doctoral dissertation in fulfilment of the academic requirements for the award of a PhD in Social and Economic Ethics of the above-named university.

Your diligent completion of the questionnaire would be highly appreciated.

Yours very sincerely,

Emmanuel Franklyne Ogbunwezeh

1.	**General moral principles (3.2)**

1.		**Yes**			**No**		
		+2	+1	0	-1	-2	
(3.2.1)	*As a matter of principle, people should help protect the natural resource base, on which the lives of future generations will depend (+2 = Strongly yes, -2 = Strongly no).*						
Please give reasons for your answer:							

1.1		**Relevant**			**Not relevant**		
		+2	+1	0	-1	-2	
(3.2.1.2/ 3/1+ 3.2.8.5)	Is it relevant to ask, whether companies profit from executions and the displacement of ethnic groups (+2 = Totally relevant, -2 = Totally not relevant)?						
Please give reasons for your answer:							

2.			Yes			Not		
			+2	+1	0	-1	-2	
(3.2.2)		*As a matter of principle, people should not cause or inflict pain (+2 = Strongly yes, -2 = Strongly no).*						
Please give reasons for your answer:								

2.1.			Relevant			Not relevant		
			+2	+1	0	-1	-2	
(3.2.2.2+ 3.2.8.2)		Is it relevant to ask, whether international companies supply dangerous products that are prohibited in the home country to Nigeria where the products are considered "harmless" (toxic waste) (+2 = Totally relevant, -2 = Totally not relevant)?						
Please give reasons for your answer:								

3.			Yes			No		
			+2	+1	0	-1	-2	
(3.2.3)		*As a matter of principle, people should not constrain the capability of others (+2 = Strongly yes, -2 = Strongly no).*						
Please give reasons for your answer:								

4.			Yes			No		
			+2	+1	0	-1	-2	
(3.2.4)		*As a matter of principle, people should deprive no one of their freedom or opportunities (+2 = Strongly yes, -2 = Strongly no).*						
Please give reasons for your answer:								

4.1.			Relevant			Not relevant		
			+2	+1	0	-1	-2	
(3.2.4.1)		Is it relevant to ask, whether companies tolerate heavy child labour (+2 = Totally relevant, -2 = Totally not relevant)?						
Please give reasons for your answer:								

4.2.			Relevant			Not relevant		
			+2	+1	0	-1	-2	
(3.2.4.2+ 3.2.5.2/4)		Is it relevant to ask, whether companies create working conditions detrimental to the family (+2 = Totally relevant, -2 = Totally not relevant)?						
Please give reasons for your answer:								

4.3.		Relevant			Not relevant		
		+2	+1	0	-1	-2	
(3.2.4.3/ 4/6)	Is it relevant to ask, whether companies cooperate with countries in which ethnic, political or religious minorities or women are systematically oppressed (+2 = Totally relevant, -2 = Totally not relevant)?						
Please give reasons for your answer:							

4.4.		Relevant			Not relevant		
		+2	+1	0	-1	-2	
(3.2.4.5+ (3.2.3.2/1/ 3.2.5.3))	Is it relevant to ask, whether international companies attempt in an aggressive manner to impose their own methods and values on Nigerian people (+2 = Totally relevant, -2 = Totally not relevant)?						
Please give reasons for your answer:							

4.5.			Relevant			Not relevant		
			+2	+1	0	-1	-2	.
(3.2.4.9/7/8+ 3.2.8.8/9)		Is it relevant to ask, whether companies in Nigeria buy up patents not to use them but to keep competitiors off the market (+2 = Totally relevant, -2 = Totally not relevant)?						
Please give reasons for your answer:								

5.			Yes			No		
			+2	+1	0	-1	-2	.
(3.2.5)		*As a matter of principle, people should deprive no one of their pleasure in something (+2 = Strongly yes, -2 = Strongly no).*						
Please give reasons for your answer:								

5.1.		Relevant			Not relevant		
		+2	+1	0	-1	-2	
(3.2.5.1)	Is it relevant to ask, whether companies show respect for indigenous traditions, rites and festivals (+2 = Totally relevant, -2 = Totally not relevant)?						
Please give reasons for your answer:							

6.		Relevant			Not relevant		
		+2	+1	0	-1	-2	
(3.2.6)	*As a matter of principle, people should not deceive or defraud (+2 = Strongly yes, -2 = Strongly no).*						
Please give reasons for your answer:							

6.1.			Relevant			Not relevant		
			+2	+1	0	-1	-2	
(3.2.6.1.+ 3.2.1.4)		Is it relevant to ask, whether companies create with their products an higher impression on quality than they actually posess (+2 = Totally relevant, -2 = Totally not relevant)?						
Please give reasons for your answer:								

6.2.			Relevant			Not relevant		
			+2	+1	0	-1	-2	
(3.2.6.2)		Is it relevant to ask, whether bribery of politiciens and decision makers in companies exist (+2 = Totally relevant, -2 = Totally not relevant)?						
Please give reasons for your answer:								

7.		Yes			No		
		+2	+1	0	-1	-2	.
(3.2.7)	*As a matter of principle, people should keep their promises (+2 = Strongly yes, -2 = Strongly no).*						
Please give reasons for your answer:							

7.1.		Relevant			Not relevant		
		+2	+1	0	-1	-2	.
(3.2.7.2)	Is it relevant to ask, whether companies honour contracts and guarantees even though a situtation of economic dependency of the country exists (+2 = Totally relevant, -2 = Totally not relevant)?						
Please give reasons for your answer:							

8.		Yes			No		
		+2	+1	0	-1	-2	.
(3.2.8)	*As a matter of principle, people should respect the property of others (+2 = Strongly yes, -2 = Strongly no).*						
Please give reasons for your answer:							

8.1.			Relevant			Not relevant		
			+2	+1	0	-1	-2	
(3.2.8.1)		Is it relevant to ask, whether local products are displaced from the market by international companies (+2 = Totally relevant, -2 = Totally not relevant)?						
Please give reasons for your answer:								

8.2.			Relevant			Not relevant		
			+2	+1	0	-1	-2	
(3.2.8.3/4+ (3.2.3.3/5))		Is it relevant to ask, whether there is any protection of nature and biological diversity by companies (+2 = Totally relevant, -2 = Totally not relevant)?						
Please give reasons for your answer:								

8.3.			Relevant			Not relevant		
			+2	+1	0	-1	-2	
(3.2.8.6/7)		Is it relevant to ask, how companies react to questions concerning personal property that was annexed in the past and given to companies (+2 = Totally relevant, -2 = Totally not relevant)?						
Please give reasons for your answer:								

9.			Yes			No		
			+2	+1	0	-1	-2	
(3.2.9/1)		*As a matter of principle, people should obey the law (+2 = Strongly yes, -2 = Strongly no).*						
Please give reasons for your answer:								

9.1.			Relevant			Not relevant		
			+2	+1	0	-1	-2	
(3.2.9.2/3)		Is it relevant to ask, whether companies respect the code of ethics prevailing in the specific industry (+2 = Totally relevant, -2 = Totally not relevant)?						
Please give reasons for your answer:								

10.			Yes			No		
			+2	+1	0	-1	-2	
(3.2.10)		*As a matter of principle, people should not subject anybody to moral obligations beyond their ability to fulfill them (+2 = Strongly yes, -2 = Strongly no).*						
Please give reasons for your answer:								

10.1.			Relevant			Not relevant		
			+2	+1	0	-1	-2	
(3.2.10.1)		Is it relevant to ask, whether companies show consideration for employee groups requiring protection (handicapped, children, women) (+2 = Totally relevant, -2 = Totally not relevant)?						
Please give reasons for your answer:								

2.	Anthropologically given motivational factors

1.			Yes			No		
			+2	+1	0	-1	-2	
(3.1.4)		Competition and solidarity are two mutually conflicting factors driving actions of companies (+2 = Strongly yes, -2 = Strongly no).						
Please give reasons for your answer:								

2.			Yes			No		
			+2	+1	0	-1	-2	
(3.1.5)		Unlimited expansion and self restraint are two mutually conflicting factors driving actions of companies (+2 = Strongly yes, -2 = Strongly no).						
Please give reasons for your answer:								

3.			Yes			No		
			+2	+1	0	-1	-2	
(3.1.3)		Self-glorification and low profile are two mutually conflicting factors characterizing the image of companies to the society (+2 = Strongly yes, -2 = Strongly no).						
Please give reasons for your answer:								

4.			Yes			No		
			+2	+1	0	-1	-2	
(3.1.2.)		Close-mindness and openness are two mutually conflicting factors driving actions of companies (+2 = Strongly yes, -2 = Strongly no).						
Please give reasons for your answer:								

5			Yes			No		
			+2	+1	0	-1	-2	
(3.1.1)		Responsibility and right of the stronger are two mutually conflicting factors driving the actions of companies (+2 = Strongly yes, -2 = Strongly no).						

Please give reasons for your answer:

3.	Orientations and virtues

1.	Orientations		Relevant			Not relevant		
			+2	+1	0	-1	-2	
(3.3.1)		Is it relevant to ask, whether companies impose moral constraints on their actions (+2 = Totally relevant, -2 = Totally not relevant)?						

Please give reasons for your answer:

2.	Orientations		Relevant		Not relevant			
			+2	+1	0	-1	-2	
(3.3.2)		Is it relevant to ask, whether companies impose limits on their actions, which are conducive to a harmonious co existence with others (+2 = Totally relevant, -2 = Totally not relevant)?						
Please give reasons for your answer:								

3	Virtues		Yes		No			
			+2	+1	0	-1	-2	
		The following items are desirable virtues in their own right (+2 = Strongly yes, -2 = Strongly no):						
	1	Truth telling						
	2	Justice						
	3	Prudence						
	4	Courage in the sense of steadfastness						
	5	Peacefulness						
	6	Sense of proportion and restraint						
Please give reasons for your answers:								

4	Virtues		Yes			No		
			+2	+1	0	-1	-2	
		The following items are desirable virtues to the extent that they are practiced in the service of higher moral principles. To the extent that they are placed in the service of low moral principles, they stop being virtues (+2 = Strongly yes, -2 = Strongly no):						
	1	Dilligence						
	2	Punctuality						
	3	Cleanliness						
	4	Orderliness						
	5	Obediance						
	6	Flexibility						
	7	Mobility						
	8	Empathy						
Please give reasons for your answers:								

Bibliography

Achebe, Chinua. 1983. The Trouble with Nigeria, Enugu, Fourth Dimension Publishers.

Adams, Patricia. Odious Debts: Loose Lending, Corruption and the Third World's Environmental Legacy. London, Earthscan. 1991.

Ali Akpajiak & Toni Pyke. Measuring Poverty in Nigeria, Oxfam GB, 2003

Aliber, Michael. Poverty Eradication and Sustainable Development, Cape Town, Human Sciences Research Council. 2002

Armendariz de Aghion, Beatriz. & Jonathan Murdoch. the Economics of Microfinance, Massachusetts Institute of Technology Press, 2005

Atasoy, Yildiz and William K. Carroll, (eds.) Global Shaping and its Alternatives, Garamond Press, December 2002

Balogun, M. Jide & Yolamu, R. Barongo(eds.) Wealth Generation for Poverty Eradication in Africa: Role of State and Non-State Actors, Nairobi, ICIPE Science Press, 2007

Balz, Bernd-Christian, Ethisch-ökologische Geldanlage: Eine kapitalmarktorientierte Analyse, Frankfurt am Main, IKO Verlag, 1999

Berger, Peter & Luckmann, Thomas. The Social Construction of Reality, New York, Doubleday & Company, 1967

Brenner, Philip, Borosage Robert & Weidner Bethany (eds.) Exploring Contradictions: Political Economy in the Corporate State, New York, David McKay Company, inc., 1974

Chang, Ha-Joon. Bad Samaritans: The Guilty Secrets of Rich Nations and the threat to Global Prosperity, London, Random House, 2008

Christian Aid, 2004, Behind the Mask. The Real Face of Corporate Social Responsibility, London.

Chua, Amy. World on Fire: How Exporting Free-Market Democracy Breeds Ethnic hatred and Global Instability, London, Arrow Books, 2004.

Clark, Gregory. A Farewell to Alms: A Brief Economic History of the World, Princeton, Princeton University Press, 2007

Clapp, Jennifer. 1998. The Privatization of Global Environmental Governance: ISO 14000 and the Developing World. Global Governance 4 (1998). 295-316

Collier, Paul. The Bottom Billion: Why the Poorest Countries are Falling and what can be done about it. New York, Oxford University Press, 2007

Cusumano, M.A, and Markides, C.C. (eds.) Strategic Thinking for the Next Economy, San Francisco, MITSloan Management Review, 2001

Csikszentmihalyi Mihaly, Good Business: Leadership, Flow and the Making of Meaning, London, Hodder & Stoughton, 2003

De Botton, Alain. The Consolations of Philosophy. London, Penguin Books, 2001

Davidow, William. H & Malone, Michael. S. The Virtual Corporation: Lessons from the World's Most Advanced Companies. New York, Harper Business, 1992

De Soto, Hernando. The Mystery of Capital: Why Capitalism Triumphs in the West and Fails Everywhere Else. London, Bantam Books, 2000

Diamond, Jared. Collapse: How Societies Choose to Fail or Succeed, New York, Viking Books, 2005.

Diamond, Jared. Guns, Germs and Steel: A Short History of Everybody for the last 13,000 years. London, Vintage Books, 1998

Didsbury, Howard Jr. (ed.) Thinking Creatively in Turbulent Times, Bethesda Maryland, World Future Society, 2004

Dorr, Donal. The Social Justice Agenda: Justice, Ecology, Power and the Church, Dublin, Gill and Macmillan Ltd, 1991

Döpfner, Claudia. Zur Glabuwürdigkeit ethisch-ökologischer Geld-und Kapitalanlagen: Eine theologisch-ethische Untersuchung vor dem Hintergrund der Frage nach der Glaubwürdigkeit der ökonomischen und monetären Strukturen, Frankfurt am Main, IKO Verlag, 2000

Easterly, William. The Elusive Quest for Growth: Economists' Adventures and Misadventures in the Tropics,

– The Whiteman's Burden: Why the West's Effort to Aid the Rest have Done So Much Ill and So Little Good New York, Oxford University Press, 2006

Ellul, Jacques, The Technological Society, New York, Vintage Book, 1964

Elkington, J., Cannibals with Forks: The Triple Bottom Line of 21st Century Business, Oxford (Conscientious Commerce). 1999.

Feather, Frank & Mayur, Rashmi (eds.) Optimistic Outlooks, Toronto, Global Futures Network, inc.,1982

Friedman, Milton. Capitalism and Freedom, Chicago, University of Chicago Press, 1982

Friedman, Thomas. The Lexus and the Olive Tree. New York, Anchor Books, 2000.

– The World is flat: A Brief History of the Globalized World in the 21st Century, London, Penguin Books, 2005

Galbraith, J.K. The Economics of Innocent Fraud, London, Penguin Books, 2004.

Garvey, James. The Ethics of Climate Change: Right and Wrong in a Warming World, London, Continuum Books, 2008.

Global Marshall Plan Initiative (Hrg.) Impulse für eine Welt in Balance, Hamburg, 2005

Grieble, Peter. Ethisch-Ökologische Geldanlage: einflusmöglichkeiten durch Beachtung von ethisch-Ökologischen Gesichtspunkten bei der Anlage von Geld. Frankfurt am Main. IKO-Verlag, 2001

Hall, Edward. T. Beyond Culture. New York, Anchor Press/Doubleday, 1977

Hancock, Graham. Lords of Poverty. London, Macmillan, 1991

Harford, Tim. The Undercover Economist. London, Abacus Books, 2006

Harper, Malcolm (ed.) Microfinance: Evolution, Achievements and Challenges, London, ITDG publishing, 2003

Harris, Nigel. The End of the Third World, London, Penugin Books, 1986

Harvey, D. The Third World in Global Development, London, Macmillan, 1987

Heilbroner, Robert & Lester Thurow, Economics Explained, New York, Touchstone Books, 1994.

Hein,Volker: Staaten, transnationale Unternehmen und Nichtregierungsorganisationen in Konflikt um biologische Ressourcen, Frankfurt am Main, Institut für Sozialforschung, 2000.

Henderson, David. (ed.) The Fortune Encyclopaedia of Economics, New York, Warner Books, 1993

Hertz, Noreena, I.O.U. The Debt Threat and Why we must Defuse it, London, Harper Perennial, 2005

Hobsbawm, Eric. The New Century, London, Abacus Books, 1999.

Hoffmann, J., Ott, K. & Scherhorn, G. (Hrsg.) Ethische Kriterien für die Bewertung von Unternehmen. Frankfurt am Main. IKO-Verlag, 1997

Hoffmann, J. Die Vernunft in den Kulturen, Frankfurt am Main, IKO-Verlag, 1992

Hoffmann, J. Der Mensch zwischen Gesellschaflichen Plausibilitäten und Glaubensgewissheit, Verlag Steinkopf, 1986

Huntington, Samuel. The Clash of Civilizations, London, Simon &Schuster, 1996

Ike, Obiora & Ndidi-Nnoli Edozien. Development is About People; Business is about Ethics, Enugu, CIDJAP Publications, 2003.

Jahn, Franziska. Zur Qualität von Nachhaltigkeits-ratings: Zwischen Anspruch und Wirklichkeit, Frankfurt am Main, IKO Verlag, 2004

Jay, Anthony. Management and Machiavelli: An Inquiry into the Politics of Corporate Life, New York, Bantam Books, 1969

Karioki, James (ed) Mazrui, Ali: A Tale of Two Africas Nigeria and South Africa as Contrasting Visions, London, Adonis &Abbey Publishers Ltd, 2006

Karl Jaspers. The Future of Mankind, Chicago, University of Chicago Press, 1958

Kebede, Messay. Africa's Quest for a Philosophy of Decolonization New VIBS, 2004

Kinoti, George. Hope for Africa and what the Christian can do, Nairobi, AISRED,1996.

Klein, Naomi. The Shock Doctrine. London, Penguin Books, 2007.

– No Logo. London, HarperCollins, 2001.

Knopp, Guido. Hitlers Managers, München, Goldman Verlag, 2007

Kovel, Joel. White Racism: A Psychohistory. London, Free Association Books, 1988.

Lasch, Christopher. The Culture of Narcissism, New York, Warner Books, inc. 1979

Langdon, Steven. Global Poverty, Democracy and North-South Change, Garamond Press, 1999

Lever, Lawrence. The Barlow Clowes Affair, London, Macmillan, 1992

Linden, Eugene. Affluence and Discontent: The Anatomy of Consumer Societies, New York, The Viking Press, 1979

Krugman, Paul. Pop Internationalism, Cambridge Massachusetts, MIT Press, 1999

Krugman, Paul. The Accidental Theorist and Other Dispatches from the Dismal Science, New York, W.W Norton and Company, 1998

Lindahl, Claes. Wealth of the Poor: Eliminating Poverty through Market and Private Sector Development, Stockholm, Sida, 2005

Lorenz, Konrad. Behind the Mirror: A search for the Natural Histroy of Human Knowlegde, New York, First Harvest Books, 1978

Mack, Timothy C. (ed.) Hopes and Visions for the 21st Century, Bethseda-Maryland, World Future Society, 2007

Maier, Karl. This House has Fallen, London, Spectrum Books. 2000

Makil, Agi, James Ethisch-okologische Bewertung von Unternehmen in Indien auf Basis des Frankfurt-Hohenheimer-Leitfadens und des Corporate Responsibility Ratings-Prufung der interkulturellen Brauchbarkeit vom Frankfurt-Hohenheimer-Leitfaden und des Corporate Responsibility Ratings fur die Messung und Forderung von Nachhaltigkeit im Indischen Kontext: Doctoral dissertation submitted to the Faculty of Catholic Theology of the Johann Wolfgang Goethe University, Frankfurt am Main,2008

Manji, Firoze. The Missionary Position: NGOs and Development in Africa. In: International Affairs 78 3 (2002) 567-83, http://www.fahamu.org/downloads/missionaryposition.pdf

Mazrui, Ali. Cultural Forces in the World Politics, Nairobi, Heinemann, 1990

Mazrui, Ali & Mutunga, W. (eds.) Governance and Leadership: Debating the African Condition, Asamara, Africa World Press, inc. 2003

Mazrui, Ali & Mutunga, W. (eds.) Race, Gender, and Culture Conflict: Debating the Africa Condition, Asamara, Africa World Press, inc. 2004

McHale, John. The Future of the Future, New York, Ballantine Books, 1969.

McMurtry, John. Unequal Freedoms: The Global Market As An Ethical System, Garamond Press, June 1998

Meadows, Donella and Co. The Limits of Growth: A Report for the Club of Rome's Project on the Predicament of Mankind, Massachusetts Institute of Technology, 1972

Meredith, Martin. The State of Africa: A History of Fifty Years of Independence. London, Simon & Schuster, 2006.

Mofid, Kamran. Globalisation for the Common Good, London, Shepheard & Walwyn, 2000

Myrdal, Gunnar. Asian Drama: An Inquiry into the Poverty of Nations Vol 1-3, New York, Random House, 1968

Nnoli-Edozien, Ndidi. Ownership and Management Structures in the Economy: African Traditional Values Applied to Modern Issues of Sustainability and the Corporate Governance Function. Enugu, CIDJAP Publications, 2007

Onwuka Dike, Kenneth & Ekejiuba, Felicia. The ARO of South Eastern Nigeria 1650-1980, Ibadan, University Press Limited, 1990.

O'Brien, Justin. Wall Street on Trial, West Sussex, John Wiley & Sons Ltd, 2003

O'Shea, James and Madigan, Charles. Dangerous Company: Consulting Powerhouses and the Businesses they save and ruin, London, Nicholas Brealey Publishing, 2002

Peters, Thomas & Robert Waterman, Jr. In Search of Excellence: Lessons from America's Best-Run Companies, New York, Harper & Row, 1988

Perkins, John. The Confessions of an Economic Hit Man, San-Francisco, Berrett-Koehler Publishers, 2004.

Project group Ethical-Ecological Rating/oekom research AG (eds.) Ethical-Ecological Rating: The Frankfurt Hohenheim Guidelines and their implementation via the Corporate Responsibility Rating. Munchen, oekom Verlag, 2003.

Rawls, John. A Theory of Justice, Oxford, Oxford University Press, 1999.

Read, Carveath. Man and His Superstitions, Guernsey, Cambridge University Press, 1925 (1995 Edition).

Reich, Robert. Supercapitalism: The Battle for Democracy in an age of Big Business, London, Icon Books, 2009

Ries, Simon. 2001. Intercultural Assessment of Sustainability: Intercultural Adaptability of oekom research AG's corporate responsibility rating (CRR)

According to the Criteria of Social and Cultural Sustainability. http://www.enodo.de/downloads/Intercultural_assessment_of_sustainability.pdf accessed on the 2nd of September, 2008

Reisch, Lucia (ed.) Ethical-ecological Investment: Towards Global Sustainable Development, Frankfurt am Main, IKO Verlag, 2001

Rist, Gilbert. The History of Development: From Western Origins to Global Faith, London, Zed Books Ltd, 2002

Rotberg, Robert. Crafting the New Nigeria, Confronting the challenges, Colorado, Lynee Reineer Publishers, 2004

Rwomire, Apollo (ed.) Social Problems in Africa: New Visions. London. Praeger Publishers, 2001

Sachs, Wolgang & Santarius, Tilman (eds.) Fair Future: Resource conflicts, Security and Global Justice, London, ZED Books, 2005

Schumacher, E.F. A Guide fort he Perplexed, London, Abacus Books, 1978

Schneider, Armin. Wege zur verantwortlichen Organisation: Die Bedeutung der ethischen und theologischen Perspektive für die Qualität der Organisations- und Personalentwicklung, Frankfurt am Main, IKO Verlag, 2005

Schneider, Hans-Albert. Ethisches Rating: Begründung Bewertungsmöglichkeit Evaluation, Frankfurt am Main, IKO Verlag, 2001

Sen, Amartya. Development as Freedom, Oxford, Oxford University Press, 1999

Smith, Adam. The Wealth of Nation, London, Everyman's Library, 1970

Stiglitz, Joseph. Globalization and its Discontents, London, Penguin Books, 2002

Stiglitz, Joseph. The Roaring Nineties: Why we're paying the price for the greediest decade in history, London, Penguin Books, 2003

Soyinka, Wole. The Open Sore of the Continent, New York, Oxford University Press, 1996

Sütterlin, Sabine. Mein Wort Zählt: Mikrokredite-Kleines Kapital-grosse Wirkung, Verband Entwicklungspolitik deutscher Nichtregierungsorganisation (VENRO), 2007

Toffler, Alvin. Powershift: Knowledge, Wealth and Violence at the Edge of the 21st Century, New York, Bantam Books, 1990

Torekull, Bertil. In Quest of a Company Soul, Stockholm, Streiffert & Co. Bokförlag HB, 1987

World Commission on Environment and Development, Our Common Future, Oxford University Press, Oxford1987.

Journals

1. Journal of Microfinance, http://www.lib.byu.edu/dlib/spc/microfinance/
2. Stanford Journal of Microfinance, Inaugural Issue, Vol.1, 2008. http://www.stanford.edu/group/publicknowledge/cgi-bin/ojs/sjm-journal
3. Journal of Markets and Morality, Vol. 9 No.1, www.marketsandmorality.com
4. Journal of the Globalization for the Common Good. http://lass.calumet.purdue.edu/cca/jgcg/
5. World Development Vol. 29, No. 1

Papers

1. Ogbunwezeh, Emmanuel Franklyne. Africa: The Ontology of Failed States. http://www.dawodu.com/ogbunwezeh1.htm
2. Olomola, A.S, Social Capital, Microfinance Group Performance and Poverty Implications in Nigeria, Ibadan, Nigerian Institute of Social and Economic Research (NISER), not dated
3. Osinubi, S.T., Macroeconomic Policies and Pro-Poor Growth in Nigeria, A paper presented at the World Institute for Development Economics Research (WIDER) conference on Inequality, Poverty and Human-Well being, Helsinki, Finland, 30-31 May, 2003
4. Xavier Sala-i-Martin and Arvind Subramanian, Addressing the Natural Resource Curse: An Illustration from Nigeria (How Can Nigeria Address the Natural Resource Curse?) IMF Working Paper, May 2003
5. Thomas, Saji., & Canagarajah, Sudharshan: Poverty in a Wealthy Economy: The Case of Nigeria. IMF Working Paper, July 2002

Legitimacy: the Treasure of Politics

Tage Kurtén / Lars Hertzberg (eds.)

Legitimacy: the Treasure of Politics

PETER LANG
Frankfurt am Main · Berlin · Bern · Bruxelles · New York · Oxford · Wien

Bibliographic Information published by the Deutsche Nationalbibliothek
The Deutsche Nationalbibliothek lists this publication in the Deutsche Nationalbibliografie; detailed bibliographic data is available in the internet at http://dnb.d-nb.de.

The publication of this volume
has been sponsored by the Research Institute
of the Åbo Academy Foundation.

Cover Design:
© Olaf Glöckler, Atelier Platen, Friedberg

ISBN 978-3-631-61883-7

www.peterlang.de

TABLE OF CONTENTS

CONTRIBUTORS

Lars Hertzberg, (b. 1943), PhD (Cornell/1970) is professor emeritus in philosophy at Åbo Academy University. He has done work on the philosophy of language, philosophical psychology, moral philosophy and Wittgenstein.

Olli Lagerspetz, (b. 1963), PhD (ÅAU/1996) is Senior Lecturer of Philosophy at Åbo since 2005. He was the Head of Philosophy in 2007-2010. Lagerspetz has studied at Åbo and at Urbana-Champaign, Illinois. In 1992-1998, Lagerspetz was Lecturer of Philosophy at the University of Wales, Swansea. He has published a book on the concept of trust and a book (in Swedish) on the clean and the dirty, as well as articles on ethics, philosophical anthropology, and the philosophy of mind.

Tage Kurtén, (b. 1950), Dr Theol (ÅAU/1982) is professor in Theological Ethics and Philosophy of Religion at Åbo Academy University. His main fields of study has been philosophical presuppositions of academic theology, ordinary life-views, especially conditions for religous life in late modernity, and questions concerning ethics, law and religion.

Ville Päivänsalo, (b. 1972), Dr Theol (Helsinki/2005), serves currently as Acting University Lecturer in Theological and Social Ethics at the University of Helsinki. He specializes in social contract theories, global justice, and the ethics of human development. His research interests also include Christian ethics, especially as related to Lutheran tradition, and business ethics.

Martin Scheinin, (b. 1954), Dr Iuris (Helsinki/1991) is Professor of Public International Law at the European University Institute (Florence). His main research interest include the constitutionalization of international law, through the increasing normative importance of universal human rights and the operation of international courts and other independent mechanisms of compliance control; and legal constraints on the use of new technology in surveillance and counter-terrorism.

Pamela Slotte, (b. 1973), Dr Theol (ÅAU/2005), is a post-doctoral research fellow at the Erik Castrén Institute of International Law and Human Rights and at the Centre of Excellence in Global Governance Research at the Faculty of Law,

University of Helsinki. Her fields of study include global ethics, political theology, as well as questions concerning ethics, law and religion. Her current research focuses on the concept of religious freedom in international law.

Mats Lindfelt, (b. 1970), DrPol (ÅAU/2007), wrote his doctoral dissertation on the normative status of fundamental rights in the EU legal order. His research intrest include european constitutionalism, interaction between different legal orders and human rights related issues. He is currenlty working as the head of academic affairs at Åbo Akademi University.

Joakim Molander, (b. 1968), PhD in Philosophy (ÅAU/2002). Both his dissertation thesis (Straffets grammatik - the Grammar of Punishment) and post doc research has been on philosophy of law and ethics. Since 2002 he has written commentary, reviews and essays on these topics in one of Sweden's large newspapers, Svenska Dagbladet. In August 2011 he will take up the position of counselor and head of Swedish development cooperation at the Swedish embassy to Rwanda. Previous work experience includes three years as first secretary at the Swedish embassy to Bosnia and Herzegovina.

Heidi Jokinen, (b. 1979), MTheol (ÅAU/2004), is a doctoral student in Theological Ethics and Philosophy of Religion at Åbo Academy University. She is currently finishing her doctoral dissertation, in which she studies victim - offender mediation in criminal cases as a conflict resolution method in a late modern society. Her fields of study include issues concerning reconciliation, forgiveness and punishment.

Lise Kanckos, (b. 1977), MSocSc (ÅAU/2003), MTheol (ÅAU/2006), is a doctoral student at the Department of Sociology at Åbo Akademi University. She is currently working on her doctoral dissertation, in which she studies discourses on religion and the best interests of the child in parliamentary debates on assisted reproduction in Finland. Her fields of study include sociology of religion, and issues concerning politics, ethics, gender and reproduction.

Malena Björkgren, (b. 1978), Dr Theol (ÅAU/2009), wrote her doctoral dissertation on domestic violence as moral and societal problem. Her research interests include feminist theology, morality and language. She is a minister in the Evangelical Lutheran Church of Finland.

INTRODUCTION

Tage Kurtén

> "Legitimacy is one of those beautiful words which the human mind cannot link with any conception but which, considered simply as words, have a power infinitely greater than any human conception." (Simone Weil 1987.)

These poetic words written by Simone Weil during the Second World War catch some main themes of the articles in this volume. This book is a study of the concept of legitimacy. The authors are united in the conviction that there is not only one correct way of defining this concept. At the same time the importance of legitimacy is recognized. The legitimacy is seen as "the treasure of politics", to quote Weil once again.

"Legitimacy" has been much discussed, not least among political scientists and in political philosophy. So why do we write another book on the matter? The present authors are convinced that there are still aspects of legitimacy that are neglected in the studies done on this concept. Some of these aspects can be elaborated further through a trans-disciplinary discussion like the one carried on in this volume.

Some of the ways the legitimacy of political decision-making and of governance are understood focus on the quality of the authorities whose legitimacy is being discussed. One could for example think of Max Weber's threefold way of understanding legitimacy as dependent upon tradition (a historical criterion), the extra-ordinary qualities of the ruler (a criterion of personal character), or upon legality (a formal and procedural criterion).

Common to such ways of defining legitimacy is an element of externalisation: the question of legitimacy can be settled by pointing to certain objective criteria, external to the individual making legitimacy judgements. In contrast to this the articles in this volume emphasize the character of legitimacy as something primarily dependent, not upon the nature of governments, politicians or court judges, but upon the people subject to the actions of such authorities. Although there are some minor differences in emphasis among the present authors, legitimacy is throughout the volume seen as something expressed by the people governed, by the members of political communities. For the most part such expressions concern something relational. Legitimacy judgements are mostly made implicitly. Legitimacy can thus primarily be seen as an important aspect of the relation between members of the society and the authorities, between the citizens and the state.

Some of the articles in the volume maintain that the legitimacy of an authority is normally taken for granted. This goes especially for the relatively stable societies in Northern Europe. The average member of such societies reveals her/his confidence in the way public matters are being handled by simply taking part in the daily life of her/his country. It is only when something happens which makes one feel discontented, uncertain or alienated in the society in which one lives that feelings and thoughts challenging the authorities arise.

It is the conviction of the present authors that, both in Europe and in the global village as a whole, we currently experience large changes on several levels both of society and of culture. These changes are shaking the trust people normally have in their own country and in its authorities. (In a newly published book many of these changes are presented and discussed: Christoffersen et al. 2010.)

It seems obvious that Western culture, for one thing, is undergoing a development which is changing its mental framework in a radical way. Sometimes it is called a shift from a modern to a late modern society and culture. Many things taken for granted in the modern era are currently being critically examined, such as the secular outlook on life as well as uncritical belief in science, technocracy, and unlimited economic growth. This critical attitude is evident in increasing public debate on moral and religious matters. Sociologists talk about "post-secularity" and "the return of religion".

These elements are associated with overall globalisation of the life of states as well as of individuals. The increasing mobility of people between countries changes the cultural and religious landscape in many ways. Clashes between Muslim immigrants and Christian traditions in European countries during the last decades are but one illuminating example. Changes in mentality also concern gender questions and the way modern governance is perceived. One of the most profound changes due to globalisation is the emerging of transnational political units, like the United Nations and the European Union.

Changes of this kind all seem to give rise to challenges to the legitimacy of the traditional nation states of Northern Europe. The present volume studies the concept of legitimacy in this context.

The texts in the book result from a research project on "Legitimacy and Morality", most of which was financed by the Academy of Finland from 2005 to 2008. The research group consists of philosophers, human rights scholars, and theological ethicists. The texts mirror the different approaches of different academic traditions. However, they are united by a common interest in highlighting legitimacy questions related to the currently ongoing changes in, primarily, European societies.

The present collection of articles contains both philosophical and theological studies focusing on language and on conceptual problems. Other articles study concrete historical phenomena. Current societies are studied on many different levels starting from the UN and the EU and ending in discussions concerning conflicts between individuals.

In "Legitimacy and the political community" Lars Hertzberg makes some philosophical remarks about the concept of legitimacy in relation to some other politically central concepts such as political community, the state and its justification, citizenry, public affairs, representation, and justice. One main point lies in his distinction between legitimacy claims and legitimacy assertions. Legitimacy claims are expressions of a person's commitment to a state authority of some kind, while legitimacy assertions are (external) observations concerning the degree to which the members of a political community hold such commitments.

Peter Winch, in his political philosophy, brought some fresh aspects into the understanding both of political authority and of the study of politics, not least through his book *The Idea of a Social Science* (1958). The views presented in this volume have close affinities with Winch's understanding of legitimacy. His ambition was to develop Ludwig Wittgenstein's insights in new settings. Winch never wrote a monograph on political authority, but over the years he devoted a number of essays to the topic. Olli Lagerspetz, in "Peter Winch on political legitimacy", sets out to bring together Winch's thoughts on the subject. The picture that Lagerspetz presents emphasizes the "grammatical" background assumptions in every normative stand on political authorities. Rather than formulating normative assessments on rational grounds, Winch in his political philosophy describes the political culture as it is expressed through and in political processes. He points out that the existence of legitimate authorities –VI stryker: "acceptance of the authorities" is normally taken for granted. It is part of life in the political community in question, not something that has been decided upon in advance. This implies that the legitimacy of, say, a certain state is always dependent on the historically contingent culture within that state. Lagerspetz presents Winch's use of concepts like political authority (in discussion with Hobbes and Rousseau), 'habits of obedience', political education, reasons, truths and symbolic language, and finally oppression, justice and particularity. He finds it impossible to summarize Winch's final position in a straightforward way. During his final years, Winch was still developing his position. He was more inclined than before to emphasize the contingent character of political consent, which was related to his developing views on the role of logic. Lagerspetz traces this development in part on the basis of manuscript notes from Winch's lectures and seminars.

The arguments developed by Hertzberg and Lagerspetz are philosophical. In the Western history of ideas, however, philosophical and theological discussions have been closely intertwined for two thousand years. In their joint article, "Legitimacy, trust and religion in a Nordic perspective", Tage Kurtén and Ville Päivänsalo discuss the role of religion, and especially of the Nordic Lutheran tradition, for legitimacy assessments. When Nordic societies are changing from modern mono-religious and mono-cultural societies into multicultural ones, parts of traditional Lutheran thought seems to become outdated. If that is so, the Nordic, mainly Lutheran, Churches will have to change their self-understanding in order to adjust to the changing situation. Only so can they contribute to society's legitimacy discourse in the face of new challenges, such as issues raised by gender or by the growing number of immigrants with non-Christian religious backgrounds.

Martin Scheinin and Pamela Slotte, in "Captain, firebrigade or icebreaker? Political legitimacy as a rationale in human rights adjudication", point to a problematic feature of court authority based solely upon consent. In their article they study how the legitimacy of international human rights courts can be questioned by authorities acting as representatives of nation states, not as individual members of the political bodies in question. In an interesting overview of the historical development in Europe from the time the European Court of Human Rights came into existence in the 1950's onwards, they show a development from suspicion and hesitation on the part of the states involved towards the current situation where HR Courts are seen as legitimate juridical bodies, with jurisdictions covering formerly autonomous nation states. One important development seems to be the fact that individual citizens of the member states are now able to appeal to these international courts. This fact in combination with an understanding of human rights as overriding the authority of the State could be seen as important ingredients in the legitimacy of such courts.

In Slotte's and Scheinin's essay the perspective differs in an interesting way from the one present in the three foregoing essays. In the latter it is primarily the relation(s) between individual citizens and different authorities that are (is TOM: VI sätter pluralis!) discussed in relation to the concept of legitimacy. National state bodies of course differ in character from individual community members. The essay by Slotte and Scheinin presents the interesting case where the HR Court is one step ahead of the legislative bodies of nation states – for example in questions concerning sexual minorities and their right to marriage and to a family life protected by the state. It would be a serious challenge to the legitimacy of the HR Court if the human rights of citizens in different member states were treated differently because of variations in the relevant national legislation. However, this is exactly what sometimes happens.

In this volume legitimacy is primarily understood as a relational concept. It concerns the way individuals subject to someone's rule relate to those who rule them. In individual states this has mostly meant the way citizens relate to different political and governmental authorities. International treaties and the development of transnational organizations like the United Nations and the European Union have, however, changed the picture. In his article, "Legitimacy, constitutionalism and European integration", Mats Lindfelt describes how the decisions made on a European level, both through the EU Court of Justice and through the European Commission, Council, and Parliament, have to face legitimacy challenges on two levels. Different institutions on the member state level (such as governments, courts, public servants) have to accept and follow European decisions and agreements. However, citizens of member states are also supposed to give their allegiance to policies on a European level. One problem, according to Lindfelt, is that "EU citizens are the subject and effect of EU law but are not, however, the authors of the law". This manifests itself as a democratic deficit, with consequences for the legitimacy of the construction of the EU. This phenomenon has been clearly reflected in a range of political parties critical of the EU in most European member states from the founding of the EU until the time of publication of this book (2011).

Some of the articles study the role of political communities in relation to the legitimacy of a state body more closely. The authority of political leaders is dependent upon their ability to come to grips with tensions within the society in question. Such an ability can be seen as an important part of the making of a just and legitimate society. Ville Päivänsalo discusses this in relation to some writings by Martha Nussbaum. Joakim Molander, in his article "Reconciliation, transitional justice and the legitimacy of the state", approaches such tensions through the concept of reconciliation. In his essay, taking examples from South Africa and Bosnia and Herzegovina, he presents different conceptions of reconciliation. Although the reconciliation work in South Africa, for example, strove for peace between different groups, he finds that reconciliation involves personal subjects and relations between persons in a way that cannot be totally neglected in a society aiming at peaceful coexistence. Providing such coexistence seems to be a *condition sine qua non* for the legitimacy of the state after times of traumatic conflict.

With a theme close to that of Molander, Heidi Jokinen, in "The quest for legitimacy in conflict resolution through restorative justice", analyses the relatively new phenomenon of victim-offender mediation within the Finnish justice system. She considers this emerging example of restorative justice a reaction against some unsatisfactory features of modern criminal court practice.

Restorative justice is seen as a way of coping with a jurisprudence found to be illegitimate in the eyes of both victim and offender.

Lise Kanckos and Malena Björkgren are taking a more sociological approach. In "Legitimacy challenges in gender politics – challenges to political legitimacy in parliamentary debates concerning LGBT rights, assisted reproduction and domestic violence", they build their concept of legitimacy on Habermas while taking in account some central points made by Hertzberg and by Kurtén and Päivänsalo in this volume. Their study shows how a new emphasis on the role of (autonomous) women in the Finnish society challenges many phenomena in society formerly seen as legitimate. This concerns questions like equal rights for same-sex couples, non-violence within the families, and equal rights to assisted reproduction. These are all examples of questions previously perceived as belonging to the private sphere. During the last decades they have, however, moved into the public sphere and become objects for public political discussion. In a country like Finland these questions are still highly controversial. The question of legitimacy in relation to them is therefore somewhat double-edged, dividing people into conservatives and liberals. The examples discussed by Kanckos and Björkgren show how changes in public debate have obvious consequences for the legitimacy of the authorities trying to keep the community and its public discourse together.

In stable democratic welfare states such as the Nordic societies during the latter part of the previous century, legitimacy could for the most part be taken for granted. What the studies in the present volume show is that this "treasure of politics" is very fragile. Legitimacy is understood as a gift which the citizens bestow on the authorities, rather than a means that the authorities can use in order to remain in power. This stresses the role of the citizens rather than of the authorities. Questions of legitimacy can therefore concern radical criticism of the current political system and of different political and governmental solutions. Legitimacy aspects have helped the present authors to highlight some of the most urgent political issues Nordic Europe today.

LEGITIMACY AND THE POLITICAL COMMUNITY

Lars Hertzberg

The legitimacy perspective

The contention of this essay is that claims concerning legitimacy and illegitimacy play a constitutive role in political discourse, a role that has not been sufficiently noted in political philosophy. One way of understanding what we mean by a state, a "body politic", I would argue, is that it is *an organization with regard to which questions of legitimacy may be raised*, whether explicitly or implicitly, even if, in prosperous or peaceful times, the issue may not actually arise.

Let us, to begin with, distinguish between two ways in which statements concerning legitimacy may be used. They may either be made *on behalf of* the political community to which the speaker belongs, or they may be made *about* some community, whether by its members or by someone who is not a member. I shall call the former *legitimacy claims* and the latter *legitimacy assertions*. A legitimacy claim has something of the character of a promise: it expresses the speaker's commitment to submitting to the authority in question, while at the same time exhorting her fellows to undertake the same commitment – an exhortation for which she will normally be expected to give reasons. In making a legitimacy assertion, on the other hand, I am purporting to describe conditions holding within a community, based on evidence of the legitimacy attitudes held by the members of the community. A legitimacy assertion need not involve any political commitments on the part of the speaker. Statements concerning legitimacy may also take a negative form: thus, by making a negative legitimacy claim, I withhold my commitment, whereas a negative legitimacy assertion records the prevalence of such claims in the community.[1]

---

1 In some cases states and international organizations are called upon to take a stand on the legitimacy of a foreign state or regime. Thus, in 1971 the U.N. had to choose between regarding the People's Republic of China or the Republic of China (Taiwan) as the rightful representative of China. However, such issues are usually derivative from the legitimacy conflicts that exist within states.

To acknowledge the *sovereignty* of a political community is to acknowledge the fact that matters of legitimacy are ultimately to be resolved by the members of the community.[2]

Legitimacy claims will not necessarily make use of the *word* "legitimacy". In fact, as will be argued later, legitimacy attitudes may also be expressed without any use of words; in that case, we might speak of manifestations of legitimacy (or illegitimacy). Legitimacy assertions, on the other hand, will always be explicit.

Legitimacy and illegitimacy claims may vary in scope. They may concern the system of government or some aspect of it, the current holders of political power or their representatives, e.g. the court system, or particular measures undertaken by them, such as taxation and legislation, the allocation of public funds, etc. These different types of claim are interdependent: legitimacy will normally be conferred on the present holder of office by the legitimacy of the system; on the other hand, an office holder by his misuse of power may undermine the legitimacy of the system itself. (Thus, a corrupt court system or corrupt law enforcement agencies will naturally undermine respect for the law.) Similarly, there may be mutual dependence between the legitimacy of particular official measures and that of the current office holders or of the system itself. And so on. For the most part, I shall not explicitly distinguish between these types of legitimacy claim, trusting the context to make it clear, as far as necessary, what type of claim is in question.

There are some closely related expressions that may be used in discussions of legitimacy. Someone who considers the government of her country legitimate may be said to give it her *allegiance*, or she may also be said to acknowledge its *authority*, or to *assent* to its exertion of power.

The suggestion that legitimacy claims have a central role in political thought is not a new one. It enters in social contract views of the state, like those of Hobbes, Locke and Rousseau. On the other hand, legitimacy issues are brought up by David Hume in his critique of the social contract views[3], as well as by Henry David Thoreau in his argument that in certain situations citizens may have a duty of civil disobedience.[4] Among more recent philosophers, legitimacy has been fruitfully discussed, for instance, by Simone Weil[5], Elizabeth Anscombe[6], Peter Winch[7], D. Z. Phillips[8] and Olli Lagerspetz[9]. (In some of

2 Families are in some ways analogous to political communities. In most cultures, the family holds a position of sovereignty, limited only by legal constraints. Outsiders do not, normally, "have a say", for instance, concerning the raising of children, the relations between husband and wife, etc.

3 Hume 1993a and 1993b.

4 Thoreau 1849.

5 Weil 1987.

6 Anscombe, "On the Source of the Authority of the State", in Anscombe 1981.

7 Primarily Winch 1991 and 2002.

8 Phillips 1996, Chap. 9, and 1999, Chap. 5.

these cases, however, as I hope will be clear, the view taken of legitimacy is problematic.) My account is largely influenced by that of Winch, although deviating from his in some respects.[10]

A distinctive feature of legitimacy claims, then, is that they are made by individuals (subjects, citizens[11]) who live under the purview of a political system, as an expression of their stand on the system itself or on those presently in power. In this respect, they differ from judgements, say, concerning the degree of democracy or equality within a political system, its observance of human rights, etc, which are not, as it were, "position-dependent" in the way legitimacy claims are: the latter types of judgement can be made equally by those who are directly concerned by the system and by those who are not. In this way, human rights criticisms may constitute a challenge to the sovereignty of a state by external groups. This may give rise to tensions between the recommendations of international human rights institutions and the national authorities of individual countries. Ensuring that those recommendations are implemented may require anchoring them, as far as possible, in the existing legal practices of those countries.[12,13]

A clarification is needed here. One often encounters arguments of the form: "Democracy and human rights are essentially bound up with Western civilization, and they simply cannot be exported to other political cultures. Hence outsiders are not really in a position to pass judgement concerning them." Claims like these will of course sometimes be advanced in blatant defence of brutal dictatorships, but they may also have more serious intent. Thus, they may mean that assessments of the level of democracy in a certain culture cannot meaningfully be made without taking into consideration the social, political and cultural conditions of the society in question. In other words, the question of what constitutes democracy varies with the cultural background, and it would be naïve, say, to expect the exact type of constitution, the very same party system, the election processes with which we are familiar to be experienced as legitimate (let alone the only legitimate form of government) in every society. Democracy, we might say, is not a surface feature, nor is there a sharp line distinguishing states that can from those that cannot be considered democratic.

Then again, a different type of reminder may be in place for those who are eager to export democracy. It might be important to point out that democracy is

---

9 Lagerspetz 1998, Chap. 7; 2004, 1299-1317.

10 For an account of Winch's views on legitimacy, see Olli Lagerspetz' contribution to the present volume.

11 In the sequel, I shall, for the most part, use the word "citizen" to refer to the members of a political community, although the term strictly speaking would only apply in democratic states.

12 On these issues, see the contribution by Martin Scheinin and Pamela Slotte to this volume.

13 Such external challenges to state sovereignty are not unique to the modern era: a rather more effective precedent can be found in the pope's power, in the Middle Ages, to impose an interdict on a recalcitrant country, thus suspending all public worship and sacraments.

not a necessary condition for legitimacy. The fact that a ruler has not been chosen by popular vote does not automatically imply that he will or should be considered a usurper of power. In fact, until a little more than a hundred years ago, most European nations did not have a system that we would be ready to call democratic. Thus, by contemporary standards, the Scandinavian monarchies of the 19th century would probably be considered fairly despotic. Even so, governments enjoyed varying degrees of legitimacy, just as democratically elected governments presently do. (Later on, I shall argue that free debate and elections are not *sufficient* for legitimacy.)

Perhaps it will be argued that legitimacy as I am outlining it here, no less than democracy and human rights, is a Western notion. It is true that I am mainly using contemporary Western states as centres of variation in trying to map out the characteristics of legitimacy discourse. Yet I would maintain that legitimacy considerations have *some* role in anything we are able to recognize as a political community. In fact, I believe the dimension of legitimacy to be an important element of the very notion of a political community.

Legitimacy and the justification of the state

The point that legitimacy claims are made by members of the community has important consequences for an issue that has long been debated by philosophers: what has been called the question of the justification of the state; or, as Elizabeth Anscombe calls it, the question of the source of the authority of the state, or, as it has also been put, the question what reason we, as citizens, have for submitting to the power of the state. The question, it would appear, arises in the following way: as citizens of a state we habitually submit to various obligations imposed on us by the authorities, whether it is a question of abstaining from unlawful conduct, conforming to official decrees and regulations, or paying taxes, etc. In many cases we do this even when it is against our own wishes or interests. What reasons could we possibly have for acting in this way?

What the legitimacy perspective entails is that our reason for conforming is simply that we regard certain measures of the state as actions legitimately undertaken by a legitimate authority. There is something we hold to be a reason for conforming which is peculiar to the relation we hold to our state. In other words, in considering something an expression of the state's authority we in that very fact judge it to be justified. To ask for a justification for the state's power, hence, is to ask for a justification of this system of justification. But such a request is not intelligible.

We might, of course, have other reasons for conforming to the state's commands: say, the fear of getting caught for cheating on our taxes, etc; but then we would not be conforming to those requirements *as* commands of the state. These reasons would be external to politics. Unless there were widespread conformity of the former kind, however, there would be no political entity, no state. On the other hand, if we do not see the government or its decisions as legitimate, we do not have any reason to conform to them *as* decisions of the state (though we may conform, say, out of fear). Of course, even in the cases in which we do accept the authority of the state's decisions, we may, say, exceed the speed limit; in doing so we may be yielding to temptation or be moved by some overriding concern.

Political philosophers have frequently thought of the state's authority as derivative. Contract theorists see it as conditional upon a commitment undertaken by the citizen. Another strand of thought considers the state's authority to be based on the citizens' need for physical protection.[14] Hobbes manages to have it both ways: the authority is based on a contract, which itself derives its binding force from the need for physical protection.[15] Perhaps a modern variant of the protection view is the idea that the state's task is to ensure the material well-being of the citizens; this sometimes takes the form of regarding the state as a giant corporation which should be managed accordingly.

All such accounts share the assumption that legitimacy consists in some feature possessed by a system of rule. Any such assumption clashes with the point for which I have been arguing, according to which legitimacy claims can only meaningfully be made by those whose allegiance is in question (just as it is ultimately up to each single individual to decide whether he or she is satisfied with something or other: your satisfaction cannot be derived from some impersonal principle). In other words, legitimacy claims cannot be second-guessed on the citizens' behalf whether by a political philosopher or by anybody else. Thus, the claim that someone is bound by an undertaking by earlier generations, as held by adherents of social contract theories (whatever else is problematic about this notion[16]) is logically distinct from that person's own assenting to the state's authority, and hence the latter cannot be reduced to the former. Nor can assent be reduced to the judgement that, for whatever reasons of security or economy, it would be advisable for this or that citizen to give his allegiance to the state. All kinds of grounds or inducements may be provided, but the individual citizen must herself take the conclusive step, or refuse to take it. Furthermore, if it is to be a genuine expression of political allegiance (rather than simply personal satisfaction), the step must be undertaken on behalf of the community.

In brief, then, there can be no *external* justification for the state's authority, and the *internal* justification is already given with the notion of political authority.

14 E.g. Anscombe 1981.
15 There seems to be an analogous duality in Rawls's idea of the original position.
16 For criticisms of this view, see Hume 1993b and Phillips 1996.

In what follows, I shall discuss some distinctive features of the concept of legitimacy, illustrating them with examples of conflicts from the contemporary political scene. First, I discuss expressions of legitimacy in the life of the individual citizen. After that I relate it to the concepts of political community, public affairs and political representation. My suggestion is that these concepts are mutually dependent. By means of the examples I try to show how issues of legitimacy enter into our everyday political concerns in a variety of ways.

Legitimacy and the citizen

The clearest manifestation of allegiance to the state is one's assenting to decisions even when they run counter to one's own wishes or interests. In normal conditions, most citizens obey most of the laws of their state, and by and large pay the taxes they are obliged to pay, without any serious attempts at sabotaging the system. This is true to some degree even in cases in which they would have a good chance of getting away with breaches of the law. Of course most citizens disobey *some* laws, and *some* citizens disobey a great many laws, but without the voluntary cooperation of most citizens in most cases, it would become hard or even impossible for the state to wield power. Nor do we simply obey the law ourselves, but we demand obedience from our fellow citizens. The citizens' allegiance also means that they assent to decisions made in their name concerning other citizens (e.g. the decisions of the criminal courts), or other states or individuals (declarations of war, interventions in the affairs of other countries, the treatment of refugees, the giving or withholding of foreign aid, etc). Furthermore, a person's allegiance to the political system, or to the present rulers, shows itself whenever she, on her part, invokes the law or calls on the authorities for help, say, in getting protection against a crime or in seeking redress. Again, allegiance may be manifested by citizens coming to the defence of the political order against internal or external enemies, sometimes even endangering their lives or health in doing do.

Taking a stand on the legitimacy of a regime is not just giving vent to one's own feelings or wishes. What legitimacy claims I can intelligibly make (i.e. which judgements of mine can be understood as legitimacy claims) is conditioned, though not determined, by the facts. There are two sides to this, one substantial and one formal. On the substantial side, a legitimacy claim may be supported by appeals to a government's good qualities: say, to its ability to restore the honour of the nation or to raise the standard of living, to its power to protect the citizenry, to its justice, etc. Very often, these appeals will take the form of apologetics: it will be pointed out, say, that, although the government has been acting ruthlessly towards its internal or external enemies, it was forced to do so to in order to stave off threats to the prevailing order.[17] On the formal side, the appeal may be to the way in which the present rulers acceded to power (through legal succession, election, etc). Obviously, in assessing the legitimacy of one's government, one may sometimes have to weigh substantial and formal considerations against one another.

It is important to note that, for me to recognize something as grounding a legitimacy claim, I myself would not have to agree with it. Grounds are important for the sake of *identifying* something as a legitimacy claim, not as a condition for *approving* it. As was said, legitimacy claims are to be made by the individual citizen: no grounds, however compelling, can force an individual to embrace a legitimacy claim or to withdraw it.

Although in grounding a legitimacy claim one is speaking on behalf of he community, this does not mean that one must submit to common opinion or to the majority view. In fact, one can even speak as a solitary voice (just as one may stand alone in *rejecting* the legitimacy of a regime), but this will only be intelligible if one can make good the case that one is speaking on behalf of the others: one might do so, for instance, by arguing that one's fellow citizens have been misled or that they are deceiving themselves.[18] On the other hand, one cannot defend one's position simply by arguing that this or that group with which one is in disagreement does not count, unless one is prepared to make the case that it does not truly belong to the community. Whether one's claims, in denigrating the positions taken by one's fellow citizens, are accepted or not will, of course, depend on the reactions of one's interlocutors. There can be no standards to be specified once and for all for deciding matters like these. Putting forward, contesting and debating legitimacy claims is part of the political life of the community; they are not matters that can be decided in advance of political debate.

It is important to distinguish the question of citizens' allegiance from the question of the popularity of a regime. As is well known, the approval ratings of some American presidents have fallen far below 50 percent, as in the cases of Harry Truman, Richard Nixon or George W. Bush, without its being concluded that they are usurpers and should step down. Only Nixon was thought to have forfeited his claim to the office, and that was for legal reasons, not because of his impopularity. In fact, it could probably be argued that during most of the history of the state, rulers have been rather impopular; or rather, for most of this time the question has not even been raised. Probably it is only in the time of the nation state that there has come to be an expectation that rulers should be admired or loved by their peoples. But this does not mean that they were lacking in legitimacy in the past.

17 The reasons given, of course, may not always be sincere.

18 This is one reason why elections cannot automatically be assumed to resolve matters of legitimacy.

Manifestations of deficient legitimacy may vary from tax evasion or a more general lack of respect for law and authority, over civil disobedience to passive or active resistance, rebellion and civil war. The legitimacy of the government may be divided or selective, it may extend to some aspects of political power but not to others. Tax laws often enjoy a lower degree of legitimacy than, say, the penal code. (Here, one should probably distinguish between legislation that invites active resistance, and which, accordingly, may reflect unfavourably on the legitimacy of the lawmakers, and laws that meet with widespread public indifference, such as current laws outlawing internet piracy.)

The balance between legitimacy and illegitimacy is affected by what might be called centrifugal and centripetal forces. Conflicts between social or ethnic groups or perceived injustices may tend to dissolve the legitimacy of the political system or the current government in the eyes of parts of the population or all of it. On the other hand, the strongest legitimacy-raising force is an external threat. The Nazi political philosopher Carl Schmitt went so far as to argue that the presence of a common enemy is a necessary condition for the existence of a political community.[19] The importance of an external threat was made palpably evident after the al-Qaida attack on the World Trade Center on 11 September, 2001. George W. Bush had been elected president with a minority of the popular vote and after a challenge to the vote count. However, eight months into his first term the attack occurred; not only did this send his approval rating soaring from 51 percent to 85 percent in a week[20], but, more importantly, it brought an end to the questioning of the legitimacy of his presidency. (In this case, indeed, his improved approval rating has to be understood, not as a response to his actual performance, but rather as an expression of the need to rally around the leader in times of threat, i.e. in this case it was obviously a measure of legitimacy rather than popularity.)

In fact, no regime can be totally devoid of legitimacy: if it were, then, even if it continued to wield power, this would no longer be political power, but an exertion of brute force.

Political community

Legitimacy claims are made in the name of a community. The question of the legitimacy of a regime is the question of its licence to act as the representative of a collective which understands itself as a political community. (The notion of political community seems to be missing in social contract accounts of the state.)

---

19 http://www.ou.edu/cas/psc/bookschmitt.htm (accessed on 18 April, 2009).

20 See http://www.presidency.ucsb.edu/data/popularity.php (accessed on 6 November, 2008).

The question of who belongs to a political community may itself be a matter of political controversy. The legitimacy of a regime may be divided if different groups in its territory do not regard themselves as constituting one community. There are several examples of this in the Balkans. Thus, the Kosovar Albanians, having felt excluded from Serb society, withdrew their allegiance to the Serbian regime in Belgrade in the 1990's. This was part of the process leading to civil war in 1999, and later to the secession of Kosovo from Serbia.

What, then, determines what constitutes a community? There can be no fixed criteria, since whatever criteria are proposed may be rejected by some or all of the individuals concerned, as the final arbiters. The idea of a political community seems to presuppose that for most members, identification is voluntary and spontaneous. There may be a tension between the way the members of a group regard themselves and the way they are regarded by others. A group seeking acceptance may be rejected, as were the Jews in 1930's Germany and Austria. Similar tendencies may be found in the response of the majority population in many European countries to certain groups of immigrants (or, on a much weaker scale, on the part of some Finnish-speaking Finns in relation to Swedish-speaking Finns in Finland).

The concept of citizenship originated in the Roman republic. Its significance lies in its reflecting and codifying a pre-existing relation of membership. However, the schematic nature of a legal notion like citizenship does not always reflect the actual nuances of a situation. In a time of extensive migration, large groups of non-citizens may come to constitute important contributors to the life of a community without being granted the formal status of membership. (Cp. illegal aliens in the United States, *sans papiers* in France, generations of migrant workers in Germany.) The right to citizenship may become a matter of debate when opposed by nationalistic and xenophobic politicians.

On the other hand, when a group strives to establish a political identity of its own, that striving may be rejected by those with whom it lives in political union. There are several instances of this on the contemporary scene. The Serbs in Montenegro regard their country as part of Serbia; the Montenegrine majority, however, overruled them in declaring independence. The Kurds in Turkey consider themselves as a separate people with a claim to sovereignty, while the Turkish government regards them as a Turkish people, "Mountain Turks". The Tamils in Sri Lanka are struggling for independence, against the resistance of the Lankese government. Among the Basques of Spain there is disagreement between the majority that apparently wants to remain part of Spain, and the radical minority that is pressing for Basque independence. In issues like these, there can be no question of deciding who is right by some kind of "objective" standards. Nor can it be settled by vote, for the question turns, precisely, on who is to have a vote in the matter. Yet the issue is important, for unless the community is largely voluntary, no such thing as democratic representation seems to be possible. If the issue is to be solved rather than simply suppressed, it can only be solved by negotiation.

A community, once acknowledged to exist, is usually given the opportunity to decide where it is to belong: is it to remain, or become, independent, or is it to remain part of, or join, some larger political community? There are several instances in which countries that are democratically governed have yet denied a portion of their country the right to secede. The U.S. Confederation is probably the most fateful example of this type of conflict, although the South's demand for independence was undermined by its failure to acknowledge the rights of the black population (the slaves).

One might ask whether the idea that some group can forcibly be made to submit to or remain under the rule of a regime that has no legitimacy in its eyes can be reconciled with the idea of a democratic government. Even if the group is allowed to elect its own representatives, the political system in which those representatives are called upon to function is not expressive of a community in which that group sees itself as having a stake. The idea of democratic representation here becomes a formal matter, without connection to the idea of legitimate government. An example of this occurred in 1921 when the Åland Islands were made part of Finland rather than Sweden, which is what an overwhelming majority of Ålanders would have preferred[21]. (Over time, however, the Ålanders have reconciled themselves with being part of Finland, though with a degree of autonomy.)

In demanding that Hong Kong be made part of the Chinese mother country in 1997, or in refusing to accept the sovereignty of Taiwan, the argument of the People's Republic of China has been that the populations of these areas is Chinese, thus advancing what might be called a metaphysical claim against their right to self-determination; by calling the claim metaphysical I mean that it is presented as grounded in some given facts independently of the choices of the people concerned. "Chineseness" does not, on the other hand, seem to matter where the demands for autonomy by the Tibetans or the Uigurs are concerned. The Chinese leadership is hardly unique in this respect, however. Governments tend to adopt whatever political principles are best suited to their present goals. Another instance of this is the European Union's and the United States' refusal even to discuss the independence of the Georgian secessionist regions of South Ossetia and Abkhasia, only a few months after agreeing to acknowledge the independence of Kosovo. Considerations of justice may be a factor in politics, but they rarely triumph unless they have power on their side.

The issue of community may also give rise to controversy of a different form: there may be competition between different levels of community. Here,

21 One of those who prominently resisted the cause of Åland was a Finnish philosopher, Edward Westermarck. His concern was that ceding the islands to Sweden would have undermined the position of the Swedish-speaking minority in mainland Finland.

what is at issue is not the question of belonging as such, but its political significance. When Finns are critical of the country's membership of the European Union, or when Americans reject the authority of the United Nations, the basis of these attitudes is not that they do not consider themselves to be Europeans or citizens of the world, respectively, but the fact that they are not willing to regard this level of community as a significant political level.

Just as there are no objective criteria for deciding who belongs to a people, there are none for what levels of community can rightly be considered political. What seems to be occurring is that there is a tendency towards splitting up the levels of political authority, states delegating some of their sovereignty upward, to inter-state organizations, and some of it downward, to regions. Inter-state authorities are not, as such, a new phenomenon: we may think about the Delian League under the leadership of Athens in the 5th century BC, the German-Roman Empire in the middle ages, the papal church, the caliphate in Baghdad, the British Commonwealth, etc.[22]

Public affairs

Not everything that happens among the members of a political community is seen to be a matter of concern to the community. Thus, in most contemporary states, it would be considered to be out of the question for the authorities to decide what people can eat or how long they should sleep, even though there may be a consensus that it would be good for people on the whole to eat healthier food or to sleep more than they usually do. We consider these matters to be private. What matters are private or public is not given once and for all. It is ultimately a matter of political culture: the community designates various matters as being within or outside the scope of public concern.[23] (In fact, at the beginning of the 21st century, a gradual shift appears to be taking place in the Western world towards treating certain aspects of health as matters of public concern, as when employers place restrictions on the smoking habits or weight of employees, or when it is proposed that public health benefits should be made conditional on beneficiaries abstaining from unhealthy practices.)

In most European countries, high culture has traditionally been a matter of public concern. There are ministries of culture, universities have predominantly

---

22 We should note that political community as such does not entail any specific emotional bonds. The idea that it should do that presumably arose with nationalism and the nation state, helped along by rulers who followed the precept "Unite and conquer!"

23 Philosophers have debated the rightful limits of political authority; consider, for instance, the debate between Robert Nozick, who argued that the state should limit itself to securing the basic physical conditions of social life, "the nightwatchman state", and John Rawls, who maintained that the state should facilitate the equal distribution of wealth in society. See Rawls 1971; Nozick 1974.

been state-funded, and public service broadcasting has held a prominent place, even though there is currently a movement to question or at least diminish public involvement in higher education, research and broadcasting. The American tradition has been different in this respect. There, high culture is very largely a matter for for the private domain. There is no department of culture or any "cultural politics" on the federal or state level. Many of the leading universities are privately owned (even if they receive some public funding), and non-commercial broadcasting is small, being financed primarily through private donations.

The status of religion and sexual life has undergone particularly large variations during the modern era. Not very long ago, they were central matters of public concern. This is evidently connected with the role that religion and the family used to have in maintaining the unity of society. In centuries past, freedom of religion was anything but self-evident in most European countries. During the era of Lutheran orthodoxy in Sweden in the 17th century, church-going was considered a public matter. People who missed church on Sunday could be sentenced to the pillory. Layman preaching and heresy were severely sanctioned by the state. The situation is rather similar in such Muslim states as Iran or Saudi Arabia today.[24]

Adultery was still criminalized fairly recently in Finland, and still is in other parts of the world (including some U.S. states). During the apartheid regime in South Africa, the authorities considered it a public matter who had sexual intercourse with whom: intercourse between individuals of *different races* was punishable. On the other hand, sexual intercourse between individuals of *the same sex* has been criminalized in several countries; this was the case in Britain, for instance, up until the 1960's. In some Muslim countries, homosexual intercourse is a capital offence to this day. Sexual orientation seems to remain the last bastion of those who view sex as a matter of public concern: in many countries, resistance to same-sex marriage is strong. But on the whole, in Western Europe and North America, sex is today among the most private aspects of life.

As a general rule, the state has been held to have a right and a duty to intercede against actions that are harmful to others. But there have been exceptions to this rule on both sides. Violence on the part of the head of

24 It is true that religion assumed an important political role in the West around the turn of the millennium. However, its role is ideological rather than official: there have been no calls for mandatory church membership or legal supervision of church attendance. In fact, the ideological role of religion seems directly connected with the presence of variations in religious outlook. It is just *because* not everybody is a born-again Christian, for instance, that one may find it important, in a political context, to emphasize one's own membership in that group. It is not by chance that the ideological role of religion has been has been weaker in Europe than in the United States, where it has never held an official position. Similarly, in the United States with its large religious variety religion has been prominent as a dimension of social identity.

household against his wife, children and servants (not to speak about slaves) has been tolerated, and still is, I would imagine, to a larger or lesser degree, in large parts of the world. This is an expression of the fact that the family (if correctly and lawfully constituted) is considered a sovereign unit. The fact that violence within the family is increasingly frowned upon seems to be an expression of a more individualistic view of society (as is, of course, the privatization of religion and sexuality). A clear expression of this is the fairly recent criminalization, in some countries, of corporal punishment of children and of marital rape.

On the other hand, in most countries *some* actions that are directly harmful or dangerous only to the agent himself are regulated by law: e.g. the use of drugs, driving without a seatbelt or without a motorcycle helmet. Citizens are considered to have both a right and a duty to intervene in order to prevent suicide; suicide attempts have been punishable offences, e.g. in Britain (they still are in India). It is interesting to note that when the use of seatbelts became mandatory, the vote of individual members of the legislature, in some countries, was considered to be a matter for their own conscience: group discipline was not enforced. The fact that special provisions were made in such a comparatively unimportant matter seems to indicate that what was at stake was not a political decision in the ordinary sense but one concerning the limits of the political sphere. This sphere seems a continual matter of controversy in the West (cp. the ongoing debates about the legality of prostitution, cannabis, chewing tobacco, gambling, etc.).

The controversy between pro-life and pro-choice advocates concerns whether a foetus is to be considered a subject of rights, enjoying the protection of the state. This, clearly, is not a matter that is to be resolved by medical criteria alone, but ultimately depends on the outlook of citizens. The large attention given to the Terri Schiavo case in Florida in 2005 can also be seen as a battle between two political cultures: while the more conservative politicians thought the decision on whether to terminate her life-support was a matter of public concern, liberal politicians argued that the decision should rest with her legal guardian. What we have here is a clash between what might be called a more communitarian world-view (regarding matters of life and death as belonging to the public sphere) and a more individualistic world-view (emphasizing the private nature of those decisions).[25]

25 One might observe that the individualist tendency goes in opposite directions with regard to to issues like abortion and euthanasia on the one hand, and domestic violence and corporal punishment on the other hand. In the former case, the sovereignty of the family is emphasized, in the latter case that of the state.

Representation

To consider the rulers of one's community legitimate is to consider them rightful representatives of the community. This means that one accepts their right to pass decisions in the community's affairs.

Citizens, in deeming their government legitimate, consent to *its acting and speaking in their name*. The government's authority derives from its being seen as the representative of the community. It was an expression of this when protesters against the Iraq war were carrying signs with the slogan "Not in my name"; they were trying to withdraw the licence of the state to wage this war in their name. This form of protest, in a sense, is more radical than simply saying "Stop this war!"

What it means for a government to be the representative of a community is not to be confused with the notion of *"representative government"*. Democratic elections are a comparatively recent way of grounding the representativity of a government, but there have, through history, been other ways of transferring legitimacy, e.g. in hereditary monarchies, etc (not to mention the unusual way in which the Dalai Lama has traditionally been selected in Tibet).

On the other hand, a ruler who has come into power through dubious or downright illegal means may yet gain legitimacy through his handling of power or because of the pressure of circumstances (again, George W. Bush's first presidential period is an illustration of this).[26] Then again, a ruler who has had power bestowed upon him through legitimate procedures may lose his legitimacy by mismanaging power. In this way, a ruler's legitimacy may be dependent on a balance between formal and substantial aspects.

It should be emphasized that an election cannot be *the ultimate source* of the legitimacy of a regime. For one thing, as was said, for an election to be seen as the legitimate expression of the will of a community, those who participate will have to see themselves as *forming* a community. Otherwise the election will be a senseless number exercise. But furthermore, the form of the election must be acceptable to the electorate. Also, since an election is an actual procedure occurring in time, the electorate must have confidence that the spectacle in which they are participating is a genuine election. Hence they have to trust those who organize it. Accordingly, an election can only have a legitimating function if it is held within a system which already enjoys legitimacy independently of

26 Interestingly, during the 2011 uprising in Arab countries, it was argued that monarchical rulers tended to possess a higher degree of legitimacy than presidents. Obviously, the reason was that they at least enjoyed a traditional form of inherited legitimacy, whereas the presidents' claims to legitimacy were simply staked on their having been chosen through what were in most cases sham elections. Here one is also reminded of Napoleon's observation that while the Austrian and Russian emperors had inherited their crowns and thus did not have to prove their legitimacy, he had to stay victorious in battle to retain his. – J. M. Coetzee's novel *Diary of a Bad Year* contains an interesting suggestion concerning the origins of political power in struggles between rival robber gangs.

this. There have been several examples in recent years of an election, in the absence of this trust, failing in its intended aim of giving legitimacy to the party officially designated as the winner. (Serbia in 2001, the Ukraine in 2004, Kenya and Zimbabwe in 2008, Moldavia in 2009.)

Whatever electoral procedures are adopted, they will inevitably be *conventional*: they are the result of a choice between various conceivable alternatives. The legitimacy of the outcome does not depend on its being a correct representation of the public will, but on the degree to which it is accepted as such by the members of the community. Indeed, the notion of a public will, I would argue, has no sense except in relation to procedures that are accepted as ways of expressing that will. Among these conventions are rules defining voting rights and the ways in which votes are translated into seats: whether there is a majority system or a proportionate system, and if the latter, what method of assigning seats will be used; whether there will be a barrier rule requiring a minimum proportion of votes for a party to have representation; how the seats assigned to a party will be awarded to individual candidates; how electoral districts are drawn up[27]; how the legislature is constituted; what the electoral terms are and whether there is a limit to the number of terms; whether there is an institution of recall; how the relation between the legislative and the executive functions is regulated, etc.

The legitimacy of the electoral system, then, does not depend on some supposed correspondence between the representatives elected (or the decisions made) and the public will. Rather, the will of the community is expressed through the adoption of a procedure which is in itself accepted as legitimate. To the extent that a procedure allows for a radical deviation between election results and predominant opinions, its legitimacy will of course be fragile. An example of this is the American presidential election system, where a candidate may lose in spite of gaining the majority of popular votes. (What has lent this a measure of acceptability is the notion that the president is elected by the states, not by the electorate in aggregate.[28]) The degree of legitimacy will largely depend on the strength of existing tensions in the society, what were above called centrifugal forces. The sharper the tensions, the harder the test to the system.[29] If the tensions are sharp enough, there simply is no peaceful solution

27 The practice of gerrymandering may be held to undermine the legitimacy of political elections. "**Gerrymandering** is a form of redistribution in which electoral district or constituency boundaries are manipulated for electoral advantage. Gerrymandering may be used to help or hinder particular constituents, such as members of a political, racial, linguistic, religious or class group." (http://en.wikipedia.org/wiki/Gerrymandering, accessed on 13 November, 2008.)

28 The system is apparently changing, more and more states adopting a system of proportional distribution of electors. See http://nationalpopularvote.com/s, accessed on 20 April, 2009.

29 A case in point was the referendum concerning membership in the EU held in Finland in 1994. The opponents of membership, having lost the election, claimed that those who had

since the parties see no reason for voluntary submission; if the tensions are weak, the procedure does not much matter.

Legitimacy and justice

Does legitimacy entail justice? Simone Weil speaks with reverence about legitimacy in the opening of her text on the legitimacy of the French provisional government:

> Legitimacy is one of those beautiful words which the human mind cannot link with any conception but which, considered simply as words, have a power infinitely greater than any human conception.[30]

It is not quite clear what Weil means by saying that the human mind cannot link legitimacy with any conception, but what she might have in mind is the point made here by saying that there can be no prior or external constraints on what government the citizens of a state may come to consider legitimate. On the other hand, one might wonder why this fact should render legitimacy *beautiful*. Later on she gives a characterization that might seem to be at odds with the claim that legitimacy cannot be linked with any conception:

> If the ruler is motivated by concern for justice and the public good; if the people are confident of this and have reasonable grounds for expecting it to continue, if the head of government does not want to hold on to power except for as long as the people retain his confidence[31]: that is legitimate government.

This formulation gives room for an outside judgement: for the government to be legitimate it must actually be motivated by a concern for justice and the common good. On this reading, it is not sufficient that the people are confident that it is: their confidence must be justified. In other words, the people might be mistaken about the legitimacy of their government. Perhaps Hitler's Third Reich would be taken to be a case of this, especially in the period before the outbreak of war. The regime managed to restore both the material prosperity and the national pride that had been shattered in the aftermath of the First World War. However, both the economy and the pride were built on shaky foundations: on inflationary economic policies and foreign policy gambles. One might well assume that if Hitler's policies and plans had been generally known, support for his policies would have dwindled (as it did when he started the war). What Weil

---

abstained from voting, as well as children, earlier generations, etc, should have been counted among the opposing votes.

30 Weil 1987, p. 87.

31 This should evidently read: "for as long as he retains the people's confidence".

appears to be suggesting is that he did not, in fact, enjoy legitimacy even during the time when he was enjoying powerful support.

The problem with Weil's claim is that it is not clear whether she is discussing legitimacy claims or legitimacy assertions. If she is laying down conditions for legitimacy *assertions*, i.e. for the sociological claim that a government is actually enjoying legitimacy, it is hard to see why this should be dependent on *the observer's* judgement about the quality of its motivations. On the other hand, if she is laying down conditions for legitimacy *claims*, this too is problematic, since, as I have tried to argue, the power to make such judgements cannot be limited in advance. At most, she might be pointing to an internal relation between the concepts legitimacy, justice and public good: i.e. she might be saying that for someone to consider his government legitimate *means* that he holds it to be motivated by those concerns. This reading could, conceivably, be made to square with her formulation. (The reference to people's confidence could then be understood as indicating the fact that a person's legitimacy claims must take account of his fellow citizens' attitudes.)

Someone might think that the remark could have a third meaning, however: it might be thought to address the question when a government can *truly* be said to be legitimate, i.e. when a judgement of legitimacy can truthfully be made, independently of the attitudes actually held by the people concerned. Perhaps Weil, confusedly, thought of herself as making such a claim. But what could be its force? At most, one might express the wish that the people concerned would adopt such and such standards in assessing the legitimacy of their government. But this does not alter the fact that the matter is up to them. There is no question of legitimacy independent of the judgement of those who form the community. That is what political sovereignty signifies.

References

Anscombe, G. E. M.

1981 On the Source of the Authority of the State. In Anscombe, *Ethics, Religion and Politics.* Oxford: Basil Blackwell.

Coetzee, J. M.

2007 *Diary of a Bad Year.* London: Random House.

Hume, D.

1993a Of the First Pinciples of Government. In Hume, *Selected Essays.* Oxford University Press.

1993b Of the Original Contract. ibid.

Lagerspetz, O.

1998 *Trust: The Tacit Demand.* Dordrecht: Kluwer

2004 National Self-Determination and Ethnic Minorities. *Michigan Journal of International Law* 25, 1299-1317.

Nozick, R.
1974 *Anarchy, State and Utopia.* Oxford: Basil Blackwell.

Phillips, D. Z.
1996 *Introducing Philosophy.* Oxford: Basil Blackwell.
1999 *Philosophy's Cool Place.* Ithaca: Cornell University Press.

Rawls, J.
1971 *A Theory of Justice.* Cambridge, MA: Harvard University Press.

Thoreau, H. D.
1849 Civil Disobedience. The text can be accessed, e.g., at http://thoreau.eserver.org/civil.html.

Weil, S.
1987 The Legitimacy of the Provisional Government. *Philosophical Investigations* 10, 87-98 [originally published in 1957].

Winch, P.
1991 Certainty and Authority. In A. Phillips Griffiths ed., *Wittgenstein Centenary Essays.* Cambridge University Press.
2002 How is Political Authority Possible? In *Philosophical Investigations* 25, 20-32.

PETER WINCH ON POLITICAL LEGITIMACY

Olli Lagerspetz

Introduction

Peter Winch (1926 – 1997) had a life-long interest in political philosophy. *The Idea of a Social Science*,[1] the book that won him early fame in 1958, was hailed as a contribution to political philosophy[2], although it focused on the methods and epistemology of social studies. Between 1958 and 1972, Winch published a number of essays explicitly devoted to questions about political authority.[3] In the late 1980's, he returned to that theme after an interval of several years.[4] On the other hand, he never published a book on the topic, even though he was known to have plans to do so.[5] In any case, his published essays together with his lectures and seminars give us an idea of what the book might have been like.[6] Even in such truncated form, this work is extremely interesting, as it represents a new take on a perennial theme: the justification of political authority. Instead of proposing a direct answer to that general question, Winch shifts the emphasis to the idea of the political as such. Thus he wants to get at

1 ISSc. For a list of my abbreviations of Peter Winch's works, see the literature list.

2 "For it is far and away the liveliest and most cogent of the responses yet made to that staid official judgement of some years ago, that political philosophy must now be presumed dead." – *The Times Literary Supplement*, quoted on the dustjacket of ISSc (1963).

3 Especially, Authority; Authority and Rationality (henceforth: A&R), Man and Society in Hobbes and Rousseau (MSHR), and Nature and Convention (N&C). The two latter essays are included in *Ethics and Action* (E&A).

4 See especially, *Simone Weil – The Just Balance* (SWJB), Certainty and Authority (C&A), and the posthumously published lecture 'How is Political Authority Possible?' (HPAP).

5 Communication with D. Z. Phillips and Lars Hertzberg.

6 See the list of unpublished sources. I am making use of my extensive (at times almost verbatim) notes from Winch's lectures and postgraduate seminars at the University of Illinois at Urbana-Champaign in the Fall term of 1990 and at Åbo in September, 1993. Their wording has obviously gone through the filter of my brain. And they represent the perspective of a student, not that of a close friend or colleague. I hope this essay to be, in a small way, an acknowledgement of my great debt to Peter Winch as a teacher.

the root of the more superficial, normative issues. Among those more superficial issues is the search for guidelines for what kinds of exercise of authority are rationally acceptable.

For Winch, political philosophy is primarily not a normative inquiry, hence his conception is not in line with what political philosophers are frequently expected to do. He investigates the background that must be in place *before* meaningful normative debate begins.

On the other hand, I will argue that also Winch's search for the grammar of the political has a normative aspect, recognisable but not fully developed. The difference between his inquiry and normative political philosophy in general lies, perhaps, in the sense in which the latter looks for accounts of political legitimacy and justice that hold *ahead of* any political process. The political process is, on that conception, merely one way of imposing the rational ideal on a society. Winch thinks, instead, that the process itself – political culture – is of importance. Its outcome and its forms will be historically contingent, but the fact that there *is* a political culture is constitutive of the meaning of legitimacy in the relevant society. There are nevertheless limits to what kinds of process in a society we can recognise as expressing its prevailing sense of legitimacy; for instance, limits to acceptable methods of producing persuasion.

Winch is concerned to describe the general place of political authority in human life, trying to outline the ways of living that make both the justification of political authority and challenges to it meaningful enterprises. The classical normative questions of political philosophy need to be addressed in the context of underlying issues about the nature of practical rationality. Practical rationality, in turn, has deep connections with the nature of human relationships. Thus, by 'practical rationality', Winch does not mean a certain faculty that individuals possess to a greater or lesser degree, the ability to make correct deductions from ends to means and vice versa. It includes the entire web of practices and ways of thinking that constitute human agency; including our ways of speaking about this, or what he often calls 'grammar' –

> 'grammar', springing from the nature of the life a man leads with other men, according to which he can formulate the difficulties which arise in the course of such a life and attempt to overcome such difficulties.[7]

As he also puts it,

> Because of the way concepts are formed and applied, and because of their connection with action and the aspirations and values that go with action, the world of which we are aware is one that is impregnated with values. That is to say, our

7 MSHR, 96 – 97.

> concepts, which give this world its shape, are unintelligible except as concepts exercised by beings whose common life exhibits certain aspirations and values.[8]

The ambition to develop Ludwig Wittgenstein's insights in new settings constitutes a persistent feature of Peter Winch's work, both in political philosophy and elsewhere.[9] Winch often develops his views by way of expositions of, and juxtapositions of, central authors of the Western philosophical canon. The political philosophers to whom he constantly returns are Thomas Hobbes, Jean-Jacques Rousseau, Simone Weil, and Socrates as depicted in Plato's early and middle dialogues, especially in *Gorgias*. This should, however, not obscure the fact that Winch is very much his own man. His interest does not lie in scholarship but in relevance for the issues he is addressing.

Despite the long time span there is a basic unity of approach both with regard to arguments and material. Below, the argument in the published material is presented in rough outline. The second half of the essay is devoted to the ways in which Winch's thought was developing and expanding in the 1990's. On the whole I will stick to his own arguments and formulations. However, due to the less systematic character of the sources, my own contribution will be more pronounced later in the essay, especially in the last section.

How is Political Authority Possible?

Peter Winch gave his main question a self-consciously Kantian formulation: *How is political authority possible*?[10] As with Kant, the phrasing indicates a seemingly inherent conceptual difficulty. It identifies a concept that obviously exists but which apparently *should not exist* if a received view on rational agency were to be upheld.

Obedience to authority means that the agent carries out some task, not because of some desire of his or her own, but due to someone else's demands. On the other hand, to obey is not simply to yield to superior force. The agent's recognition of an authority as legitimate implies that his or her obedience is, in some sense, voluntary.[11] However, someone might maintain that 'voluntary obedience' is a contradiction in terms. On a widely held view on the nature of agency, a rational agent will not voluntarily do anything except what the *agent* has good reasons to do. In the philosophy of action, the problem emerges from the description of 'reason for action' as the end product of a combination of

8 SWJB, 115.
9 See Lassman 2000, 129: "Winch's work is the best indication that we have of what an approach to political philosophy inspired by Wittgensteinian ideas might look like."
10 Seminars on Authority 1993, p. 1; HPAP, title. See also A&R, p. 11, C&A, p. 224.
11 See also MSHR, 100.

beliefs and desires. I have no reason to act unless I have the appropriate desire, which then constitutes the ultimate motivating force.[12] But if it is my desire to act, why call it obedience? And if I have no desire, why act at all?

Thomas Hobbes identified the paradox in the *Leviathan*; indeed that book as a whole is an extended attempt to solve it. For Hobbes, a command "is, where a man saith, *Doe this* […] without expecting other reason than the Will of him that says it". However, "the proper object of every mans Will, is some Good to himselfe".[13] Thus two questions are raised: *Why* should anyone voluntarily obey someone else's commands; and more radically, how is the *concept of* voluntary obedience possible? Winch points out, however, that Hobbes and most other contract theorists tended to assimilate the two questions.[14]

For Hobbes, who advanced a view on motivation as a causal force[15], the paradox of obedience is enhanced because of the generally presumed impossibility of causation at distance. The other person's motives are supposedly causal forces operative within that individual. But I can be moved to action only by causes that operate within *me*.

At this juncture, it will be natural to look for the ultimate reasons for the agent's compliance in some *long-term* interest. Compliance might be explained when the agent has "*consented* to be subject to someone's authority for the sake of long-term concerns of his or her own".[16] The political contract tradition constitutes an attempt to assimilate political authority to such cases. Hobbes famously argued that only a political contract or 'Covenant' provides the individual the escape from an anarchic state of nature, where life is otherwise bound to be "solitary, poore, nasty, brutish, and short".[17]

Hume, in his essay 'Of the Original Contract', raises two arguments against contractual approaches.[18]

He points out that no one believes this in real life. We do not think the legitimacy of the political system to which we belong is derived from our consent. On the contrary, we consent because we already perceive the system as legitimate.

More importantly, he claims that the idea of a contract is, in any case, open to the same challenge that gives rise to the original problem. Also our duty to fulfil our promises (for instance, made in the context of a contract) implies that we may be required to act contrary to our present interests and desires. For this reason, Hume classified both political loyalty and the keeping of promises

12 C&A, 223 – 224.

13 Hobbes, *Leviathan,* Ch 25, 303 [131 – 132], quoted in A&R, 11, MSHR, 101, C&R, 224, Seminars on Authority 1993, 2.

14 Seminars on Authority 1993, 1.

15 Hobbes, *Leviathan*, Pt I Ch 6.

16 C&A, 224.

17 Hobbes, *Leviathan*, Ch. 13, 186 [62].

18 Hume 1970. Hume's essay is dicussed in A&R and C&A.

as "artificial virtues".[19] The very view on motivation that creates the apparent need of a contract theory also implies that "allowing oneself to be constrained by one's *past* promise is just as irrational as allowing oneself to be constrained by the will of another".[20] Hence the original problem remains untouched. Winch points out that the issue has both a 'sociological' and a 'philosophical' aspect.[21] There is the question what considerations could persuade rational beings to get started with the practice of keeping promises. And there is the question what it can *mean* to be 'bound' by one's commitments.[22]

With Hobbes, the problem surfaces in the question how the Covenant, which supposedly makes both organised society and promising possible, can be based on a mutual promise. On the Hobbesian view, force and *fraud* characterise human interaction in the state of nature.[23] Hobbes's solution consisted in the imposition of an enforcing agency, the Sovereign. However, Winch argues that, while the enforcing agency would presumably solve the sociological question how to maintain order, it would not introduce the *concept* of being bound by one's word.

Winch's discussion of the Hobbesian take on political authority – much less my exposition here – does not constitute a detailed and documented refutation of Hobbes' work. Other interpreters have emphasised the aspects of Hobbes' work that relate it to 17th-century ideological debate.[24] As far as I am aware, Winch has not commented on alternative interpretations of Hobbes. He has simply taken hold of a form of argument that recurs in political philosophy but which found an unusually lucid expression in Hobbes.

Winch's responses to the problem of motivation involve, in a sense, a revision of the order in which social life is conceptualised. The original dilemma arises from a conception where the absence of any commitment on the part of the individual is the starting point. That conception creates the need for an account of how the solitary individual reaches out to others and establishes mutual obligations. Winch's view implies, on the contrary – if I understand him correctly – that we are committed to one another from the outset. Our commitment to stick to our words is not an additional element mobilised at certain untypical occasions, say speech acts involving some equivalent of 'I promise'. It is, instead, part and parcel of what it means to address someone meaningfully. The distinction between truth an falsity – even in cases of *de facto* solitary exercise of rationality – is, in itself, but an aspect of the norm of truthfulness. "[A]dherence to the norm of truthfulness *goes along with* the

19 Hume 1986, III. II.II ('Of the Origin of Justice and Property'), III. II.V ('Of the Obligation of Promises'). Cf. Winch, Lectures on the Philosophy of Law and of the State 1988, 38-9.
20 HPAP, 29. Also see C&A, 227.
21 HPAP, 27.
22 See also, e.g., Watson 2006.
23 Hobbes, *Leviathan*, Pt I Ch 13, 188 [63].
24 Skinner 1996; Skinner 2002; MacPherson 1962, 18, 22.

distinction between true and false statements; without the one there could not be the other".[25]

Certainty and 'Habits of Obedience'

In line with Hume's essay (and his own work on understanding other cultures) Winch is sceptical of the idea that specific procedures – such as the existence of an elected legislative assembly – could constitute the universally valid conditions for political legitimacy. What is legitimate depends on the prevailing culture of political thinking, which will be historically contingent.[26] In Hume's own society, hereditary monarchy with severely limited male suffrage was the accepted norm. But we can go along with saying that this was a legitimate form of government at the time without agreeing that it would be so today.

Winch, following Hume, argues that consent indeed is a source of political legitimacy, but not in the sense that the contract theorists like to think. We grow into ingrained "habits of obedience".[27] This means that our political thinking, from the start, involves acceptance of the possibility that someone else may be in a position of authority. Challenges to a government on the basis of its illegitimate character presuppose the idea of *legitimate* political authority. This will even be true of convinced anarchists, who in fact think of the government differently from how they would relate to a Mafia-like protection racket.[28]

> There is a range of normal behaviour and normal ways of speaking and arguing which is necessary if there is to be such a position as that of "exercizing state authority" for anybody to occupy. [...] [T]alk about "legitimacy" or otherwise of régimes [...] is actually in large measure constitutive of the relation between state and citizen and, moreover, an important area within which human rationality is exercized.[29]

Following Hertzberg's analysis in the present volume[30], we can sum up this position by saying that the idea of a *political* life in a society involves the idea of there being the position of *legitimate authority* for someone to occupy.

On Winch's view, political authority is a special case of the general role of authority in human life.[31] The apparent paradox of political authority is a

25 N&C, 62.
26 SWJB, 185 – 186; Seminars on Authority 1990. Also see Hertzberg, in the present volume.
27 C&A, 228.
28 A&R, 18. For a related point, see ISSc, 52 - 53: 'The Anarchist', who makes a point of challenging all conventions, will also be following rules in doing this.
29 A&R, 19.
30 See the article by Lars Hertzberg in this volume.
31 "To understand how political authority is possible, we should try first to understand the central role played in *all* education by response to adult authority on the part of children". – HPAP, 32.

special case of the problem of how our acceptance of other people's authority is to be reconciled with rationality.

At this juncture, he brings in a perspective from Wittgenstein's *On Certainty*.[32] Wittgenstein starts from the observation that there will be statements that we will not doubt. I will not doubt that all humans have brains[33] or that the world is more than 150 years old.[34] These statements look like contingent truths. But my confidence in them is not based on some undisputable *empirical* evidence. Any supporting facts I might muster could be doubted more easily than the general conclusions. (Indeed I would find it hard to believe alleged disconfirming data precisely because of the perceived impossibility of the scepticism that they would entail. Thus the general conclusions support the would-be proofs, not the other way around.) At the same time it is difficult to see how I could lead a normal life at all if I were constantly to raise doubts of this general character. For instance, historical inquiries would never come off the ground if it was agreed that the world *might* have simply popped into existence a few years ago, complete with fake memories and records. Wittgenstein argues that my absence of doubt here is "not, so to say, hasty but excusable: it is part of judging".[35]

I build up my world picture by listening to others and generally believing them. But even my disbelief presupposes trust in other directions. For instance, I learn to check up on dubious information against alternative sources. My rational thinking on the whole is characterised by my membership in a "community [...] bound together by science and education".[36] – Thus thinking is in an important sense a communal endeavour. Human beings, by sharing a 'grammar' by which they conceptualise their world, also relate to one another.[37] The unity of human society is 'a unity essentially involving *concepts*'.[38] This spontaneous unity contrasts with Hobbes' conception according to which unity must be brought about through the imposition of a Sovereign.

Winch points out that, in growing into the life characterised by this predicament, children will take the authority of their parents, teachers, and books for granted. This means that, in many cases, no question arises for the children about the correctness of what the adults tell them. And this is "quite continuous with" children's natural tendency to do what adults tell them to do, "a response which cries out to be called an acceptance of adult authority".[39] The fact that we do things simply because others expect us to is not a departure from

32 Wittgenstein 1972.
33 Wittgenstein 1972, § 159. Cf §§ 281, 284.
34 Wittgenstein 1972, §§ 138, 182–192.
35 Wittgenstein 1972, § 150.
36 Wittgenstein 1972, § 298, quoted in C&A, 232.
37 As Winch puts it in ISSc, 121: "the social relations between men and the ideas which men's actions embody are really the same thing considered from different points of view".
38 Authority, 99.
39 C&A, 231.

rationality. It is an important, indeed constitutive, form that practical rationality takes, not only in children but perhaps even more so in adults. To submit to an authority is not to be subjected to power, to an alien will.[40] In conclusion, Winch writes:

> The notion of practical reason itself requires at many points a recognition of the authority of others that is *primitive*. Once this is accepted the notion of the state's authority is freed from the requirement to satisfy conditions that are in fact unsatisfiable.[41]

Legitimacy and Political Education

The argument clears the concept of authority of the sense of paradox attached to it. But it does not entail that our primitive acceptance of authority commits us to accepting *political* authority. In his earliest formulation of the argument, Winch had made that assumption which he subsequently withdrew.[42] In order to constitute a full response to the question how political authority is possible, the general description of the role of authority in practical rationality must be supplemented with an elaboration of its relation to a life that involves a political setting.

In the essay 'Man and Society in Hobbes and Rousseau', Winch connects this issue to Rousseau's discussion of civic virtue and its formation in education.

In opposition to Hobbes, Rousseau maintains (in Winch's formulation) that "an undertaking 'simply and solely to obey' […] could only yield a relation *antithetical* to the political relation" between citizen and sovereign.[43] That relation requires, on the contrary, active citizens prepared to exercise judgement about the justice of social arrangements.[44] A genuinely political relation between citizen and the state involves exercise of sovereignty – self-legislation – by citizens. It is not grounded on a contract, lying in a dead past, by which they have signed away their freedom. "Power can be transmitted, but not will".[45] In Rousseau's ideal society, the social contract provides a framework for the citizen's continuous exercise of will *in the present*. It allows for the transformation of their particular wills into a collective 'general will'.

---

40 Authority, 100.

41 C&A, 235.

42 See Authority, 105: 'the fact that one is a social being, engaged in rule-governed activities […] is in itself sufficient to commit one to the acceptance of legitimate political authority'. In his 1967 postscript to a reprint of the essay originally published in 1958, Winch calls this 'quite [a] false remark' (p. 110).

43 MSHR, 103, emphasis added.

44 MSHR, 108.

45 Rousseau 1967, *The Social Contract*, Book II, ch I, quoted in A&R, 15, MSHR, 103.

However, according to Rousseau, the citizens' expression of their wills must have certain characteristics in order properly to qualify as an exercise of the general will. Their thinking about the questions on which they are called to deliberate must be informed by a concern for the good of the community.[46] The term 'general will' is not commonly accepted in political philosophy, but the conceptual point that Rousseau is making is a straightforward one. In order to say that *a group*, not only the majority of its individual members (or indeed all of them), holds this or that view, we must assume that the individual members have considered the issue from (what they think is) the point of view of the group as a whole.[47]

Rousseau recognises that these habits of thinking can only result from a particular kind of training. Thus *Émile* is a natural continuation of his thoughts on civic virtue.[48] As all human societies are riddled with injustices, education must above all equip us to recognise and react to unjust social arrangements when we see them.[49]

Winch contrasts Rousseau's view on the role of education with that of Hobbes. Hobbes describes the management of society as a *science* based on deduction from general principles.[50] Civil unrest can be forestalled by teaching politicians the elements of this science. Arguably, the Hobbesian conception of social life is at bottom a non-political or anti-political one. It is an attempt to reduce justice to legality[51] and political questions to questions of expediency. In the parlance of today, we might describe the contrast as one between conceptions of politics as based, respectively, on 'civil society' and 'social engineering' or 'managerialism'.[52]

Winch clearly thinks that the choice between the two conceptions is not arbitrary. Rousseau describes an aspect of the grammar of political life that Hobbes has missed.

It seems to me that the discussion reviewed in this section suggests two characteristics of legitimacy claims. Those claims arise within a political culture; that is, a setting where individuals see themselves as called to voice their views, not only as individuals, but also in their capacity of members of a

46 Rousseau 1967, Bk IV, ch. I. Rousseau speaks of the voters expressing their views of what is "advantageous to the state". The "state" is, in Rousseau's terminology, the political community as a whole while "government" refers to the administrative apparatus.

47 See Lagerspetz 2004, 1301 – 1302.

48 There is also a problem involved. On Rousseau's view, social life is essential to humans, but it has also a corrupting influence on us. Rousseau avoids the problem by letting Émile grow up in an isolated country setting.

49 MSHR, 108.

50 Thomas Hobbes, *Behemoth*, Dialogue IV. Quoted in C&A, 235, MSHR, 90, seminars on Authority 1993, 21 September.

51 MSHR, 107.

52 Winch's arguments in ISSc already indicate scepticism towards the idea of scientifically based social engineering.

community.[53] Secondly, a legitimacy claim is a claim that relates entitlement to position of authority to a conception of justice.[54] Considerations of legality or expediency are not enough. These qualitative requirements are important, because they imply constraints on when we can correctly describe someone as making a claim about legitimacy.[55]

Aristotelian and Socratic Reason

In the late 1980's, Winch returned to the question of political authority. There is an obvious continuity with the earlier work but also – especially in the unpublished material – attention to previously underdeveloped themes. The following sections will discuss the new directions his thought was taking.

Some of the new impulses are indicated in the self-critical preface appended, in 1990, to a new impression of *The Idea of a Social Science*. It highlights Winch's changing approach to the role of rules in human conduct. He is criticising his earlier self of "an over-idealization of logic".[56] He had also underestimated the role of conflict and divergences of opinion in social life. Despite the fact that his book had included important arguments to the contrary,[57] he had been implicitly assuming that conceptual difficulties can be resolved by an appeal to "a formal system"; in this case, "a system of modes of social life, each with criteria of intelligibility peculiar to itself".[58] By way of analogy, Winch might have said the corresponding thing about the position of 'grammar' in his his properly political philosophy. In 1972 Winch had written, in 'Authority and Rationality':

> What we can understand as a possible mode of intelligible […] human conduct […] *is* limited by the grammar […] which we have acquired in our commerce with actually existing institutions and forms of behaviour. A grammar can be extended and

53 Also see Hertzberg, the present volume.

54 Also see SWJB, 185 – 186.

55 Suppose I believe a government has stimulated economic growth in my country. In themselves, such beliefs do not constitute support for my (let us assume) simultaneous belief that it is the legitimate government. These issues are analytically distinct, even if it may sometimes be difficult to treat them separately. Economic policies are in many ways connected to questions of justice, as they affect the distribution of resources and the rights and duties of those concerned. Hence ostensibly economic arguments often involve explicit or tacit ideas about justice.

56 Preface, xvi.

57 In particular, the discussion of 'What the Tortoise said to Achilles', ISSc 55 – 57.

58 Preface, xvi. – By this, Winch had also unwittingly given some leeway to a standard objection raised to *The Idea of a Social Science*. According to that objection, Winch had claimed that various forms of culturally determined 'grammar' constitute self-contained cultural bubbles beyond external assessment or critique. (I regard the objection as mistaken, but this essay will not be the place to criticise it.)

> developed, but there are limits to what changes will be *counted* as extensions and developments of a grammar.[59]

To be fair, Winch is not saying here that grammar cannot be criticised or changed. In fact he explicitly says in the essay that our grammar of political thought is historically contingent. His formulation nevertheless gives the impression of a system with limits closed in advance; moreover, a system to which every member stands in the same kind of relation. In his later work he says more explicitly that rule-governed behaviour is not completely determined by rules. To follow a rule is to exercise one's *judgement* in certain ways.[60] What *is* excluded by grammar is something we find out by trying to express the things we think we want to say and *seeing whether* we can endorse the new expressions as sensible.

In the 1990's, Winch addresses the variety of ways in which the roles of logic and reasoning have been understood. He demonstrates this by way of a comparison between Socrates and Aristotle. Aristotle regarded logic as the science dealing with formal relations between propositions. What on this view guaranteed the 'authority' of logic was the fact that it was "guided [...] by the rails[61] mapped out" by "the constraints of *how things are*"[62]. However, Socrates is offering a different conception of reasoning - and this is the conception that Winch defends. "Logic", on the Socratic conception, is a comprehensive description of the reasoning that takes place between human beings: of what kinds of argument are valid, acceptable, and meaningful. The assessment of arguments involves the requirement that the interlocutors mean what they say and are genuinely concerned for the substantial issues being discussed. *Formal* logic, as a discipline, takes hold of certain features of correct reasoning, trying to capture them in rules, but it does not constitute an independent source of authority apart from the validity already present in the things we say.

> In *Gorgias* the *authority* carried by Socrates's arguments is *the authority of Socrates, the man.* And this is emphasized in the dramatic structure of the dialogue. Or rather, it is *the authority carried by the spectacle of a certain type of life, which Socrates both exemplifies and describes.*[63]

It is a rival view, not an unsophisticated version of the formal science brought to greater perfection by Aristotle. However, Aristotle's view on logic has largely

59 A&R, 17.
60 Seminars on Authority 1990.
61 Cf. Wittgenstein 1953, I § 218.
62 The Authority of Reason, 2, 3.
63 The Authority of Reason, 4 (italics in the original). Cf Ethics and Value Theory, 28.8.1990.

prevailed in philosophy.[64] It is already present in Plato's later dialogues, including the bulk of the *Republic*, where the personal voice of Socrates is in effect substituted by universally valid prescriptions of Reason. It is also expressed, according to Winch, in Hobbes's description of proper political thought as a science. Winch illustrates the distinction further with reference to R. M. Hare's 'universal prescriptivism' put forward in his *Freedom and Reason*.[65] According to Winch, Hare holds that we are free to choose our principles, but then need to "feed them into a logical machinery".[66] Hare depicts the alternative as intellectual anarchy.

Winch thinks such approaches render the 'consent' invoked in contract theories largely illusory. Their basic principles are usually assumed to be extremely general and next to self-evident for rationally self-interested agents, and the rest of the argument follows the rails of the deductive procedure. Winch insists, instead, that genuine consent must have something contingent about it: it is what people as a matter of fact agree to.[67]

In mainstream political theory, politics is frequently depicted as the method of arbitrating between the interests of individuals or other agents. These interests are by and large treated as preexistent. What is effectively ignored in these approaches is the fact that the question what *is* in our interest is, in itself, a question for genuine politics to examine. On a contrasting view that Winch attributes to Socrates, politics is the pursuit of the good of human beings, which takes the form of a cooperative dialogical examination. "Genuine concern for the good of human beings is expressed, characteristically, in the kind of dialogue between few persons where the parties are made to examine themselves". [68] In *Gorgias*, Socrates describes himself, for the same reason, as "the only or almost the only Athenian living who practices the true art of politics".[69]

But Winch realises this will raise the question of how such dialogue, suited for face-to-face interaction, could be reproduced in the context of political decision-making. The difficulty is especially obvious in times of crisis, but in fact it exists all the time. There is an inherent tension in the Socratic view on politics; expressed in the later part of the *Gorgias,* and in the parable of the Cave

---

64 Winch also points out that 'Wittgenstein, so Rhees says, used the term "Aristotelian logic" (with which he contrasted his own way of treating logic) to *include Frege and Russell!*" – The Authority of Reason, 3.

65 Hare 1963.

66 Seminars on Authority 1990.

67 Seminars on Authority 1990; SWJB, 184 (à propos of the role of 'contract' in Rawls). Also see Lassman 2000, 134. – There is perhaps a parallel with Winchs's emphasis, in CWUO, on the importance, in intercultural understanding, of *getting along* with each other as opposed to his earlier concentration on identifying the rules according to which the other person is acting.

68 Ethics & Value Theory, 27.9.1990.

69 Plato, *Gorgias*, 521d.

in the *Republic*.[70] The philosopher who has seen the light and returns to report about it is completely unable to convince those who still sit inside the cave. In order to convince the multitude, the philosopher needs to turn into the kind of person whom he or she wants to convince, thus defeating the philosopher's original purpose.[71]

Politics, Truth, and Symbolic Language

In Winch's contrast between Socratic and Aristotelian reason, the personal and contingent character of practical rationality is emphasised – the variations that had earlier tended to slip out of sight under the general cover of 'grammar'.

For instance, the roles of images in arguments may go beyond their use as illustrations. An image may be constitutive of a way of thinking; a form of reasoning is to be understood in its light. Winch argues, paraphrasing Wittgenstein:

> One of the most important facts of human life is that certain pictures force themselves upon us. Thinking very characteristically depends on such pictures. The pictures must be respected and not treated as superstition![72]

This is not to say that the inherited picture must always be accepted; this is also seen in Winch's phrasing. A picture may 'force itself' on us and impede clear thinking. The employment of imaginary examples may be one way to question its self-evident status. New images may initiate new ways of reasoning.

Socrates' description, in *Gorgias,* of how the soul stands trial in the afterlife is one such case.[73] The point of evoking the image of a trial is not to establish a supernatural deterrent. He invites us to see our present lives in a light where we can see why justice can be a central concern in someone's life. It is analogous to the use of abstract geometry for the clarification of empirical spatial relations.[74] – Similarly, Rousseau's social contract is not mainly a blueprint for a future society. It is an object of comparison, designed to help us get sight of crucial features of the grammar of political life.[75]

---

70 Plato, *Republic*, Book VII. Winch develops this in Ethics & Value Theory. See esp. 27.9.1990.

71 Also see Rousseau, *Émile*, Book I, quoted in MSHR, 98: "In order to make them behave according to your wishes, you have to behave according to their wishes. As soon as you have to see with others' eyes, you have to will their wills."

72 Seminars on Authority 1990. - Winch is obviously developing Wittgenstein's views here. Cf. Wittgenstein 1980, 83e.

73 Plato, *Gorgias*, 523 – 527.

74 Ethics & Value Theory, 27.9.1990.

75 Cf.Rousseau's (1967) motto for the Discourse on the Origin of Inequality (taken form Aristotle's *Politics*, Book I Ch II): *Non in depravatis, sed in his quae bene secundum naturam se habent, considerandum est quid sit naturale.*

Winch also cites Wittgenstein's comment on Spengler's use of images.[76] In his *Decline of the West*, Spengler described certain simple images as prototypes (*Urbilder*) of a given culture. He claimed that seemingly disparate cultural phenomena within the Apollonic, Faustic, etc. cultures were somehow expressions of the prototype of their respective culture.[77] Wittgenstein thought Spengler had misunderstood the role of the prototype in his own thinking. The existence of a prototype is not demonstrated by objective resemblances between existing cultural phenomena and the prototype. Instead, "the prototype characterizes the form of Spengler's argument".[78] It is Spengler's way of drawing attention to aspects of cultural expressions that he thinks are important or revealing. "The prototype is something that is being offered to you and you must find out whether you find it illuminating".[79] An honest argument "makes it clear that this *is* a form of persuasion. It has the form, 'Look at things like this and see if it does not make things clearer'".[80]

Already in "Authority and Rationality", Winch takes up Weil's insistence on the contingent character of the symbolic language that expresses the citizens' relation to politics. Weil writes, of various forms of political institution,

> They are analogous to love letters, to exchanges of rings, and other tokens between lovers. In certain circles a woman would not regard herself as truly married were she not to wear a golden ring. The conjugal bond does not of course consist in the ring. But all the same it is needful that women who feel this way should wear a ring.[81]

I *can* see political authority as legitimate when I have access to a political culture, a living symbolic language that relates the citizens to the state. The importance of following particular electoral procedures lies primarily in the fact that they express a prevailing understanding of the legitimate relation between the rulers and the ruled. Its legitimising role is contingent on the political thinking within the community.[82]

On the other hand, the images, language, and arguments that have previously expressed our sense of legitimacy may lose their hold on us. This

76 Seminars on Authority 1990, last session. The reference is to Wittgenstein 1980, 14.

77 Spengler 1921, e.g., 8 – 9, 67, 243. – Thus there is a deep connection "between differential calculus and the principle of the dynastic State at the time of Louis XIV, between the ancient *polis* and Euclidean geometry, between the spatial perspective of Western oil painting and the overcoming of space by means of railways, telephones and long-distance weapons, between counterpoint in instrumental music and the economic credit system" (Spengler 1921, 8, trans. OL).

78 Seminars on Authority 1990, last session.

79 Seminars on Authority 1990, last session.

80 Seminars on Authority 1990, last session.

81 Weil, 'La légitimité du gouvernement provisoire', in *Écrits de Londres*, quoted in A&R p. 17. A slightly different translation is found in Weil 1987, 88.

82 As Hertzberg points out in this volume, election results are liable to be contested when the political system as a whole is in crisis.

happens, for instance, because of general cultural changes or because of their misuse in propaganda. Weil claimed this had happened in pre-war France, where a system of democratic elections existed alongside pervasive cynicism and distrust of politics:

> Practically no Frenchman approved of Daladier's usurpations. Practically no Frenchman became indignant about them. It is the feeling for legitimacy which makes us indignant about usurpations.[83]

At Winch's seminar, this was compared with a contemporary example:

> Corruption in society and language go together. E.g., 'Left' vs 'Right' in American politics: supposedly the 'Left' are the people who agree that the government should take money from people and do things with it. The 'Right' disagree.[84]

As the terms 'left' and 'right' were trivialised, rational public discussion of the general goals of politics had become almost impossible; at the same time this corruption of language was itself the symptom of a decline of public political thought.

This opens up questions about different ways of producing persuasion; in Socratic terms, the distinction between genuine politics and false semblances of it.[85] Despite the openness of the concept of rationality, which allows for various methods of persuading, we still do (and must) distinguish between legitimate and illegitimate instances of this. One illegitimate method, particularly rife in political philosophy, consists in denying that one is engaged in persuasion but merely in a neutral exercise of rationality.[86] – In a political context, a certain rhetoric may involve pitting one section of the population against another. That would count against its legitimacy.[87] The *mindlessness* of public support for a cause also counts against its being a genuine expression of people's sense of legitimacy.[88] These examples remind of Socrates, in the later part of *Gorgias*, criticising contemporary politicians for catering to the worst instincts of the populace.

---

83 Weil, quoted in MSHR, 107. Cf Weil 1987, 88.

84 Seminars on Authority 1990. – This remark was made at the seminar in a discussion with Lynette Reid. I am unable to recall whether it was Reid or Winch who first brought up the example.

85 Plato, *Gorgias*. Cf. also the general contrast made in the dialogue between genuine activities and their false semblances.

86 Seminars on Authority 1990.

87 Seminars on Authority 1993, 21.9.1993.

88 Winch made a reference to the first Gulf War. He was thinking over these issues at the outbreak of the war, at a university campus where disproportionate interest in spectator sports seemed, for some people, seamlessly to blend into support for the first war in history to be enjoyed on television.

These reflections express the assumption that saying, of a group of citizens, that they view a political measure as legitimate is more than just saying they support it. It is to claim that their views are informed by what they perceive as justice and public responsibility.

To think politically is to relate oneself to society and to reflect on one's own role in it. A political culture needs a symbolic language suitable as a vehicle of such thought. In his 1990 seminar, Winch used Václav Havel's essay 'The Power of the Powerless'[89] (written in 1978) to discuss ways in which the individual's relation to politics may be corrupted when that language has lost its meaning. He agreed with Havel that many of the features he is citing may also be found in liberal societies; such as the use of legitimising myths in the discourse that mediates between the rulers and the ruled.

Havel describes a shopkeeper in East Bloc Czechoslovakia placing in his window the slogan: 'Workers of the world, unite!'. He puts up the sign – which has probably arrived from a central warehouse together with the onions and carrots –simply because that is expected. Havel writes:

> Let us take note: if the greengrocer had been instructed to display the slogan, 'I am afraid and therefore unquestionably obedient', he would not be nearly as indifferent to its semantics, even though the statement would reflect the truth. [...] [H]is expression of loyalty must take the form of a sign which, at least on its textual surface, indicates a level of disinterested conviction. It must allow the greengrocer to say, 'What's wrong with the workers of the world uniting?' Thus the sign helps the greengrocer to conceal from himself the low foundations of his obedience, at the same time concealing the low foundations of power. It hides them behind the facade of something high. And that something is *ideology*.[90]

Ideological excuses become the bridge through which the power structure approaches the individual and vice versa. The message of the sign is directed upwards, towards the greengrocer's superior. The main conflict takes place *within* the individual – who must choose to display or discard the sign – not between different social groups.[91] Against conformism, Havel raises the possibility of 'living within the truth': rejecting ritual, discovering one's authentic thinking. It has a political significance, not because it is inherently oppositional, but because of the context of 'post-totalitarian' society (Havel's term) where it is bound to lead to conflict. 'Living within the truth' arises out of what a person *normally* does – as a greengrocer, poet, brewery worker and so on – when the requirements of 'life itself' (Havel's term) conflict with prescribed behaviour. – Winch was on the whole impressed by Havel's analysis, although

89 Havel 1990. – Winch also discusses Havel in Introduction, 12 – 16.
90 Havel 1990, 42.
91 Seminars on Authority 1990.

he thought the essay ignored some of the complexity of determining what it is that 'truth' requires of us.[92]

In sum, the material with which Winch was working in the 1990's raises the disquieting possibility of a third alternative beyond legitimacy and illegitimacy. The discourse in which ideas of legitimacy are formulated may lose its hold on us. Conceptions of legitimacy are culturally specific, but it is imaginable that citizens no longer generally think of their relation to the state in these terms at all. Exactly when this may be said to happen is a question of both degree and context. In any case, there are characteristic ways in which words and phrases may be emptied of their original meaning.

Oppression and Justice

In *The Idea of a Social Science*, Winch had compared social relations with "exchange of ideas". In 1990, he accuses himself of painting a "cosy" picture that ignores the "*fragility* of the ethico-cultural conditions which make such an exchange of ideas possible".[93] Treatises on political philosophy tend to presume the possibility of rational deliberation free of constraint. In his work on Wittgenstein's *On Certainty*, Winch went some way towards demonstrating the importance of relationships of dependence in the development and exercise of rationality. Yet even those forms of dependence belong to a setting where everyone at least potentially participates in a community of equals.

But interpersonal relations also come in the form of conflict, oppression and exclusion, something probably endemic to every society. Political philosophy should not only consider the ideal case of unconstrained dialogue, but also our possible choices in the face of an oppressive or unresponsive political system.

In the 1990 Preface, Winch speaks of "the enormous *contrast* between human relations ruled by ideas of justice and those governed by force".[94] He notes the work of Jürgen Habermas "though his way of treating [these questions] would not be mine".[95] More importantly, he refers to his freshly published book on Simone Weil who, "as it seems to me, has done more than anyone to reveal the depth of such issues".

Weil explores the differences between oppression and legitimate hierarchical relationships. On her view, obedience is not one aspect of an oppressive relationship, but rather oppression and obedience stand in contrast to one another. Obedience implies consent while oppression implies dismissal of

92 Seminars on Authority 1990.
93 Preface ..., xvii.
94 Preface ..., xviii.
95 Preface ..., xviii. Cf. ATP, where Winch takes issue with some views of Karl-Otto Apel, many of which have inspired Habermas. See Lassman 2000, 137.

the question of consent. Thus oppression stands to obedience as rape stands to love.[96]

The two key Weilian concepts in this connection are probably 'the power to refuse' and 'justice as a supernatural virtue'. Weil was disturbed by what she saw as a human natural tendency towards oppressive attitudes. In an unequal power relationship, the stronger party is tempted to turn the other into an object, a thing. Most vividly, she describes this in her discussion of Achilles in the *Iliad*. For a moment, Achilles is moved by Priam pleading for mercy; then he impatiently pushes him aside as if a dead object, a mere obstacle.[97] But according to Weil, human life also involves a conflicting impulse: the power to refuse to go along with the objectifying impulse. "[I]t happens, although extremely rarely, that a man will forbear out of pure generosity to command where he has the power to do so".[98] Weil calls this impulse supernatural, as it conflicts with a natural human tendency to view the world solely from one's own point of view, reducing other people to opportunities and obstacles.[99]

Weil, in Winch's analysis, holds forth the possibility of conceiving of justice as a perspective that goes beyond the bargaining scenarios that recur in mainstream contract theories. The consent of the other is sought as an end in itself, not for prudential reasons only.[100]

However, Winch takes exception to Weil's claim that this perspective must be alien to normal human intercourse.[101] This connects to Winch's insistence on the sui generis, primordial character of our reactions to human beings.[102] These are natural responses, ones from which ethical concepts (such as that of 'being a neighbour to someone') subsequently develop. Cruel impulses, too, are only intelligible because they are responses to fellow humans (or other living beings), not towards objects.[103] It is, for instance, significant that Priam is, in a sense, defiled – which cannot be said of a rock removed from a piece of waste ground.[104] In this sense, Priam is *not* turned to a thing.

Justice and Particularity

Winch is sceptical of the chances of defining central concepts of political philosophy – such as 'justice', 'consent', or 'legitimacy' – in the abstract, regardless of the cultural and political conditions in which they have a role. This

96 Weil, 'Are We Struggling for Justice', quoted in SWJB, 106.
97 Weil, 'The Iliad: Poem of Force', quoted in SWJB, 148.
98 Weil, 'Waiting for God', quoted in SWJB, 205.
99 Note the Hobbesianism of this picture of human beings as obstacles.
100 SWJB, 187 – 188; Lassman 2000, 136.
101 SWJB, 190.
102 See the essay 'Who is My Neighbour?' in TTMS.
103 SWJB, 154.
104 SWJB, 154.

criticism targets much of mainstream political philosophy; including, for instance, Rawls' thought experiment where a 'veil of ignorance' is assumed. In the original situation, as described in *A Theory of Justice,* the would-be members of the ideally just society are supposedly ignorant of the place they will personally occupy in it, and even of important facts about their own selves, their life plans and their conception of the good. Yet they are expected to be familiar with 'the general facts of human society'.[105] The objection is that the meanings of the concepts in terms of which human society can be conceived depend on their concrete applications – which, however, the model deliberately has blotted out.

The search for universally valid definitions of social justice represents an attempt to move the issue into an objective rational realm outside politics. Arguably, it may obscure the fact that different agents will stand in different relations to society. Genuine political debates typically involve conflicting views on what exactly *is* included under the headings of 'political questions' or 'justice'. The meanings of 'justice' in a particular linguistic community are brought out in the ways in which members of that community go about arguing about the justice of particular actions and policies; the ways in which, for instance, we are outraged at injustices. In his essay on Hobbes and Rousseau, Winch writes,

> Conceptions of justice are only developed through discussions of injustices. Men capable of becoming citizens must then receive an education which enables them to understand what those injustices are, an education which consists not merely in inculcating a 'science' of what human relationships necessarily are, but rather in creating human beings of a sort who will be capable of discerning qualitative distinctions between different types of human relationship and who will therefore be capable of entering into such relationships.[106]

This kind of education and subsequent social engagement will necessarily involve disagreement. The responses that constitute one's political consciousness crucially concern injustices in one's own society. However, those are arrangements whose primary beneficiaries tend not to perceive them as unjust. Arguably, the meaning of 'justice' only unfolds in a discussion where one's own, possibly controversial, views are brought up. In an essay that partly overlaps with the present discussion in both its themes and conclusions, Peter Lassman writes,

> One important and often overlooked part of Winch's work is his stress upon the ways in which [...] the reality of deep disagreements belongs to our concept of poli-

105 Rawls 1971, 137 (§ 24). – Peter Winch, personal communication with the author, January 1991.

106 MSHR, 108 – 109.

> tics […,] the way in which [the domain of the political] is, in part, constituted by deep and, possibly, irreconcilable conflicts.[107]

In the beginning of his posthumously published lecture 'How is Political Authority Possible?', probably held in 1988, Winch observes that perhaps the most interesting contributions to political philosophy have been written in the course of arguing for specific political causes.

> This situation suggests the possibility that the question 'what political authority is' gains its sense from a context of particular political concerns, concerns which, of their nature, will not be shared by everybody and will be opposed by the concerns of others.[108]

He continues, disappointingly, "I am not going to discuss that interesting possibility here". However, the material with which he subsequently worked – by Havel, Weil, and Socrates/Plato – was written by thinkers trying to get to grips with corrupting tendencies within particular societies.

Winch's general discussion of the idea of legitimate political authority suggests that its possible applications cannot be cast in concrete by the imposition of criteria identified, as it were, ahead of the relevant political and cultural processes in each society. If the criteria are local rather than universal the further elucidation of the concept of legitimate authority must be done by way of examining its historically contingent applications.

What will that inquiry be like? Lars Hertzberg argues in the present volume that a distinction must be made between legitimacy assertions and legitimacy claims.[109] Legitimacy assertions are factual statements about the legitimacy claims that the members of a given society generally make. They do not commit the speaker to a normative position but they are, roughly, sociological statements about prevalent attitudes in a particular society towards given authorities.

But the proposed distinction does not seem to me quite clear-cut simply because the *investigator's* position is not clear-cut. The sociological examination of prevailing views on legitimacy in a society must presuppose that we are able to *recognise*, say, a mode of discourse in a society as expressive of the members' conceptions of political legitimacy. But our 'ability' to do this equals our preparedness to *go along with* certain descriptions.[110] Thus we must

---

107 Lassman 2000, 134.

108 HPAP, 20.

109 See the article by Lars Hertzberg in this volume.

110 As Winch put it in a different occasion, "What a man finds it possible or impossible to say, the difficulty or ease with which he can combine diverse ideas, are important indications of the kind of man he is. [...] It is not just a mechanical exercise in which the work has, as it were, already been done in a hidden realm by logic and simply needs to be revealed to view." – See 'Darwin, *Genesis* and Contradiction' (included in TTMS, 132-139), 138.

ask ourselves: is the debate that, in a given society, gives rise to claims about entitlements to power positions, sufficiently closely related to recognisable ideas of legitimacy? Does it reflect an understanding of the state as a political community? Are its arguments related to ideas of justice?

Consider the question whether popular craving for a 'Leader', as in interwar Europe and present-day Russia, constitutes an expression of a people's sense of political legitimacy. Or is it something else; perhaps – as Weil would have maintained – a symptom of the loss of the feeling for legitimacy in the societies involved? To change the example slightly: Does the popularity of the British National Party in certain neighbourhoods in Britain reflect the wish for a political alternative or is it, instead, a rejection of politics altogether?[111] Addressing such questions will involve a characteristic dialectic between relevant sociological facts and our own inclination to recognise some expressions of opinion, but not others, as genuine political arguments. Our inclination to say the one thing or the other is personal but not arbitrary.

It will obviously also depend on the context. For instance, Weil's harsh comments on pre-war French society were intended to contribute to a future reconstruction of Europe. She was not only commenting on the thinking of her fellow Frenchmen; she was *addressing* them.

The dialectic involved here is very similar to the process of inquiring whether a person really means what he or she is saying. We will not always take people's expressions of desire at face value. This is obvious in the case of children. Responsible parents treat some of their children's utterances not as wishes but as starting points for further probing. This also happens when people's explicit desires have unwelcome implications of which they are unaware. You might hope for an inheritance until you realise it is implicitly to hope for someone to die. *Gorgias* shows such dialectic in action. Socrates distinguishes between a person's genuine and apparent will. What a person really wants is discovered and confirmed by means of self-examination in dialogue with others. But it is also significant that Socrates would simply not accept certain utterances as genuine expressions of a person's will. Thus he holds it unthinkable that anyone could willingly harm himself or herself. And he maintains that no one who really understands the choice would choose to commit rather than suffer an injustice. Connecting to Socrates' argument here, Winch repeatedly stressed the role of shame in the dialectics of *Gorgias*. Socrates made Gorgias, Polus, and Callicles see they could not seriously hold the views they were advocating without turning into persons that they would not want to be.[112]

---

111 Suggestion by Philip Hutchinson, in discussion, 28 March 2009. – In his biography of Hitler, Joachim Fest (1973) connects the rise of Fascism in Germany with the traditional German concept of *Bildung* that idealised the unpolitical man. The Leader was seen as providing an opportunity for society to do without politics altogether.

112 Ethics & Value Theory.

But this is not an uncommitted inquiry in the traditional sense. It is committed to an understanding of the nature of the human good. And it is committed to the good of the person with whom Socrates is talking, the person whom he wants to draw into the dialogue.

The present essay cannot end with a summary of Peter Winch's final position on legitimacy. This last section has rather been my commentary, supported by textual evidence, about the direction where his thought seemed to be moving. I do not think it is obvious whether his take on legitimacy was normative or descriptive; or rather, it is not obvious that the dichotomy is helpful in this case. His work certainly involves a *description* of a certain mode of living and relating to political authority. His descriptions of the grammar of political life, the arguments that I have been reviewing, constitute the exposition of an ideal of a civil society. The implicit argument against rival ideals (including social engineering and managerialism) is not that those ideals are necessarily incoherent, even if they sometimes are. Crucially, they do not capture the form of life that the reader would recognise as properly political. Moreover, the life they do depict would strike us as alien and impoverished.[113] Winch presented a conception according to which the human good is best pursued in a setting where citizens freely develop their ideas of justice in genuine dialogue. It is a society where a symbiosis, or mutually reinforcing relation, obtains between their ethical concerns and the political discourse. It allows and encourages us to 'live within the truth'.

Bibliography

Works by Peter Winch:
(a) Published

A&R
1972 Authority and Rationality. *The Human World* No. 8, August 1972, 11 – 21.

ATP
1979 Apel's 'Transcendental Pragmatics'. In S.C. Brown, ed., *Philosophical Disputes in the Social Sciences*

Authority
1972 Authority. In A. Quinton, ed., *Political Philosophy*. Oxford Readings in Philosophy. Oxford: Oxford University Press, 97 – 111.

113 Cf ATP, 61; Lassman 2000, 137. This apparently does not exclude the possibility of a culture where the alien form of life is the normal life and whose members, like Wittgenstein?s cave man, would not find it uncongenial. Only, that is not the culture of Winch or his readers.

First published in *Proceedings of the Aristotelian Society* 32, 1958-9, 235 – 240.

C&A
1990 Certainty and Authority. *Philosophy* (supplement) 1990, 223 – 237. Republished in A. Phillips Griffiths, ed. (1991), *Wittgenstein Centenary Essays*. Cambridge: Cambridge University Press, 223 – 238.

CWUO
1997 Can We Understand Ourselves? *Philosophical Investigations* 20 (1997), 193 – 204. First published (in Swedish translation by Alexander Motturi and Anna Hallberg) as 'Kan vi förstå oss själva?' *Glänta* 1-2 /1995, 99 – 106.

E&A
1972 *Ethics and Action.* London: RKP.

HPAP
2002 How is Political Authority Possible? Ed. D. Z. Phillips. *Philosophical Investigations* 25 (2002), 20 – 32.

ISSc
1963 *The Idea of a Social Science and Its Relation to Philosophy*. London: RKP, first published in 1958.

Introduction
1990 Introduction. In I. Maclean, A. Montefiore, & P. Winch, eds., *The Political Responsibility of Intellectuals.* Cambridge: Cambridge University Press, 1 – 16.

MSHR
1972 Man and Society in Hobbes and Rousseau. In *Ethics and Action.* London: RKP, 90 – 109. First published in M. Cranston & R. Peters, eds. (1972). *Hobbes and Rousseau: a collection of critical essays.* New York: Doubleday.

N&C
1972 Nature and Convention. In *Ethics and Action.* London: RKP, 50 – 72. First published in *Proceedings of the Aristotelian Society* 60 (1960), 231 – 252.

Preface
1990 Preface to the Second Edition. In Winch, *The Idea of a Social Science and Its Relation to Philosophy*, Second Edition. London: RKP, ix – xviii.

TTMS
1987 *Trying to Make Sense*. Oxford: Blackwell.

SWJB
1989 *Simone Weil: "The Just Balance"*. Cambridge: Cambridge University Press.

(b) ***Unpublished (on file with the present author)***

Winch, P
1988 Lectures on Philosophy of Law and of the State 1988. Manuscript, The University of Illinois at Urbana-Champaign, (ii+) 74 pp. Distributed to students at Illinois in 1990.
ca. 1993 Reason, Will & Representation in Rousseau. Lecture Notes, 5 pp. Distributed to students at Åbo in 1993.
ca. 1993 The Authority of Reason. Lecture Notes, 7 pp. Distributed to students at Åbo in 1993.

(c) ***Notes from Lectures (on file with the present author)***

Winch, Peter/ Lagerspetz, Olli
1990 Seminars on Authority. The University of Illinois at Urbana-Champaign. Notes taken by O. Lagerspetz, 39 pp.
1990 Ethics & Value Theory. The University of Illinois at Urbana-Champaign. Notes taken by O. Lagerspetz, 72 pp.
1993 Seminars on Authority. Seminars 13 & 21 September 1993 at Åbo. Notes taken by O. Lagerspetz, 6 pp.

Other Literature

Fest, J
1977 *Hitler*. London: Penguin Books. Translation of (1973) *Hitler – Eine Biographie.* Frankfurt a. M.: Propyläen Verlag.

Hare, R M
1963 *Freedom and Reason.* Oxford: Clarendon Press.

Havel, Václav
1990 The Power of the Powerless. In Václav Havel et al., *Living in Truth*, ed. Jan Vladislav. London: Faber & Faber, 36 – 122.

Hobbes, T
1839 *Behemoth*. In T. Hobbes, *The English Works, vol. VI.* London: Bohn. (*Behemoth.*)
1981 *Leviathan.* London: Penguin. First published 1651. (Page numbers in brackets refer to the original edition.) (*Leviathan.*)

Hume, D

1970 Of the Original Contract. In *Hume's Ethical Writings*, ed. A. MacIntyre. London: Collier-Macmillan, 255 – 273.

1986 *A Treatise of Human Nature*. London: Penguin Classics. First published 1739 – 1740.

Lagerspetz, O

2004 National Self-Determination and Ethnic Minorities. *Michigan Journal of International Law,* 25 (2004), 1299 – 1317.

Lassman, P

2000 Politics and 'the Fragility of the Ethico-Cultural'. *History of the Human Sciences* 13 (2000), 125 – 139.

MacPherson, C B

1962 *The Political Theory of Possessive Individualism.* Oxford: Oxford University Press.

Plato

1952 Gorgias. In *The Dialogues of Plato*. Trans. Benjamin Jowett. Chicago: Encyclopaedia Britannica, 252 – 294. (*Gorgias.*)

1952 The Republic. In *The Dialogues of Plato*, trans. Benjamin Jowett. Chicago: Encyclopaedia Britannica, 295 – 441. (*Republic.*)

Rawls, J

1971 *A Theory of Justice*. Cambridge, Massachusetts: Harvard University Press.

Rousseau, J-J

1967 *The Social Contract and Discourse on the Origin of Inequality*. New York: Washington Square Press.

1992 Emile. London: Everyman's Library, J. M. Dent & Sons.

Skinner, Q

1996 *Reason and Rhetoric in the Philosophy of Hobbes.* Cambridge: Cambridge University Press.

2002 *Visions of Politics: Volume III: Hobbes and Civil Science.* Cambridge: Cambridge University Press.

Spengler, O

1921 *Der Untergang des Abendlandes.* Band I. Gestalt und Wirklichkeit. München: Oskar Beck.

Watson, G

2006 Promises and Reasons. Paper at *Georg Henrik von Wright - Reason, Action and Morality* Memorial symposium at Åbo, 26 May 2006.

Weil, S
1987 The Legitimacy of the Provisional Government. Trans. Peter Winch. *Philosophical Investigations* 10 (1987), 87 – 98.

Wittgenstein, L
1980 *Culture and Value.* Chicago: The University of Chicago Press.
1972 *On Certainty.* New York: Harper & Row.
1953 *Philosophical Investigations.* Oxford: Blackwell.

LEGITIMACY, TRUST AND RELIGION IN A NORDIC PERSPECTIVE

Tage Kurtén and Ville Päivänsalo

What role can religion possibly play when it comes to the legitimacy of a democratic system of governance? In this article we explore the manner in which the Nordic societies, where religion is returning to the public sphere, are currently developing. The implications of such development are discussed, including a discernment of the ways in which this development could influence issues tangential to the legitimacy of a political system. Starting with a general presentation of the Nordic, hitherto mainly Lutheran societies, we investigate the challenges inherent to their traditional self-understanding of the church through an examination of the close similarities between the concepts legitimacy and trust. Certain main features in the present late modern situation are introduced and examined through a discussion of ideas from the modern liberal thinker Martha C. Nussbaum and theologians Stanley Hauerwas and William Cavanaugh, who are both critical of the modern liberal understanding of the state.

Legitimacy and trust

A democratic state is the institution most fundamental to a democratic system of governance. There are, however, other institutional levels relevant to a democratic system, ranging from municipalities to international organisations formed through agreements among (democratic) states. As Lars Hertzberg writes in this volume, legitimacy judgements may have different objects: 'They may concern the system of government or some aspect of it, the current holders of political power, [...] or particular measures undertaken by them.'[1] While we agree with Hertzberg's understanding of legitimacy, we nonetheless suggest that

1 See the article by Lars Hertzberg in this volume.

the concept of trust can help us reveal facets of legitimacy that are otherwise hardly noticed.

In those instances when a political body is seen to be legitimate, it would appear that a state of affairs exists where this body is fully accepted, that is to say it is not questioned. One can thus say that legitimacy resembles a relationship of trust. The legitimacy of a state, a political system and so forth can be perceived as one aspect of a trustful relationship between a citizen or group of citizens and the institutions involved in a democratic system. When citizens consider a state or its representatives legitimate, this can usually be discerned in these individuals expressing confidence in relation to said state and its associated public authorities. This can be described as a non-coerced acceptance of a system and its rulers. As regards trustful relationships between human beings, the manners in which trust and confidence manifest themselves in relation to a state vary across cultures and communities. A political system can therefore exist in many different forms yet still be found legitimate by the members of that political community.

Trust in its most profound sense is seldom explicitly expressed. It is instead tacit.[2] Trust in a relationship is for the most part taken for granted – as it is when an individual feels confident in the company of another individual.[3] In that legitimacy is analogous to trust, legitimacy *judgements* are comparatively rare. In normal circumstances legitimacy is *shown*, not explicitly communicated.

This should not, however, imply that the legitimacy of a political system is independent of other factors. We maintain that individuals' life-views, whether religious or non-religious, play an important role in determining what kind of state or political system is considered legitimate. These are not two separate issues, a certain life-view (religious conviction, philosophical system or the like) and the acceptance of a state as legitimate. Instead the acceptance of a system as legitimate must be seen as component of an individual's life-view. If citizens cannot endorse the legitimacy of a prevailing regime from the standpoint of their life-views, the bonds of trust between the citizenry and the state disintegrate. The primary causes for such can, in principle, lie either in the system of government or in a particular way of life, for example when individuals refuse to affirm a particular system. It is more likely, however, that a whole range of factors influence and cause this break down.

In a democratic society, citizens normally accept the state and the political decisions associated with the state, including the individuals occupying governmental, administrative or political positions. Through such acceptance, citizens express their trust in the state and thus the legitimacy of the rule of law

2 See Løgstrup 1962, 17-33; Hertzberg 1994, 124; Kurtén 2000, 103-106. See also Lagerspetz 1996, 6-10.

3 See Kurtén 2000, 98-100.

and the democratic system under which they live. Indeed, at least in the case of democracy, a trustful relationship can exist in harmony with quite vehement criticism of particular policies. Only when something occurs which disturbs the fundamental trust of citizens does the *question* of legitimacy come to the fore. Hence the legitimacy of a state, political decisions or political actors only becomes of interest when a reason arises to question their legitimacy.

Understood in this way legitimacy can also be perceived as a morally important phenomenon. KE Løgstrup provides a fundamental description of the tacit ethical demand confronting each morally sensible human being in encounters with fellow humans. Løgstrup has convincingly argued that an element of trust is embedded in most encounters between different individuals.[4] When you ask a stranger for directions to the railway station in a foreign city you trust that that stranger will not lead you astray. This type of 'trustful acting' is something that the other party cannot escape in that the trust shown is constituted by the situation and the relation. Very often trust is tacit. Individuals do not normally exclaim, 'I trust you!' out loud. However, what is most important, morally speaking, is that embedded in trust lies a demand that is demonstrated in different ways. It is a demand placed on an individual in regards to whom trust is shown. This demand is moral, inescapable and mostly tacit. It nevertheless exists in the situation.[5] We maintain that this feature of trust can also be seen *mutatis mutandis* in those relationships that affirm or disaffirm the legitimacy of a state or other political bodies. The legitimacy 'given' to a state (to politicians, public servants and the like) by its citizens thus constitutes a tacit demand that all state authorities take responsibility for the individuals showing trust towards them, that is to say those individuals providing them legitimacy.

Interpreted so, it is understood that a moral dimension exists in all state undertakings. An (implicit) demand is placed on state authorities to respond to the trust shown by citizens when citizens, through their actions, indicate that the legitimacy of authorities is taken for granted. Through their actions, these citizens justify the existence of the state and the state authorities in question.

Situations can arise in life between individuals where deep trust may transform into suspicion and mistrust. When another individual behaves in an extremely contradictory manner to what you would expect, the trust relationship is often shattered. When you discover your best friend trying to steal your car something fractures in your relationship, something that might be very difficult

4 See Løgstrup 1962, 17-33.

5 This does not imply that all individuals respond to such demands; some are capable of ignoring the demand, neither acknowledging nor wanting to acknowledge it. Nor does it imply that the trust shown will not be abused in many and perhaps very malevolent ways. The potential for evil in such situations can be partly ascribed to the inescapable element of trust shown in the primary relation.

to rectify. Normally you will at least ponder the reasons why you should once again rely upon that (former) friend.[6]

A political body can similarly lose its legitimacy. This can occur, for example, if a government does not respond to its citizens in the manner that the citizens expect. It can also occur due to changes in what can be called the overall framework in a society, such as citizens' life-views or the prevalent religion. We see that as Western societies have become more and more heterogeneous in religious terms, the connections between Western states and any particular religion have been weakened.

So far we have argued that legitimacy is linked to trustful relationships between citizens and different state authorities. Each citizen in a democratic society is, however, entitled to assert his political power by participating in elections and engaging in public discussion. Hence a sharp division between a state and its citizens is dissolved. We therefore seek to understand the relevance of trust among various social groups, whether majorities or minorities, to the legitimacy of political authority.

There are of course many factors which could be significant as regards the continuous trust that a citizen has in a state and its political system. We, however, focus in particular on the role that religion can play in the life of a democratic community.

Although the conceptual issues examined here are very similar in all of the Nordic societies, we have chosen to focus on Finland as a case study. We therefore present an overview of the relationship between church and state (religion and politics) in Finland during the past century and relate this to general development in Western Europe in Modern times. We also examine some central features in the current late modern situation and introduce a few new aspects tangential to the situation in Finland through the works of the American writers mentioned previously in the article introduction. We conclude with a discussion of the new perspectives garnered regarding the role that religion plays in the legitimisation of the Nordic-type political system.

Church and state in Finland since the Reformation

All of the Nordic countries have been dominated by a Lutheran tradition since the time of the reformation.[7] On a political level this has meant that as early as the 16th century church and state were considered separate from one other on a theoretical, theological level. The circumstances of the late medieval period,

6 Cf. Hertzberg's distinction between trust and reliance, with the former being spontaneous and the latter being in need of reasons. Hertzberg 1994, 118-120. See also Lagerspetz 1996, 40-54.

7 For the many aspects of this development and the present state in the Nordic countries concerning religion and state, see Christoffersen et al. 2010.

when church authorities exercised power to a high degree in most European countries, came to an end and the role of religion changed. Nonetheless, such development did not entail the immediate secularisation of political life and thinking. In all of the Nordic countries, Christianity in accordance with the Lutheran self-understanding was considered 'the Religion' for many centuries. This provided the church authorities considerable influence over numerous aspects of life in Nordic societies, including the Nordic people's understanding of political life. The Nordic countries were in many ways rather monocultural until the beginning of the 20th century and even in some ways still monocultural until the latter part of the same century.

A good deal of Lutheran theological thinking still assumes such a monocultural situation. The unique Nordic idea of the 'folk church' can be considered an aspect of this.[8] In the Nordic states it was important that the religious teachings of the church questioned neither the legal system nor the state itself. The state needed the church as a legitimating factor and actor. Theologically, the traditional Lutheran doctrine of the two kingdoms, the worldly and the spiritual one, has played an important role.[9]

The two kingdoms doctrine refers to the two different manners in which God rules over the world and its people. God rules the earthly kingdom through law and brutal force by using 'the sword', that is to say state and civil law. Through the sword, God battles evil: manifested in human beings as selfishness and rudeness and in social structures as injustice and oppression.

In Lutheran tradition each human being is able to achieve an external righteousness under the rule of law. Through reason each individual can achieve an understanding of justice and accept the legitimacy of a state that upholds justice. The political sector of a society is thus clearly separated from the religious realm and the church.

Law is, however, not the founding force of the church; instead the church is founded on the gospel. A member of the Christian church achieves inner righteousness before God through a gracious act by God, so receiving justification by faith. A Christian can spontaneously perform good works in faith without being compelled to do so by law. Interpreted in this manner there is no coercive power in the church, God rules through his word.

Historically, one important reason why religion lost much of its public political influence in Europe and, as a consequence, religion became a private matter was the 17th century wars in Europe, often regarded emphatically as religious wars. The religious traditions perceived as significantly attributing to the cause of these disastrous 17th century wars lost their legitimating power in

8 Two books pertaining to the folk church tradition have recently been published in Finland. See Björkstrand 2008 and Vikström 2008.

9 See Raunio 2007, 220-240. A description of this Lutheran doctrine and perspective can be found here.

the European states. Consequently, influential Western philosophers attempted to find another way of legitimating the state and political authorities through human reason. This trend has coloured Western political thought ever since. Philosophers have not, however, yet reached consensus on the matter.

Lutheran thinking has quite effectively dealt with this issue during the last few centuries. Emphasising a traditional theory of *Lex Naturae*, Lutheran social ethics perceives political questions as being linked to questions connecting all human beings through a common and consequently universal reason.[10] State authorities then, as far as they are considered rational, can rely on legitimacy support from the church and its members.

The institutional separation of state and church[11] has been followed by a more profound change in political sentiment. Questions of law and politics are seldom considered in religious terms.[12] Political language increasingly seldom includes any religious connotations. This is an aspect of the so-named privatisation of religion and the secularisation of politics, which has tended to parallel a liberal understanding of universal rationality.[13]

Currently, however, many thinkers have begun to question the idea of universal rationality.[14] Such doubt is an important feature of the emerging late modern sentiment. The mainstream discussion of the impact of criticism on universal rationality, however, has principally occurred in the Anglo-American context. In the Nordic context, consequently, there still exist plenty of related issues where Lutheran thinking has profoundly influenced the understanding of the relationship between church and state and which should thus be explored.[15]

As regards the aim of this article it is important to understand that the Lutheran theology mentioned here previously has supported the attempt by modern Nordic countries to separate state and church. Secular political philosophers have also expressed the desire to separate state and church. Until the middle of the 20th century, both secular and religious thinking supported the features central to the emergence of the modern state in the Nordic countries. In the present late modern era, however, a growing number of theologians and philosophers find it impossible to continue to support such a view.

---

10 See Svend Andersen's article "Law in Nordic Lutheranism", Andersen 2010.

11 Such a separation was near to completion in Finland with the introduction of the new church law in 1993. While in the other Nordic countries the state-church separation has not reached the level achieved in Finland, similar development is occurring throughout Northern Europe. See Christoffersen et al. 2010.

12 Hertzberg's notation in this volume that religion and sexuality currently seem to be privatised to a high degree, that is to say placed within brackets in public life, can be seen as mirroring the 'final goal' of this modern development.

13 So-named secularisation can also be seen as a development in which different sectors within a society struggle for autonomy from church authorities (and, as in many cases, also from political authorities).

14 See for example MacIntyre 1988.

15 See for example Ulrik Becker Nissen's article "Lutheran Natural Law", Nissen 2010.

The current late modern sentiment

The Nordic cultures have undergone change during the last few decades, as have all Western cultures in general. Some authors label this change 'Late modernity' as we will also. This choice underscores a situation in which central features of the modern way of thinking seem to be in decline. This is seen, for example, in political and religious life. The sharp distinction between politics and religion that has lead to a total separation between the two has been the deliberate goal of many actors in modern political and philosophical life. This trend, however, now appears to be waning. Jürgen Habermas acknowledges this when he admits that political discourse can no longer be considered entirely free from religious impact and religious overtones.[16]

The main reasons underlying this current development appear to emanate from certain features of the globalisation process and various spectacular events that have occurred during the last decade. Yet seen in a broader sense, one significant reason that stems from the changes occurring in Western countries emerges. Until recently, most Western countries have been dominated by one religion, Christianity, and one World-view, a technological-scientific view. That other world religions are seen more and more in the daily life of Western societies would appear to have radically changed the status of the thus far (pre)dominate Christian faith. Faith in the human ability to control nonhuman reality and human life through science and technology, extremely central to modernity, has also been questioned. This to a large degree stems from the perception of society that nuclear weapons and nuclear energy are dangerous and that science is incapable of handling environmental problems in a satisfactory way. Furthermore, the terrorist attacks perpetrated in the United States on 11 September 2001 (also known as '9/11') can be considered an ultimate 'eye-opening' event for thinkers such as Habermas, an event that exposes the complexity inherent in an attempt to build a political philosophy or legitimate the political arena based purely on secularised, modern reason that emanates from a kind of scientifically trained rationality.[17]

Sociologists of religion note that public discourse is currently undergoing a change. Religion is returning to the public sphere.[18] The direction that this ongoing development will or could take, however, is still open. Could religious (theological) thinking once again, as in the late medieval times, become a factor and part of a political (philosophical) discussion that strives to formulate a view which would give political life and the democratic state a theological *rationale* and thereby provide the political system theoretical legitimacy? Or does the

---

16 See Habermas 2005.
17 See also Habermas 2005.
18 See for example Heelas 1998; Hervieu-Léger 2003.

bankrupting of overtly secularised forms of contract theories (with their one-sided, secular accounts of the legitimacy of the current state) stem from a false understanding of how legitimacy can be reached? If so, how should philosophers address the question of legitimacy and understand the role of religion in late modernity?

When reviewing some of the main features of the move from a modern to a late modern sentiment, the following description emerges. Legitimacy is understood as a relationship or at least as being dependent on a relationship between a political body or political authorities and the individual members of that body, that is to say the citizens subordinate to these authorities. In general, legitimacy is more a matter of tacit trust than theoretical reflection and deliberate reasoning. Thus one can maintain that legitimacy is normally a condition that a political body and its members are in. It is only when something occurs that awakens suspicion or disappointment among members (or an individual member) that the question of legitimacy becomes explicit. Only then will the reasons for questioning a ruler, a decision or a legitimate (or illegitimate) system emerge.

One change in relation to modernity in a late modern setting appears to be the types of arguments that are likely to emerge. In that the role of religion has changed, religious arguments could become significant in a manner rarely seen in the highly modern Western societies during the latter part of the 20th century. The liberal quest for a neutral attitude towards all religion appears to be problematic.

In the next four sections[19] Päivänsalo will critically examine one example of a philosophical defence of mainstream liberalism. He begins by examining certain conceptual problems seen in Martha C. Nussbaum's view of liberalism while arguing that Nussbaum cannot fully perceive the role that religion can play in stabilising a political community. He furthermore maintains that Nussbaum fails to fully understand trust as a context-specific source of political legitimacy. In the three sections following those written by Päivänsalo,[20] Kurtén will discuss the ideas of theologians Stanley Hauerwas and William Cavanaugh, who deepen the criticism of mainstream liberalism by arguing for a relatively innovative view on religion and political life. The innovative views of Hauerwas and Cavanaugh are essential to understanding the concepts of religion and legitimacy in a late modern setting.

---

19 Päivänsalo has written the following sections: 'Liberalism, religion and late modern legitimacy', 'An American tradition of political liberalism', 'Strangers, democracy, and the emergence of trust' and 'Cracks in the trust-like legitimacy in Finland'.

20 Kurtén has written the sections entitled 'A theological critique of mainstream liberalism', 'Changing concepts - religion and politics in a new light' and 'Religion that changes the conditions for political legitimacy'.

Liberalism, religion and late modern legitimacy

Martha C. Nussbaum provides a most intriguing liberal perspective on religion in *Liberty of Conscience: In Defense of America's Tradition of Religious Equality* (2008). Nussbaum's version of liberalism strongly relies on John Rawls' pioneering *Political Liberalism* (1993), in which Rawls argues that fundamental liberal ideas can be endorsed by a broad variety of reasonable comprehensive doctrines, whether religious or non-religious. Nussbaum's extensive studies on Western antiquity provide her with impressive background knowledge of religious and political issues.[21] Especially her work *The Clash Within: Democracy, Religious Violence, India's Future* (2007) relates her ideas to a non-Western context.[22] Yet Nussbaum's account of political liberalism is notoriously Rawlsian and as such thoroughly modern.

We see in Nussbaum's *Liberty of Conscience* and *The Clash Within* that when liberals attempt to define 'reasonable' limits for religions they are unable to do so in a wholly acultural manner. Although Nussbaum has both vividly and at length written on the history of ideas, she appears to have adopted an exceedingly acultural liberalism and its relatively uniform liberal psychology. For Nussbaum, for a state to be considered legitimate both it and its background culture must be liberal. Her criteria for and definition of 'liberal' do not essentially change despite application in countries with quite dissimilar cultures and disparate contextual challenges.

Furthermore, the relationship between liberalism and trust is more complex than Nussbaum maintains. Trust cannot be brought about through a mere liberal imperative to trust. Trust instead is tacitly present in the more or less heterogeneous background culture of a society including the life-views of its citizens—otherwise it is not present at all. If trust does not exist at all in a society, problematic tensions in that society will be present.

In the West, the origin of liberalism is usually traced to the disruption of pre-modern cultural cohesion and the societal trust it maintained.[23] Hence liberalism was once able to prepare the way for a more trustful society. However, as William Cavanaugh[24] reminds us, the emerging modern state clearly held a monopoly on violence.

Nussbaum appears to assume that a self-consciously modern liberalism will always generate the societal trust needed in a society. However, if one looks

---

21 She has also authored, e.g., *The Fragility of Goodness* (1986), *Love's Knowledge* (1990), and *Upheavals of Thought* (2001a).

22 See also *Women and Human Development* (2001b) and *Frontiers of Justice* (2006). In the latter, Nussbaum sympathetically criticises Rawls' combined theory of Justice as fairness and Law of peoples for disregarding important issues related to the disabled, global justice and non-human nature.

23 For a comparison, see Amartya Sen (2005) regarding the emergence of reasonable liberalism in India.

24 See Cavanaugh 2002; 2004.

at the works of Cavanaugh and, for instance, Samuel Huntington[25] and Vandana Shiva[26], this assumption becomes questionable. Liberal accounts of the politics of equality and tolerance regarding religious issues, for example, have proven successful in many historical epochs but, without genuine support from a background culture, the power of liberal ideas is quite limited. In late modern societies these ideas do not have the privilege of being the most progressive. This development exemplifies how a feature that is unconsciously taken for granted (liberalism) can begin to be called into question. Thus the dependency that the legitimacy of the liberal state has on its background culture becomes once more clearly discernible subsequent to high modernity. Moreover, religions cannot be extracted from a background culture: they are destined to have an effect on politics through social and democratic processes.

If citizens of the United States, for instance, wanted to broadly support a liberal regime, there would be no conflict between liberalism and democracy. Yet tensions between the democratic process and liberal ideas have actually been quite common in the United States. We see then that the emphasis Nussbaum places on liberal ideas is problematic from the viewpoints of both democracy and legitimacy. Democracy provides legally established recognition of the voice of each citizen and, thereby, to the entire background culture; the concept of legitimacy calls attention to the deep, culturally specific roots of trust and thus complements the fundamentally procedural concept of democracy.

Liberal ideas such as liberty, equality, justice and reasonableness are often entwined with other moral and non-moral ideas in tremendously complicated ways. When analysing and balancing such concepts in a particular context there is no cause to decide in advance that liberal ideas should take precedence. Tragic events such as the violent episodes in Gujarat, India, and Jokela and Kauhajoki, Finland (to be discussed below) must direct us to deep analyses that reject the straightforward view that liberal ideas are the sole anchors of legitimacy.

An American tradition of political liberalism

It is conceivable that the politically liberal legitimacy of a state is found plausible in the United States because that country has a long tradition of such. In the United States political liberalism has also tended to generate trust across various religious and non-religious perspectives. Nussbaum, nonetheless, does not defend the American tradition of religious equality by presenting it as a familiar tradition from her home country but instead defends it through presumably universally valid arguments embedded in said tradition.

25 See Huntington 2002.
26 See Shiva 2005.

Consequently, she contends for example that Europeans could learn a lot from the American tradition of political liberalism.[27]

Nussbaum finds it alarming that various key representatives of the United States government have publicly endorsed monotheism.[28] She does not, however, wish to join the choir of public intellectuals that consistently denounce religion.[29] In a genuinely politically liberal spirit, Nussbaum expresses her wish to avoid 'arrogant secularism' as well as 'aggressively insular forms of Christianity' in her political liberalism.[30]

The essential concepts that Nussbaum employs to specify her position are liberty, equality (and equal respect), conscience, protection of minorities, neutrality, establishment, separation and accommodation. Nussbaum also defends a set of principles.[31] For instance, her Respect-Conscience Principle demands that the public sphere respect that citizens have different religious commitments and demands that it provide a protected space for conscience-based acts so that '*all citizens enter the public square "on equal conditions"*.'[32]

Even if we acknowledge that Nussbaum's principles are rather elegant, we must nonetheless admit that fleshing out the significance of 'equal respect' or 'equal conditions' in practice often involves highly contextual adjudication. Nussbaum's own historical analysis helps us clarify the contextual impact.[33]

In the Constitution of the United States religion clearly has special standing. The constitutional meaning of religion in the United States has been fervently discussed in connection with the exemption from military conscription that Quakers and Mennonites in the United States have been granted. The significance of this practice came under intense scrutiny during the Vietnam War when 'people were prepared to say more or less anything to avoid the

27 See Nussbaum 2008, 12-16.

28 Nussbaum (2008, 5-6) cites John Ashcroft's call for his staff to sing Christian songs each morning and George W. Bush's talks on the 'author of freedom' as cases in point.

29 See Nussbaum 2008, 10-11. Here she reminds professing public atheists such as Daniel Dennett that not all religious believers are 'dummies' and that many philosophers, including herself, are religious believers. Nussbaum (2008, 2, 14-15) is a converted Jew. Regarding the deeper significance of Judaism for Nussbaum, see for example her discussion of the music of Gustav Mahler in *Upheavals of Thought* (Nussbaum 2001a, 614-644).

30 Nussbaum (2008, 10-11) continues by asserting that this does not need to imply a literal, unconditional separation of church and state in that it would not be feasible anyway: 'Imagine what it would be like if the fire department refused to aid a burning church, if churches didn't have access to the public water supply or the sewing system, if the police would not investigate crimes on church property, if clergy could not vote or run for office.'

31 See Nussbaum 2008, 19-25.

32 Nussbaum 2008, 23. As another example, the Equality Principle states that '*all citizens have equal rights and deserve equal respect from the government under which they live.*' (The italics in both quotations are Nussbaum's.)

33 While Nussbaum (2008, 164-165) willingly recognises that interpretations of the constitutional clauses on religion have varied throughout history, she actively recommends renewed interpretations that take the guiding ideas of the American Constitution into consideration.

draft.'[34] Nussbaum courageously attempts to delineate the criteria inherent in public reason in order to clarify cases such as this. She plausibly contends that it would be practically impossible to grant conscientious objector status to any individual who refuses military conscription. The mere strength of the commitment of an individual, for example, should not make a difference; no one 'wants to give a draft exemption to someone who is intensely attached to his car.'[35] Instead, Nussbaum cites group-membership, ultimate significance and reasonableness as relevant criteria.[36]

Such a process of selecting/delineating the criteria relevant to exemption inevitably reflects the traditional culture where the discussion is taking place as well as timely challenges more profoundly than what Nussbaum admits. All of the arguments she presents rely on notoriously vague concepts. How strong must a relationship be to a traditional group to be considered strong enough? What defines the search for 'ultimate significance'? Who determines when a religious or non-religious view is sufficiently reasonable? In most societies it is of course the business of the courts to envisage practical solutions to such questions but without doubt the solutions presented are deeply influenced by interpretations of concepts that stem from the surrounding culture and political underpinnings. One of the subtle themes intrinsic to the background of constitutional argumentation and democratic politics is trust, for example as related to the fear of strangers.

Strangers, democracy and the emergence of trust

Nussbaum mentions that the fear of strangers has often been a major obstacle on the road towards full religious equality in the United States. American history provides examples of the fear of Roman Catholics, Jehovah's Witnesses and Mormons. In the case of Mormons, Nussbaum speculates that their polygamous practices are perhaps not that horrible after all and supports a rather inclusive attitude towards these groups.[37] As world religions have increasingly found their way to the United States, the accommodation process has been comparatively successful. Nussbaum emphatically maintains that the 9/11 terrorist attacks

---

34 Nussbaum 2008, 165.

35 Nussbaum 2008, 167.

36 See Nussbaum 2008, 167-174. The Quakers and Mennonites have long traditions of authoritative interpretation on this issue. Nussbaum continues by maintaining that the ultimate significance of religious concerns can be inclusively recognised not only in Theistic religions but also in Buddhism and Taoism, for example. Finally, Nussbaum takes up the search by American southern slaveholders for religious meaning as an example of an unreasonable view.

37 See Nussbaum 2008, 175-198.

generated surprisingly little hostility towards Islamic believers.[38] She regrets that European nations have typically maintained more homogeneity in the public sphere, which according to her has resulted in violence in the past and discrimination in the present.

In the late modern era, however, the homogeneous cultures of the past cannot provide the basis for political legitimacy on either side of the Atlantic. Late modern development calls forth a more heterogeneous cultural self-understanding within and across each region. The issues of religious and ethnic dissimilarity are often intertwined with the issues of economic justice and immigration, for example.[39] What seems evident is that for a trust-like legitimacy to emerge, trustful relationships among various groups that are 'strangers' to one another are sometimes needed. What seems less clear is that liberals, too, are strangers to certain groups. For non-Westerners, Westerners were originally strangers: strangers who at times have been liberators, at times conquerors and at times apt business partners. As Huntington reminds us, what Westerners herald as being universalism non-Westerners tend to see as Western and, accordingly, conductive to Western imperialism.[40] Similarly, proponents of liberal accommodation cannot simply assume that they are able to provide universal terms of accommodation and that all others should comply with their premise.

We agree with Nussbaum that as strangers become more familiar many ungrounded fears fade away and the space for peaceful coexistence and cooperation expands. However, in order to cultivate prospects for future trustful relationships, liberals must avoid promoting a liberal monoculture. A deeper analysis of the reasons underlying mistrust can on occasion highlight the importance of liberal ideas but a too programmatic approach in this respect rebuffs its own premise and is not likely to be successful under late modern circumstances.

A current issue Finns nowadays face is the challenge to accommodate immigrants into Finnish society. In certain instances the Lutheran Church in Finland has asserted its opinion on this topic, such as in 2009 when Finnish immigration officials refused to grant a residence permit to 64-year-old Egyptian grandmother Eveline Fadayel. Fadayel, who had already been residing in Finland for several years on a non-permanent status and sought to permanently reside in the country with her sons and their families, was publicly defended by Archbishops Jukka Paarma (Lutheran) and Leo (Orthodox) and also offered sanctuary by a Lutheran congregation. The archbishops stated that

38 See Nussbaum 2008, 346-350. She is of the opinion here that, in accordance with government instruction, American citizens were quite willing to distinguish between ordinary Muslims and terrorists.

39 See for example Amy Chua's (2002) discussion of affluent ethnic minorities around the world, including Chinese, Indian and Russian pioneers of economic globalisation.

40 Huntington 2002, 66.

the decision made, in this case by the Finnish Immigration Office, was inhumane and expressive of a peculiarly individualistic understanding of the significance of family.[41] Such actions do not fit into the liberal narrative, where the decline of traditional churches creates room for multiculturalism. The church instead in this instance became an advocate of multiculturalism and reproached a state that functioned on particularly Western and individualistic premises.

The question of democratic rights for cultural majorities also still remains unanswered: when the majority of individuals in a state represent a particular type of cultural inheritance should national policies disregard this majority? More fundamentally, should the liberal strategy be uniformly viewed as the best transmitter of trust when clashes among traditions occur? In *The Clash Within*, Nussbaum addresses such questions by providing an example from India.

Nussbaum discusses the Hindu right's fear of Muslims in India and finds the politics of the democratically successful Hindu party, the Bharatiya Janata Party (BJP), to be illegitimate. Nussbaum grounds her discussion in the violent incidents that occurred in the state of Gujarat, India in 2002. On 27 February 2002 it is believed that Muslims extremists attacked a train filled with Hindu pilgrims during which 58 Hindus, including 25 women and 15 children, were burnt alive in a railway coach. Nussbaum contends however that this incident might have been an unfortunate accident. Nussbaum maintains that, at a minimum, the Muslim group responsible for the incident did not attack in as organised a manner as has been officially reported and that the Hindu-sympathetic public authorities unfairly accused the Muslim group of terrorism. In the days following this initial incident, outrage among Hindus in Gujarat gave rise to mob violence that led to the death of more than two thousand Muslims. Nussbaum states that the violence was often cruel and included mass rapes and calls this second incident genocide.[42] Nussbaum's analysis of the Gujarat case reveals her effort to show that the BJP's fear of Muslims was exaggerated and wildly intolerant and violent.[43]

The BJP officially condemned the violence following the initial incident. Yet Nussbaum insists that the BJP itself is an essential part of the problem. From the viewpoint of social trust, it is noteworthy how strongly Nussbaum bases her criticism of the BJP on psychological analysis. While Nussbaum's deep analysis is illuminating it is also likely to intensify Muslim mistrust of the BJP and as such can negatively impact the peace process between Muslims and

41 Nobel Peace Prize laureate Martti Ahtisaari publicly opposed this decision as well. However, in September 2009, the Administrative Court of Helsinki upheld the decision (Finnish Broadcasting Company 2009). Nevertheless, the European Court of Human Rights ruled against the implementation of this decision. Fadayel died in Finland on 11 January 2011 at the age of 65 (Finnish Broadcasting Company 2011).

42 See Nussbaum 2007, 17-36.

43 Nussbaum (2007, 48-49) mentions Finland as one of the few countries that made 'a highly vocal protest at that time.'

Hindus. Her arrogant criticism risks unnecessarily weakening the prospects for a peaceful, democratic and trustful coexistence among the groups in question.

The Gujarat incident illustrates how deeply the concepts of trust and mistrust can be intertwined in the traditions of a particular nation or region. Without deep exploration of the root causes involved, it is not plausible to tell groups to disregard the past and begin to trust one another anew.[44] Moreover, Nussbaum's analysis reveals that when she engages in the deep analysis of root-factors her 'politically liberal' position becomes one stance among a myriad of others. Her politically liberal stance is perhaps well grounded but nonetheless subject to criticism from the standpoints of truth, morality, democracy and trust-based legitimacy. In sum, liberalism cannot generate societal trust merely from its own ideas.

Cracks in the trust-like legitimacy in Finland

The Finns have a long experience of surviving and developing as a nation and possess a tradition in which Lutheran Christianity has played a significant role. Now, when the Lutheran church has almost been completely separated from the Finnish state and the membership of the church is in decline, Finland seems to be close to the politically liberal ideal; all of the traditional privileges normally ascribed a singular religious view will soon be lost to history. Simultaneously, however, a large number of Finns are deeply concerned over what they perceive as the overwhelming power of the competitive market and the adoption in society of an ever-increasing techno-materialistic world-view: both possess religion-like features yet do not provide any ultimate meaning. Below are descriptions of two incidents that have markedly revealed the cracks that exist in the bonds of trust within the Finnish societal culture.

The most shocking outbursts of violence in Finland in recent years have been two mass school shootings by native youth. On 7 November 2007 Pekka-Eric Auvinen killed nine people including himself in Jokela, Finland while on 23 October 2008 Matti Saari killed eleven people including himself in Kauhajoki, Finland.[45] Auvinen and Saari are not the first to engage in such rampant behaviour, there are precursors abroad - in the United States and Germany. Neither Auvinen nor Saari were religiously motivated but were instead misanthropes who held strong life attitudes. A recent Finnish article in which Auvinen's Internet messages are used to elucidate his inner world is

44 Hans Küng (1990) has often emphasised that without a truthful dialogue among the representatives of different religions, the prospects for peace are not promising.

45 See for example Keskusrikospoliisi, Pääosasto 2008; *Suomen Kuvalehti* 2008.

dismal reading: he was bullied at school (as was Saari), admired Nietzschean philosophy and had recently been rejected by a (cyber) romantic interest.[46]

Whatever the primary causes for these two events, intensified competition, lack of trustful community and overtly permissive handgun legislation—common to both Finland and the United States—have certainly influenced the outcomes.[47] Following a second mass school shooting in Kauhajoki, commentators lamented how little the Finns had learned from Jokela. It was first after both of these tragedies that restrictions to Finland's liberal handgun legislation were urged. Some commentators have emphasised that Auvinen and Saari were individually responsible for their deeds while others have shifted blame for the incidents onto decision-makers. Yet virtually all have lamented that many schools in Finland lack a confidential community and that this same deficiency is also generally seen in Finnish civil society as well.[48]

These incidents have not undermined the legitimacy of the very basic socio-political structures of Finland. Many Finns however are genuinely perplexed. The traditional welfare state does not seem to provide an option for the future anymore and some native Finns are quite likely to feel like immigrants in their own country these days. Pekka Malmikunnas, an intriguing figure in Kari Hotakainen's novel *Ihmisen osa*[49] [The human lot] (2009), characterises this category of late modern Finnish identity.

The main objective of the examples from India and Finland has been to support two key points. First, deep conceptual problems exist in any attempt to define 'religion' or a 'reasonable' lifeview, and these problems have practical implications. Although clear examples of, for instance, unreasonable religions or life attitudes exist, the democratic process of identifying the criteria relevant to intolerable unreasonableness is culturally shaded.

Second, even though the liberal tradition has generated a lot of expectant trust across religious and cultural barriers, liberal ideas alone cannot produce trust-like political legitimacy everywhere. Violence is prevalent enough in the world to make trustful policies fragile, and liberal ideas have historically all too often accompanied imperialism and intolerance. This is not to imply that merciless realism would be any better as a general guideline but that the choices made in accordance with predominantly liberal, realist or even pacifist policies are more dependent on contextual challenges than Nussbaum seems to admit. Trust can be generated through liberal policies only if the relevant cultures possess the internal resources for it. It is not possible that one single set of

---

46 See Teppo Sillantaus 2008.

47 See Jokelan koulusurmat 7.11.2007: Tutkintalautakunnan raportti 2009. In respect to future guidelines, this report emphasises the prevention of marginalisation.

48 See for example Helsingin Sanomat's HS-panel (2008), where 80 representatives from Finnish academic and cultural life answer the question: 'Are politicians/decision-makers responsible for the Kauhajoki school killings?'

49 Translated as 'The human lot', Hotakainen 2009.

principles can serve as a fixed point for defining 'legitimacy,' even though in monocultural societies – whether liberal or non-liberal – this may appear to be the case. The criteria for legitimate practices and ways of life must be continuously and repeatedly determined, taking into account liberal principles as well as the cultural resources available for the formation of societal trust. And trust will always remain at least partially tacit.

A theological critique of mainstream liberalism

Both philosophers and theologians have recently questioned different features of the modern understanding of the state and state authorities. Päivänsalo has presented a critical discussion of Nussbaum's rather positive philosophical account of political liberalism in relation to religion. Kurtén will now discuss arguments by Hauerwas and Cavanaugh in order to deepen the theological view of religion and politics.

American theologian Stanley Hauerwas is an influential spokesman for those who criticise the idea of a liberal state. In the discussion of the relationship between church and state, Hauerwas criticises modern separation such as has occurred in the Nordic countries. Hauerwas maintains that the problem is not the separation in itself but the manner in which this separation is understood. Although Hauerwas writes emanating from a North American context, the conceptual problems he addresses are quite comparable to those being faced by all current Western countries, albeit with small differences.

Hauerwas examines two presuppositions in current liberal political philosophy that he finds to be problematic. The first is the distinction between the public and private spheres that has made political marginalisation of the religious sphere possible. The second is the separation of state and church, politics and religion, which results in the idea of the state being somehow superior to the church.

According to Hauerwas, the presupposition underlying the modern separation between state and religious bodies is the idea that a just and righteous state can be realised through liberal, democratic rule. The most important political questions can, consequently, be disinvolved from religious deliberations. The church can thus be considered to merely represent one voice among many that search for universally correct solutions and thereby contribute to the legitimacy of political authority. The correct solutions, however, must be independent from any specific religious outlook. What Hauerwas among others questions is the idea of a liberal state where the legitimacy of political authorities and the political decisions reached can be taken for granted due to a liberal sentiment that all citizens are supposed to embrace.[50]

50 Hauerwas 1999, 13-22.

Hauerwas still advocates a separation between church and state but not out of the belief that a democratic system and a common human rationality automatically contribute to the common good. In Hauerwas' understanding of religion, a state cannot *a priori* depend on religion to support it and provide it legitimacy. The idea of a liberal democracy being able to provide the best results, an idea still strongly supported by modern moral philosophers, has according to Hauerwas undergone an alteration in the works of postmodern thinkers such as Richard Rorty and Jeffrey Stout. Still, Rorty and Stout advocate continuing the liberal state. [51]

Hauerwas can be interpreted in more than one manner. The interpretation found to be important here is a reading where the liberal democratic state is criticised for giving the false impression that it only offers a neutral means for political decision-making. What is presupposed in this liberal idea is a faith in human ability to construct common policies on rational grounds. Decision-making, however, occurs in a political community and quite often on the nation-state level. While it is not entirely impossible that a community is capable of reaching a common understanding on shared interests, such interests are more often than not prejudicial towards or detrimental to those not belonging to the group making the decisions. [52]

In his recent work Hauerwas also criticises the modern state for its inability to avoid becoming a coercive power that decides over life and death.[53] The target of his criticism is the modern state and its monopoly on brute force. Hauerwas questions the omnipotence of every state, including those perceived to be liberal.

Perhaps we begin to wonder: what is the alternative that Hauerwas offers? One answer could be: a return to an old idea of Christian rule. Hauerwas

---

51 See Hauerwas 1999, 31-33. Hauerwas makes the following reflections on this topic: 'Should we not, as Christians, be about developing the epistemological and moral resources to save the liberal project? If we did that, might we not find ourselves in a less awkward situation by showing the church still has something to offer the world? For if a nonparticularistic account of truth is not forthcoming, are we not condemned to war between "local" polities? [...] These awkward times give us the opportunity to recover the locality of Christian salvation called the church. Without the recovery of such locality, of such particularity, we will find that we lack the means as Christians to challenge those that would make war in the name of universal ideals.' Hauerwas 1999, 35.

52 See Hauerwas 1999, 32-33. 'Ironically, since the Enlightenment's triumph, people no longer kill one another in the name of God but in the name of nation-states. Indeed I think it can be suggested that the political achievement of the Enlightenment has been to create people who believe it necessary to kill others in the interest of something called "the nation", which is allegedly protecting and ensuring their freedom as individuals. Rorty and Stout seem to suggest a more modest account of human ambitions that is extremely attractive, but one wonders if such moral modesty is capable of challenging, and in fact if it does not presuppose, our current nation-state system and the correlative assumption that war is justified in the names of such states.' Hauerwas 1999, 33. William Cavanaugh develops a similar perspective in his strikingly titled article "Killing for the telephone-company". See Cavanaugh 2004.

53 Hauerwas-Coles 2008, 1-3.

however does not advocate any such 'Constantinian' idea. Hauerwas instead is often accused of 'fideistic tribalism', in which Christians withdraw from the world.[54] Yet such criticism is also misplaced. If Hauerwas were to advocate fideistic tribalism it would make his argument rather uninteresting, in the opinion of this author.

What Hauerwas' argument underscores is the current importance of the church for any Western political community. The importance of the church does not lie in the offering of 'the correct political solutions' but instead in the presence of the church: a group of devoted Christian individuals in the public political sphere bearing witness of an understanding of life not automatically accordant with the outlook on life prevalent in a liberal society. The most important critical question concerns the self understanding of a political authority (or a political system) as being uncritically self assured. By its very existence the church represents a critique of every political authority (and political system) that is uncritically self-assured. Thus individuals representing the church equate to individuals representing a view of the world that radically questions each political body that strives for unlimited power. The only view in Hauerwas' opinion that can in the long-term counter such a yearning for omnipotence seems to be the view of a divine power greater than any self-sufficient human power. Hauerwas presents this idea in an approach where he speaks of the church as God's salvation for the political sphere.[55]

Hauerwas in this instance is in agreement with various other contemporary theological writers such as John Milbank, the Archbishop of Canterbury Rowan Williams and Hauerwas' own former student, William Cavanaugh. The following quotation from a text by Rowan Williams highlights a central point. Referring to St Augustine's discussion of the church and state in his book *City of God,* Williams writes: 'Thus if the pagan *res publica* is deficient as a commonwealth, it is not because Augustine polemically sets a standard of unattainably high righteousness of religious probity, but because a society incapable of giving God his due fails to give its citizens their due – as human beings made for the quest and enjoyment of God.'[56]

Many of us would feel at loss answering what this could possibly mean in a Finnish setting today. The religious presuppositions embedded in the quotation make it seemly incomprehensible in the eyes of a non-religious person. There is, however, a central point here. What these theologians are trying to express is that a modern faith, with a presupposed common human understanding of life in society and politics, should not be taken for granted. 'Not giving God his due' equates to the modern trust that human reason and ability are capable of building

---

54 Hauerwas 2001, 90-109.

55 'Rather it is to say that salvation is a political alternative that the world cannot know apart from the existence of a concrete people called the church.' Hauerwas 1999, 35.

56 The quotation is copied from Hauerwas 1999, 41.

a just and good society. The liberal faith in human reasonableness as *the* means whereby to make generally acceptable decisions is, consequently, seriously questioned. A state mainly grounded on such liberal faith must be considered a failure.

Changing concepts - religion and politics in a new light

In order to deepen understanding of arguments such as those put forth by Hauerwas, the manner in which William Cavanaugh describes religion in relation to the modern state is presented. William Cavanaugh is one of the contemporary theologians attempting to reinterpret Western theological history. For these contemporary theologians, the most important reappraisal concerns the Constantinian change in the relationship between the state and the Roman church.[57] Church historians usually assess the development following the rule of Constantine in the 4th century in positive terms. Certain contemporary theologians including Cavanaugh, however, maintain that problematic consequences arise from the close relationship between the church and worldly government. According to Cavanaugh, this close relationship has had long-term profound consequences both for the church and the Western understanding of the state. Seen from Cavanaugh's theological perspective, these negative consequences became palpable in modernity.

One overarching point in Cavanaugh's criticism of modernity concerns how the modern state rests on a sharp distinction between state, society and the church.[58] Cavanaugh would instead like to establish a new understanding of the church that eradicates this sharp distinction between religion and politics.

The development in modernity that accords a special body called the state monopoly over coercive power has made the authoritarian state possible, according to Cavanaugh.[59] In his view the so-named wars of religion in Europe in the 16th and 17th centuries were not primarily wars between 'religions', that is to say between different interpretations of the Christian faith. War was waged to help the modern central state 'create an autonomous political sphere from which would be excluded its greatest rival, the church. [...] what was at stake in these wars was the very creation of "religion" as a universal impulse essentially separate from an activity called "politics".'[60] The anti-clerical political endeavour underlying these wars was a fundamental force in the secularisation

57 Milbank 1997.
58 Cavanaugh 2008, 11.
59 Cavanaugh provides the military junta of Chile and its exercise of torture as an example. He could equally have presented the American Guantánamo Bay detention camp as an example. Cavanaugh 2008, 3.
60 Cavanaugh 2008, 5.

of politics.[61] Hence Cavanaugh concludes that our current distinction between politics and religion has never been *discovered* (for example by social researchers); this distinction was instead *invented* by certain key actors in a given historical situation.[62] This means that it can also be deconstructed in a new historical situation. According to Cavanaugh this is what is currently taking place in many parts of the Western world.

In Cavanaugh we find a radical rejection of the whole idea of the modern state, with its latent possibility to become totalitarian. Cavanaugh maintains that the current late modern development seems to entail a fading away of this totalitarian modern state that has been negatively defined in relation to religious bodies. This implies that the state in this current development should not be understood as resistant to change when new actors, for example religion, appear on the stage. Cavanaugh maintains that current development implies a radical change of the concept of the state and of the entire political realm.

One feature of such ongoing development is the idea, presented throughout this volume, that the legitimacy of the modern democratic state and its representatives cannot be wholly based on rational political philosophy but must be seen as something which is only expressed through and by the actions and reactions of the ordinary members of a political system, be they religious or secular.

Legitimacy understood in that manner cannot be isolated from different religious and/or moral points of view. Legitimacy of the state does not need to be defended by rational reasoning whenever it is questioned. The trust or distrust shown by individuals or smaller groups of individuals towards a state, and whereby the legitimacy of that state is expressed, can rest on many other things that individuals' consider important in their lives rather than the rational calculi (which frequently emanate from the idea of *homo oeconomicus*) favoured by political philosophers. This seems to be what Cavanaugh means when he speaks of society being more important than the state and of religion gaining a new role in present-day Western societies.

The whole concept of a political life that could still succeed in relatively completely excluding religious thinking from political decisions becomes an anomaly in this view. Seen thus, political life appears to rest on a false presumption concerning the character of the state, a presumption that, among other things, presupposes the profound Western separation of church bodies from state bodies.

If we apply this 'Cavanaughian' view to the current development in the Nordic countries, one sees that the Christian religion, and thereby the Christian

61 'The resulting appearance of the plural "religions" is said to make the secular state necessary, but in fact there is nothing inherently violent in religious pluralism and theological politics *unless* one assumes that politics means the totalising practice of the state.' Cavanaugh 2008, 5.

62 Cavanaugh 2008, 5.

church as a possible political actor, is no longer the sole religion in the social arena. The current Nordic societies are religiously and culturally divided into many different groups representing various religious and non-religious views. Furthermore, the role of church members in the various church and other religious bodies has radically changed during the last decades. No church authority, in for example the Nordic Lutheran churches, exercises any clear (religious or political) power over the members of their churches. The legitimacy of a political order must rest on the trust shown the political system by individuals representing many different views of life. These life-views are important and as such have a role to play in issues of legitimacy.

Religion that changes the conditions for political legitimacy

What Hauerwas and Cavanaugh are expressing is that the idea of a state which can remain neutral in questions concerning life and death, in other words existential questions, is impossible. The modern liberal and democratic state rests on an ideology, and this ideology does not automatically concur with other ways of understanding life such as seen in various religious traditions. Tension relating to different policies in a community appears to relate not only to concrete policy questions but also to the framework within which the political discourse takes place.

When religious ways of looking at life return to the public sphere there are no guarantees that different interlocutors will reach mutual understanding. In such a situation, the most profound means whereby to communicate is for individuals to honestly stand for what they find to be right and true without any guarantees in advance that others will agree with them. This is what Hauerwas is saying. In the Nordic setting this means that religion can be considered important for the legitimacy of the political system and political decision-making in ways that cannot be discerned in advance.

If we lose modern faith in a common rationality and in a neutral rational foundation for the rule of law, we must then accept that the legitimacy of the system within which we live and its political decision-making can be questioned in a manner that no individual can for certain predict in advance. There is no common solution that joins individuals together in a theoretically (rationally) manageable way. Consequently, the presupposition underlying the traditional Lutheran understanding of political life risks leading the Lutheran church astray.

If we cannot presuppose a common (rational) basis for life together, which traditional Lutheran Ethics has implied, what then becomes central is the articulation of the way of life we wish to embody, not the search for a supposed given truth of life in the community. Engaging in public discussion should entail an attempt to express one's own identity and not so much a search for a common (theoretical) understanding.

This ultimately means that a religious body must retain its identity as a religious body and not endeavour to adjust to the thinking of the surrounding, supposedly neutral political discourse. Through adjustment, religious tradition is in danger of loosing its religious identity and part of this religious identity can include firm opinions concerning which actions individuals should take. The following example will highlight the tension that exists between different manners of understanding the role of the church.

Lutheran tradition had for a long time led many Finns to believe that the church should neither discuss nor become involved in economic matters or more substantial political issues. The 1999 Finnish Lutheran Bishop's Conference, nevertheless, took a critical stand on the economic development occurring at the time. The Bishop's Conference issued a statement saying that they found the economic free market system, both globally and nationally, to be constructed more on greed than a mutual interest in the common good. They continued by stating that the prevalent economic policy of the time showed very little common responsibility for the worst off members of society. Representatives of the employee associations in Finland met this statement with astonishment and near anger. One of the replies from this group was that the church should concern itself with religious questions and not intervene in matters it did not understand.[63]

The reaction of the employee associations is understandable in the light of traditional Lutheran moral teaching. It is also typical of a modern understanding of life and society. Society today employs experts in all different sectors of societal life and non-experts are considered unqualified to provide opinion. This understanding is valid given the presuppositions of a modernity view of life. The example also shows how religion in such a framework can be marginalised on the grounds of principle. It is this marginalised situation of the church that current theological voices criticise. What, then, can be said about a church body such as the Finnish Lutheran Bishop's conference engaging in social discourse? Their engagement, seen in the form of a statement, can be considered an expression of the bishops' religious outlook on life. Interpreted so, their statement does not primarily seek to rationally convince each listener that their, the bishops', view is reasonable and correct. Instead the statement can primarily be considered an expression of a life-view. Their expressed stance does not necessitate agreement with their point of view. Yet neither is there anything that prevents others from listening to their voice. The manner in which politicians choose to listen to such voices is significant to the legitimacy of the politicians,

63 "Kohti yhteistä hyvää" [Towards the Common Good]; Hytönen M, Kirkko ja nykyajan eettiset kysymykset. Helsinki: Kirjapaja, Kirkon tutkimuskeskuksen julkaisuja 80. 2003, 166-170;

and thereby the state, in question, primarily in the eyes of all those agreeing with the statement made by the bishops.

Conclusions

To conclude our article we return again to where we began and ask how the socio-political role of the Lutheran church in the Nordic cultures of today can be understood and in what sense such understanding can illuminate the concept of legitimacy. As previously described, for a very long time and almost until current time the Nordic countries have consisted of extremely monocultural societies shaped by one Christian tradition, the Lutheran tradition. Among other things this has entailed the dominance of a classical Lutheran understanding of the relationship between church and state. The doctrine of two kingdoms and the distinction between law and gospel have been decisive in the manner in which the relationships between religion, ethics and law have been understood and expressed in much of Finnish, as well as Nordic, legislation.

Christians and secularised members of modern society alike have been able to together agree to accept a state and its authorities as being legitimate. A sharp separation between church and state, religion and politics has been an element of this common understanding. Yet in the late modern society currently taking shape, such separation can no longer be presumed. We appear to be encountering a changing concept of what a state is, where new features will determine the legitimacy of the state and its politics – reason and theoretical reasoning are no longer automatically the best means whereby to address instances where the legitimacy of authorities is being questioned.

The central question in this article concerns the role of the Lutheran church in the Nordic countries, and especially Finland, in these changing circumstances. Historically speaking, the Lutheran church has gradually lost influence over political life and the legislative process during the past century. The church has allowed other authorities to take over its political influence, all in accordance with traditional Lutheran theology.

This article demonstrates how the concept of trust helps discern elements that are otherwise difficult to discern in this situation and shows how those elements that are discerned in this manner constitute the legitimacy of the political system on different levels. Both trust and legitimacy are embedded in life circumstances where an individual feels confident in a concrete situation. We have highlighted trustful relationships between citizens and political authorities and among citizens themselves.

Legitimacy understood as analogous to trust helps reveal the significance of religion for political legitimacy, not least in a late modern setting. Legitimacy as one aspect of a relationship between citizens and political authorities is dependent on the life-views of those citizens. Through the manner in which citizens live, the legitimacy of political authorities is affirmed or disaffirmed. Religion is central to the manner in which religious individuals live. The same also applies *mutatis mutandis* to the role of a religious body, for example the church, in relation to politics and the state.

In four sections of this article, Päivänsalo has explored how such features have been neglected in the liberal philosophical understanding of political authorities and legitimacy. Using Nussbaum as an example of liberal understanding, Päivänsalo has demonstrated how concepts such as 'reasonableness' and 'religion' in a universal fashion are defined in the liberal tradition and how this liberal effect is limited in a late modern setting due to the contextual character of said concepts. He also has shown how mutual trust between citizens and different groups within a society must be considered an essential factor in the ability of a political system as a whole to remain legitimate. In the sections following those written by Päivänsalo, Kurtén has continued by delineating how Hauerwas and Cavanaugh offer a manner of understanding both 'state' and 'church' that implies a critical assessment of both concepts as understood in modernity.

Emanating from Cavanaugh, we can say that religion is returning to the public sphere in a manner that alters both the concept of the church and of the state. Religion and politics can no longer be understood in accordance with Enlightenment thinking, in other words they can no longer be separated. Politics must accept a much broader democratic discourse, where a common rationality cannot be presupposed. Members of the church and other members of society do not automatically share a common framework. In a Cavanaugh-inspired interpretation this implies that the church, like any other religious body, can (and perhaps should) become politically active in a manner not previously seen. We see two important aspects of this situation.

First, the church no longer functions as a political body in the same sense as in medieval times, with a politically important church authority speaking on behalf of the church. Instead religion, in so far as it can influence society, influences the development of a democratic society through religious individuals who anchor their political actions in the religious framework where they feel they belong. For example, as Cavanaugh suggests, liturgy can become important.

Second, if we extrapolate to the Finnish setting, the Lutheran church is only one of many different life-view groups in Finland despite that, as of 2010, approximately 78% of the Finnish population belongs to the Lutheran church. Accordingly, a consensus that emanates from life-views cannot be presupposed.

Generally speaking, in Finland such development will lead to patently changed conditions for the legitimacy of the Finnish rule of law. Both the issues leading citizens to question legitimacy and the way the legitimacy deficit is being addressed are changing. Religious traditions of different varieties have a part to play in this change, a fact that is more evident now than during the latter decades of the 20th century.

Late modernity appears thus to perceptibly influence the political life of the Nordic countries. If we no longer presume the modern idea of a society that is demarcated into narrow expert-led sectors, significantly more room will exist for different actors to discuss matters of common concern. There will also be considerably more space for explicit religious considerations, exhibited through the life and actions of individuals confessing different religious faiths.

In a modern society such as Finnish society in the latter half of the 20th century, the idea of a universal social ethical language, where particular religious considerations have no special part to play, has discouraged religious voices from being voiced in political discourse. Once this premise is radically challenged, the situation will have already changed. Profound change will not occur immediately, but there are many indications that we already are in the midst of such a change. This change is due to a new understanding of the church, common social life and the state and is demonstrated in the manner in which the legitimacy of political life is sustained.

Bibliography

Andersen, S

2010 Law in Nordic Lutheranism. In Christoffersen et al. 2010.

Björkstrand, G,

2008 *Framtidens kyrka. Herdabrev till Borgå stift.* [The church of the future. Pastoral letter to the Diocese of Porvoo.] Helsingfors: Fontana Media 2008.

Cavanaugh, W T

2002 *Theopolitical Imagination. Christian Practices of Space and Time.* London: T & T Clark Ltd.

2004 Killing for the Telephone Company. In *Modern Theology 20:2.*

2008 *Torture and Eucharist. Theology, Politics, and the Body of Christ.* Malden et al.: Blackwell Publishing.

Christoffersen, L & Modéer, K-Å & Andersen, S (eds)

2010 *Law and Religion in the 21st Century – Nordic Perspectives.* Copenhagen: Djøf Publishing.

Chua, A

2003 *World on Fire. How Exporting Free Market Democracy Breeds Hatred and Global Instability.* London: Arrow Books.

Finnish Broadcasting Company
2009 Hallinto-oikeus: Egyptiläinen isoäiti ei saa jäädä Suomeen (Published 4 August 2009). [Administrative court: Egyptian grandmother not allowed to stay in Finland.] Available at: http://www.yle.fi/uutiset/kotimaa/2009/09/hallinto-oikeus_egyptilainen_isoaiti_ei_saa_jaada_suomeen_977526.html (Accessed 30 September 2009).

2011 Egyptiläisisoäiti Eveline Fadayel on kuollut (Published 11 Jan 2011). [Egyptian grandmother Eveline Fadayel is dead.] Available at: http://yle.fi/uutiset/kotimaa/2011/01/egyptilaisisoaiti_eveline_fadayel_on_kuollut_2278005.html (Accessed 11 February 2011).

Habermas, J
2005 "Religion in the Public Sphere". Lecture presented at the Holberg Price seminar 29 November 2005.

Hauerwas, S
1999 *After Christendom. How the Church Is to Behave If Freedom, Justice and a Christian Nation Are Bad Ideas.* Nashville: Abingdon Press.
2001 *The Hauerwas Reader.* (Ed. by J Berkman and M Cartwright). Durham – London: Duke University Press.

Hauerwas, S – Coles, R
2008 *Christianity, Democracy, and the Radical Ordinary. Conversations between a Radical Democrat and a Christian.* Eugene (Oregon): Cascade Books.

Heelas, P
1998 Introduction: on Differentiation and Dedifferentiation. In Heelas (ed.) 1998 b.

Heelas, P (ed.)
1998 *Religion, Modernity and Postmodernity.* Oxford-Malden: Blackwell Publishers.

Helsingin Sanomien HS-raati
2008 HS-raati ei syyllistä päättäjiä koulusurmista (Published 25 September 2008). [HS-panel does not blame decision makers for school killings.] Available at: http://www.hs.fi/juttusarja/hsraati (Accessed 20 September 2009).

Hertzberg, L
1994 *The Limits of Experience.* Helsinki: Acta Philosophica Fennica. Vol. 56.

Hervieu-Léger, D
2003 Individualism, the Validation of Faith, and the Social Nature of Religion in Modernity. In Fenn RK (ed.), *The Blackwell Companion to Sociology of Religion.* Malden et al.: Blackwell Publishing.

Hotakainen, K
2009 *Ihmisen osa*. [The human lot.] Helsinki: Siltala.

Huntington, S
2002 *The Clash of Civilizations and the Remaking of World Order.* London: Simon & Schuster UK Ltd.

Jokelan koulusurmat 7.11.2007: Tutkintalautakunnan raportti
2009 Oikeusministeriön julkaisu 2009:2. [Jokela school killings 7.11.2007: Investigation Commission report 2009 Ministry of Justice, Finland publication 2009:2.] Available at: http://www.om.fi/Etusivu/Julkaisut/1232607489599 (Accessed 14 February 2011).

Keskusrikospoliisi, Pääosasto
2008 Tiivistelmä Jokelan koulukeskuksen ampumistapauksesta 7.11.2007 (Published 17 April). [The National Bureau of Investigation, Headquarters 2008 Summary of the Jokela School Centre shooting incident 7.11.2007] Available at: http://www.poliisi.fi/poliisi/-krp/home.nsf/PFBD/544F0B84A5C04A9FC225742E0029C866/$file/Jokela+end.pdf?OpenElement (Accessed 5 February 2009).

Kurtén, T
2000 Suspicion concerning world-views in *The Future of Religion – the Future of Suspicion. Proceedings of the 13th biennial European conference on the philosophy of religion.* Järvenpää, Finland.

Küng, H
1990 *Projekt Welthethos*. München: Piper

Lagerspetz, O
1996 *Tacit Demand. A Study of Trust.* Åbo: Department of Philosophy, Åbo Akademi University.

Løgstrup, K E
1962 *Den etiske fording.* [The ethical demand.] København: Gyldendal.

MacIntyre, A
1988 *Whose Justice? Which Rationality?* London: Duckworth.

Milbank, J
1997 Postmodern Critical Augustinianism: A Short *Summa* in Forty-two Responses to Unasked Questions. In Ward (ed), *The Postmodern God. A Theological Reader*. Malden-Oxford: Blackwell Publishers.

Nissen, U B
2010 Lutheran Natural Law. Thought in the Nordic countries in the 21st century. In Christoffersen et al.

Nussbaum, M C
1986 *The Fragility of Goodness: Luck and Ethics in Greek Tragedy and Philosophy*. Cambridge: Cambridge University Press.
1990 *Love's Knowledge: Essays on Philosophy and Literature*. New York: Oxford University Press, 1990.
2001a *Upheavals of Thought: The Intelligence of Emotions*. Cambridge, UK: Cambridge University Press.
2001b *Women and Human Development: The Capabilities Approach*. Cambridge, UK: Cambridge University Press.
2006 *Frontiers of Justice: Disability, Nationality, Species Membership*. Cambridge, MA: The Belknap Press of Harvard University Press.
2007 *The Clash Within: Democracy, Religious Violence, and India's Future*. Cambridge, MA: The Belknap Press of Harvard University Press.
2008 *Liberty of Conscience: In defense of America's Tradition of Religious Equality*. New York: Basic Books.

Rawls, J
1993 *Political Liberalism*. New York: Columbia University Press

Raunio, A
2007 *Järki, usko ja lähimmäisen hyvä. Tutkimus luterilaisen etiikan ja diakonian teologian perusteista.* [Reason, faith and the neighbour's good. An inquiry in the foundations of Lutheran ethics and the theology of diaconate.] Helsinki: Suomalaisen teologisen kirjallisuusseuran julkaisuja 252.

Sen, A
2005 *Argumentative Indian: Writings on Indian History, Culture and Identity*. New York: Picador.

Shiva, V
2005 *Earth Democracy: Justice, Sustainability, and Peace*. Cambridge, MA: South End Press.

Sillantaus, T
2008 Pekka-Eric Auvisen elämän viimeinen syksy. In HS Kuukausiliite 6 June. [The last autumn in the life of Pekka-Eric Auvinen. In HS

monthly supplement 6 June.] Available at: http://www.hs.fi/kotimaa/artikkeli/Pekka-Eric+Auvisen+el%C3%A4m%C3%A4n+viimeinen+syksy/1135241702685 (Accessed 4 February 2009).

Suomen Kuvalehti
2008 Kauhajoen surmaaja: Matti Juhani Saari (Published 24 September). [The Kauhajoki killer: Matti Juhani Saari.] Available at: http://www.suomenkuvalehti.fi/etusivu/uutiset-ja-politiikka/kotimaa/kauhajoen-surmaaja-matti.aspx (Accessed 5 February 2009).

Vikström, B
2008 *Folkkyrka i en postmodern tid – tjänsteproducent i välfärdssamhället eller engagerande gemenskap?* [The state church in a postmodern era - service provider in a welfare state or engaging fellowship?] Åbo: Skrifter utgivna av institutet för ekumenik och socialetik 12.

CAPTAIN, FIRE BRIGADE OR ICEBREAKER? POLITICAL LEGITIMACY AS A RATIONALE IN HUMAN RIGHTS ADJUDICATION

Pamela Slotte and Martin Scheinin

Introduction

Human rights are paradoxical. People speak in terms of human rights in situations where it would appear that the boundaries for how one individual should relate to another as a *human* being are crossed, in a manner of declaring: 'That's no way to treat a human being!' Consequently it is when something goes seriously wrong that human rights claims are voiced. In such situations human rights provide a manner whereby the harm done can be addressed and articulates that which has previously been more or less assumed. The web of relationships that enables a decent human life has broken down in some respect[1] or has, for various reasons, never been present to begin with.

Accordingly human rights are therefore supposed to articulate something that is deemed obvious, self-evident, commonsensical and unquestionable. Stating that a 'human rights violation' has occurred emanates from an assumption that a common understanding exists of what is being violated in a given situation. The assumption is made that since we are all human beings we should possess a shared understanding of human life and as such an appeal is made to a common humanity. Drawing on Roland Barthes, Zygmunt Bauman maintains that myths present history as nature. According to Bauman the task of myths is to present the humanely constructed as something irrefutable, and 'the myth of universal human rights' is no exception.[2] When human rights are invoked, the subject matter in a sense is not open to discussion.

1 Slotte 2005, 381-382. Of course, due to the power of the rhetoric in the world today, human rights may also eventually be purely used in an instrumental fashion. Here, we nonetheless wish to emphasise an 'ideal' that claims voiced in human rights vocabulary are want to.

2 Slotte, 2007a, 423; Bauman 1999, 9.

Yet human rights do not necessarily provide a definition of a 'natural' way of relating to human beings as much as they provide a platform and language for questioning and criticising what is actually taking place, thereby transcending 'natural' circumstances.[3] How something ought to be is asserted. Human rights, as ideals, anticipate something, 'They celebrate the transcendent, to-be-realized.'[4] As Costas Douzinas states:

> Human rights work in the gap between ideal nature and law or, between the existent and its transcendence.[5]

Due to the characteristics inherent in human rights parlance, human rights are perceived as standing beyond and above the political community. They are perceived as a fortification that hinders the individual from being completely overridden by communal concerns that have found expression in legislation and public policies. Such a perception is also underscored by the fact that human rights are also often invoked in exactly those situations where a clear or at least uncontested legal basis for arguing that something is a *human rights* violation does not exist. The term itself implies that, frequently enough, human rights cannot be legally enforced in that a disagreement or ambiguity exists as to which point of view the law actually represents:

> If human rights were legally enforceable, one could, and normally would, appeal to one's *legal* rights, and would not have to appeal to one's human rights. One appeals to human rights precisely when legal institutions fail to recognize and enforce them.[6]

This is also where a paradoxical facet of human rights becomes evident. We can speak of the Janus face of states: states are generally identified as both the principal protector and guarantor of human rights yet are also the principal violator of human rights. Human rights can for example be invoked when a state has not been able through legislation to accommodate the injustice and pain that certain groups of citizens experience. In such an instance the state in question has failed to sufficiently consider the needs and rights of certain individuals when interpreting what its duties amount to under a particular international human rights treaty. Yet states do enjoy certain discretion within institutionalised practices of human rights adjudication (which may be imperfect in their own significant ways) when it comes to implementing human rights, as we shall reveal in this article.

---

3 Slotte 2005.

4 Hastrup 2003, 20; Slotte 2007, 423-424.

5 Douzinas 2007,13. Douzinas concludes that the 'confounding of the real and the ideal is characteristic of human rights discourse'. Douzinas 2007, 10.

6 Cf. Freeman 2002, 10. Slotte 2007b, 90.

The paradox of a state being identified as both the principal guarantor and violator of human rights affects the human rights system in various ways. In this article we focus on how this paradox manifests itself: how human rights bodies, endowed with monitoring how states implement human rights law, are torn between affirming shared practices in regard to the interpretation of what human rights law demands in terms of state action and transcending 'the given' as a way to address the promise of 'justice' that the human rights ideal embodies. Human rights are equally 'a partially institutionalised practice and an anticipation of the future.'[7] We maintain that the concept of 'legitimacy' helps illuminate how human rights bodies actually address this paradox in their adjudicative practice.

Legalistically speaking, human rights bodies are given certain powers by states to adjudicate human rights abuses that are, by and large, perpetrated by these same states. The task of human rights bodies is also, simultaneously, the safeguarding of individuals. When safeguarding individuals, the views of a human rights body may challenge those views held by the political community of states that has established the aforementioned human rights body. Furthermore, as discussed in this article, human rights bodies are endowed with adjudicative powers by states yet often lack substantial means whereby to enforce their conclusions and judgements. Accordingly, primarily voluntary compliance with these conclusions and judgements would seem to indicate that states interpret power as being exercised by an authoritative body.[8] In other words, to paraphrase an observation made by Lars Hertzberg elsewhere in this volume, states which consider 'the government [of an international human rights body] legitimate may be said to give it [their] *allegiance*, or [they] may also be said to acknowledge its *authority*, or to *assent* to its exertion of power'.

Authority is related in this manner to how power is exercised, to the 'practice' of human rights bodies. The human rights bodies discussed in this article perform the delicate task of adjudication in awareness of the fact that their success is dependent on states trusting in their competency and voluntarily abiding by their decisions. As we shall demonstrate, the legitimacy of human rights bodies is unstable and depends on them proving themselves to be trustworthy in the eyes of the political community that they serve.

'Legitimacy' also features in the discussion of international law in other manners. A prime example relates to the conceptual legality-legitimacy pair. One contested manner of 'speaking' in terms of legitimacy is to retrospectively affirm actions, often a military intervention, that have initially defied the international legal framework and/or rules pertaining to who is authorised to act in a situation. Another obvious way of connecting legality and legitimacy to one other is to allow the latter to denote the moral validity of international norms as

7 Douzinas 2008, 13.
8 Kurtén 1998, 70.

opposed to their legal validity or legality. However, in this article, we do not focus on these ways of speaking about 'legitimacy'.

Rules that govern international relations

Let us expand on the ideas presented above and provide some general insight into the interrelationship between shared understandings, the ideal of justice that human rights embodies and political/judicial legitimacy in respect to international human rights. Mutual understanding and respect for the sovereignty of the other is a prerequisite for cooperation between states, both in regards to issues of form and substance. For example, a human rights treaty results from the joint effort of states (and other actors such as human rights NGOs or individual experts). Together states formulate legal provisions that articulate shared views on different issues. At the same time these provisions refer to something more profound than the mere will of the states involved as their normative basis. A human rights document is adopted when a majority, and primarily a large majority, of states agree to both its substance and qualification as a purveyor of human rights. A human rights treaty becomes legally binding when a state agrees to ratify the treaty and actually does so. When a sufficient number of states have completed this process the treaty enters into force. A human rights body tasked with monitoring the implementation of the treaty is also usually established as the result of such an agreement. Consequently, the human rights body will, through its actions, come to serve a political community of states.

The preparatory work associated with the discussion preceding the adoption of a treaty can prove to be an important source of law when, following its entry into force, a human rights body interprets the articles in said treaty.[9] An even more important interpretative principle in international law states that, as a point of departure, a treaty article should be interpreted in 'good faith' and that what is written should be interpreted according to the 'ordinary meaning' of the words.[10] This principle also indicates the idea that a shared understanding of life and language defines what human rights are.

During deliberation of whether a human rights violation has taken place, a human rights organ investigates, among other things, subsequent state practice in order to determine the substance of the right claimed to have been violated.[11]

---

9 The 1969 Vienna Convention on the Law of Treaties (United Nations Treaty Series, vol. 1155, p. 331), Article 32, attributes the role of 'supplementary means of interpretation' to the preparatory work of a treaty.

10 Vienna Convention on the Law of Treaties, Article 31.1.

11 When elevating state practice to qualify as a primary means of interpretation, the Vienna Convention on the Law of Treaties requires that such practice 'establishes the agreement of

It is through the incorporation of human rights law into national legal frameworks and the political decision-making processes of states that the definition of rights emerges in the form of concrete legislation regarding what is allowed, permitted or prohibited.

When adjudicating situations of perceived human rights violations, human rights bodies address all of these issues during deliberations. If a clear consensus among states is not discernable[12], the European Court of Human Rights (the Court), for example, is more likely to grant states some leeway – a so-named 'margin of appreciation' – in the interpretation of what a human right (such as the right to privacy) entails in their country.[13] The margin of appreciation indicates that a state, in certain cases and in accordance with certain clearly delineated grounds, may take economic, social and cultural factors into consideration when interpreting the manner in which its citizens enjoy the rights enshrined in the European Convention on Human Rights and Fundamental Freedoms (the ECHR). Article 8 of the ECHR provides an example of a framework for such discretion in regard to the right to private life.[14] While the doctrine of a margin of appreciation may be a specific creation of the Court, it is at the same time an expression of a more general idea of subsidiarity that is, in varying forms, universally present in human rights adjudication.

If a clear consensus on an issue among states exists, the Court will in all probability affirm this consensus in its decision on whether a violation has taken place or not. Shared state practice, then, is interpreted as expressing the shared understanding of the parties who are members to a treaty. If we extrapolate to the ECHR, these parties (those expressing a shared understanding) equate to the member states of the Council of Europe. In such situations the Court makes

---

the parties regarding its interpretation' (Article 31.3.b) instead of merely representing the practice of one or more individual states.

12 See e.g. *Cossey v. UK*, ECHR Series A (1991) No. 184, 13 EHRR 622, para. 40: 'Accordingly this is still, having regard to the existence of little common ground between the Contracting States, an area in which they enjoy a wide margin of appreciation (see the Rees judgement, p. 15, para. 37). In particular, it cannot at present be said that a departure from the Court's earlier decision is warranted in order to ensure that the interpretation of Article 8 (art. 8) on the point at issue remains in line with present-day conditions (see paragraph 35 above).'

13 See e.g. *Müller and others v. Switzerland*, Series A. (1988) No. 133, para. 35: 'Today, as at the time of the *Handyside* judgement, it is not possible to find in the legal and social orders of the Contracting States a uniform European conception of morals.' Human rights are frequently the focus of critical writings that argue that the contingent nature of all value preferences (which human rights are said to embody) effectively exposes human rights as expressive of particular rather than universal understandings of human beings and life. However, what the quotation here indicates is that an idea of value pluralism is actually inherent in human rights discourse.

14 'The extent of this margin depends on a number of criteria; the Court usually emphasises the degree of consensus among member states, and on particularly contentious issues it has indeed stepped back to await the crystallization of a common European approach and has sought to respond to political movement within the member states concerned.' Krisch 2008, 207.

reference to the prevailing conditions, attitudes and understandings in a political community that the Court, as well as the European human rights system as a whole, is to serve.

It is not always evident that justice, the ideal, will prevail when a solution to a conflict is sought by affirming the given, 'the factual', in this manner. Instead the applicants bringing a case before the Court could effectively argue that its search for resolution will affirm injustice. Here the shared, 'obvious' understanding of a certain aspect of human life is called into question and, as mentioned previously, human rights provide a manner whereby a significant claim against such state legislation and practice can be made.

The relative elasticity of what is 'correct' and 'just' is often reflected in the diversity of opinions expressed by the members of the human rights body making the decision. This is evident when the range of dissenting (or concurring) opinions that accompany various judgements are studied. The Court at times reaches a decision with the smallest margin possible. We also draw attention to later on in this article how dissenting opinions especially have become characterised as being expressive of human rights 'activism'. Judgements, in turn, are often reflective of juridical 'restraint'[15].

The judgements of the Court are 'declaratory'. The Court concludes in a legally binding manner that a state has or has not violated the ECHR. However, the Court does not possess any coercive means whereby to enforce its judgements even though the Committee of Ministers may adopt a resolution in which it criticises a state for a lack of compliance with a court judgement. Ultimately the Committee of Ministers can resort to sanctions against a non-compliant state through the auspices of the Council of Europe framework. What is most significant is that the judgements of the Court are not formally legally binding for other member states. Rather the judgements of the Court relate to a specific case in a specific state. In practice, though, the interpretations of the Court extend beyond specific, individual judgements:[16]

> Although the primary purpose of the Convention system is to provide individual relief, its mission is also to determine issues on public-policy grounds in the common interest, thereby raising the general standards of human rights and extending human rights jurisprudence throughout the community of Convention States.[17]

The fulfilment of the aim or 'ideal' of raising the general standards of human rights depends on states voluntarily complying with the guidelines that the case

---

15 Bruinsma 2008a: 'On the basis of an analysis of Grand Chamber decisions with separate opinions in the period 1998-2006 I have come to the conclusion that in the ECHR judicial restraint corresponding with the statesman's perspective prevails, and that human rights activism finds an outlet in separate opinions.' See also Voeten 2008, 422.

16 Gerards 2008.

17 *Karner v. Austria*, judgement of 24 July 2003, European Court of Human Rights, appl. no. 40016/98, *Reports 2003-IX*, para. 26.

law of the Court delineates. Hence the legitimacy of the Court within the political community of the member states of the Council of Europe is revealed through voluntary state compliance.

The independence and impartiality of the Court are important 'institutional' features that contribute to it being perceived as legitimate. 'Procedural' features such as 'the right to be heard' are important in regards to the legitimacy of the Court.[18] However, the judges of the Court are also cognisant that their authority and legitimacy relies on their not voicing views perceived as being too antagonistic in relation to member states. Voluntary compliance is thus connected to the quality and persuasiveness of the Court's interpretation of the ECHR in its judgements:

> The Court carefully has to position itself vis-à-vis the State Parties, navigating between the Scylla of providing too little protection to individual rights and the Charybdis of pronouncing judgements that are not compatible with fundamental views and legal or institutional constructs existing in a certain state.[19]

It is this last aspect of legitimacy that we primarily investigate in this article. To demonstrate how the points made thus far in this article play out in practice, we will now examine a theme addressed in other articles included in this volume, namely human rights as related to gender/sex, family and marriage, which are often described as 'sensitive' issues.[20] An analysis of the argumentation put forth in judgements related to these issues effectively shows how legitimacy forms an undercurrent when human rights bodies come into contact with the Janus face of the state.

The relevance of institutional history

In the second section we described the importance of highlighting how from an institutional perspective legitimacy forms an element in the relationship between human rights bodies and states. In this section we will explore the relevance of institutional history/memory in regards to the understanding of organisational legitimacy before investigating how the issue of legitimacy in the relationship between human rights bodies and states is realised in concrete argumentation.

---

18 Cf. Gerards 2008.

19 Gerards 2008. See also Mahoney 1990; and Bruinsma 2008b: 'In the sensitive area of human rights violations the ECHR has to steer a middle way between human rights activism and the judicial restraint of the lawyer-statesman'.

20 This is further highlighted by the fact that an *ad hoc* Grand Chamber of the Court (or before the entry into force of Protocol No. 11, the plenary chamber) has decided on several of these issues. A Grand Chamber decides cases that raise difficult interpretative questions, cases which 'seem to disclose legal inconsistencies' or 'touch on national or political sensitivities'. Gerards 2008; see also Bruinsma 2008a, 32.

How this seemingly feeds into the self-understanding of the (current) experts serving on human rights organs is discussed in section 4.[21]

The ECHR was signed on 4 November 1950 and entered into force on 3 September 1953 following its ratification by eight countries. At present 47 countries have ratified the ECHR.[22] In the discussions leading up to the adoption of the ECHR, the relationship between the national (state) and international (European) levels as regards protection and agenda setting in relation to human rights was a central issue. Both substantial and formal aspects were at stake and, as a Committee of Experts noted, the aspects were political:

> The Committee included their own 'preliminary draft convention' which they noted was 'drawn up on the basis of the Consultative Assembly's draft'. The Committee, however, pronounced itself unwilling to finally decide on the detail in which enumerated rights should be drawn or whether a Court should be included since these were fundamentally political decisions; it instead submitted alternative texts in both respects.[23]

When first drafted, it was proposed that the intention of the ECHR should be to affirm the human rights practice already *present* in EU member states – that is to say the 'natural' or 'actual' state of affairs in terms of prevailing official understanding of what a state owes its citizens:

> The [Legal] Committee unanimously agreed that for the moment, only those essential rights and fundamental freedoms could be guaranteed which are, to-day, defined and accepted after long usage, by the democratic regimes.[24]

As pertains to substance, however, the final version of the ECHR is a compromise between merely enumerating rights and highly detailed rights clauses.[25] Through the more generally formulated rights articles, one sees that a

---

21 Different legal sociological studies have been conducted that examine if (and if so when) the behaviour of the judges of the Court and experts in the Commission are influenced by their professional backgrounds and their nationality. However, the perspective on the issue put forth in this article differs from such a perspective.

22 Simplified Chart of signatures and ratifications to the ECHR, status as of: 26/4/2011. At: http://conventions.coe.int/Treaty/Commun/ListeTableauCourt.asp?MA=3&CM=16&CL=ENG (24.4.2011)

23 Janis et al. 2008, 18; 4 *Travaux Préparatoires*, 14, 16 (Council of Europe, *Collected edition of the 'Travaux préparatoires' of the European Convention on Human Rights*. 8 volumes. The Hague/ Boston/ London/ Dordrecht/ Lancaster: Martinus Nijhoff, 1975-1985. Hereafter *Travaux Préparatoires*).

24 1 *Travaux Préparatoires*, 218. A pragmatic reason existed for why this appeared to be an acceptable manner whereby to address the present political situation. 'Everyone will, however, understand that it is necessary to begin at the beginning and to guarantee political democracy in the European Union and then to co-ordinate our economies, before undertaking the generalization of social democracy.' Rask Madsen 2007, 142, quoting Pierre-Henri Teitgen, as presented in Merrills & Robertson 2001, 8.

25 Janis et al. 2008, 18; 4 *Travaux Préparatoires*, 246-248.

'space to manoeuvre' has been built into the treaty. Moreover, while the sovereignty of individual states is affirmed in regards to the protection of these rights and freedoms and the interpretation of what this protection legally and practically entails is delineated, a call also exists for the 'establishment of a collective guarantee of essential freedoms and fundamental rights'.[26] Thus the ECHR acknowledges that the Janus face of the state wishes to manoeuvre as it itself desires.

An early draft proposal of the ECHR included the right of individual petition: individuals would apply to a commission that was to be established alongside a court, with the commission being able to refer cases to the court. This was controversial.[27] It was initially believed that the establishment of a court to deal with individual petitions would challenge the 'sanctity of state sovereignty'[28] that was at stake. A court was eventually established, but the European countries were nonetheless still split over the right of individual petition. Some countries feared 'that the right of petition might easily lead to abuse, particularly in the interests of subversive propaganda'.[29] It was difficult for states to agree on the judicial jurisdiction of the proposed court. Because of the divisiveness surrounding these issues, a compromise was brokered in which both the right of individual petition and the judicial jurisdiction of the proposed court were made optional in the original version of the Convention.[30]
For a long time, many European governments shied away from these optional clauses. One could say that they were not willing to consent to being governed in the innovative manner being developed:

> Historically, the Europeans were familiar with bills of rights but, unlike the Americans, they were generally unfamiliar with judicial enforcement of those rights. Domestically, they trusted the legislative and executive branches of government rather than the judicial branch to protect fundamental freedoms.[31]

The conviction existed that it is the states themselves that are the proper subjects of international law, not individuals. States are the protectors and interpreters of rights. It was argued that when a state signs up to a treaty, it does so because its national legislation *conforms* to the treaty in question[32], that is to say human rights protection already exists in its own legal system. It was also argued that the human rights protection of a state willing to sign up to a treaty is already effective. It would appear that the ECHR is mainly perceived to be an instrument that can be wielded against threats to a liberal democratic society, a

26 1 *Travaux Préparatoires*, 216.
27 1 *Travaux Préparatoires*, 228-234.
28 Janis et al. 2008, 16. See also Rask Madsen 2007.
29 4 *Travaux Préparatoires*, 252.
30 1 *Travaux Préparatoires*, xxvi-xxviii.
31 Janis et al. 2008, 19. See also Frohwein 1984.
32 Janis et al. 2008, 20. See also e.g. Rask Madsen 2007, 153.

type of society to which the original ratifying Western European states subscribe:

> More precisely, the Convention was mainly assumed to provide the legal and political means for deterring the future rise of any sort of fascism in Europe – from within or from the outside – rather than, at least initially, being the instrument for substantially altering or unifying the practices of the legal systems in the member states.[33]

Still, little by little attitudes and actual practice changed. Countries began to recognise the right of the Commission to hear individual cases, a role it acquired in practice in 1955.[34] In 1950 doubt existed as to whether the required number of eight state ratifications delineated in the optional clause establishing a court would ever be achieved. Yet by 1958 this number was met and the Court began its work in 1959.[35] The workload of the Commission and the Court was initially relatively meagre. The Commission admitted 54 applications in the 1960s, whereof 49 were individual petitions, and the Court rendered 10 judgements after not having been referred a single case in the 1950s.[36] While the Court slowly established itself during the 1970s, the real turning point occurred in the 1980s. By May 1990, all of the members of the Council of Europe, including Finland as the newest member, had ratified the ECHR and acknowledged the jurisdiction of the Court as well as the individual right to petition. The caseload of the Commission and the Court accordingly multiplied, continuing throughout the 1990s. The membership to the Council of Europe and the ECHR had almost doubled by the late 1990s.[37]

By the late 1990s all members of the Council of Europe had consented to the two optional clauses that, with the passage of time, were perceived as legally optional yet politically non-optional. At the same time the caseload of the Court became almost unmanageable. The Commission and the Court were merged in 1998 in an attempt to reform the system, and through this reform both the jurisdiction of the Court and the right of individual petition were also made legally mandatory for any state party to the Convention. It is frequently pointed

33 Rask Madsen 2007, 140. See also Rask Madsen 2007, 144-147, for an account of what this 'mental and political externalization' meant for different member states, especially France and the United Kingdom.

34 The Commission was charged with the following task: 'On the one hand, the Commission was meant to shield the Court from a possible deluge of individual complaints, a function that also protected the traditional sovereignty of the member states. On the other hand, the Commission was meant to serve as an international institution directly accessible to individuals, a radical departure from traditional state-centred international legal process. Fashioned and acting in compromise, the Commission stood as an intermediary both between individuals and governments, and between individuals and the Strasbourg Court.' Janis et al. 2008, 25.

35 Janis et al. 2008, 70; Rask Madsen 2007, 144.

36 Janis et al. 2008, 21.

37 Janis et al. 2008, 22; Rask Madsen 2007, 154-155.

out that the Court was a victim of its own success, and the figures speak for themselves. During 2000-2005 the Court received 220254 applications, whereof 5022 are declared admissible; the Court also delivers 4954 judgements during this period of time.[38] So what does the history of the development of the Court and the Commission tell us as regards legitimacy?

> From its inception, the Strasbourg organs were dependent on a positive stance by national authorities; with no enforcement tools at their disposal, compliance had to be essentially voluntary. If the Court and Commission wanted to become influential, they needed to establish, on the one hand, their authority as impartial and trustworthy interpreters of the Convention; on the other, they had to take care not to upset national authorities so much as to provoke a backlash. This posed a dilemma, as the image of impartiality could easily be undermined by sensitivity for the concerns of particular member states, but Strasbourg managed to navigate between the two poles with great talent.[39]

The Court does not initially enjoy any self-evident legitimacy. It must *acquire* legitimacy. We may therefore speak of legitimacy in relation to the Court in terms of something that must be constructed and 'defended'. Drawing on the terminology used by Malena Björkgren and Lise Kanckos in another article found in this volume, we might speak of an unstable legitimacy. The Court needs to win the confidence and trust of the member states to the ECHR, and this is accomplished in the early days by treading carefully.[40] As noted in the quotation above, sensitivity may undermine the image of the Court as an impartial adjudicator but is nonetheless simultaneously vital to its work. Legitimacy is gained through discretion. In addition to a group of legal experts with professional academic backgrounds, the first years of the Court were 'conveniently' influenced by the strong presence of a group of legal experts with a background in diplomacy[41]:

> Its [the ECHR system's] initial operation was dominated by a group of high-level legal experts who managed to both develop its legal functionality and appear unthreatening to central national political interests. These jurists deployed a tacit understanding of the relationship between law and diplomacy, using the latter when

38 Janis et al. 2008, 21, 23; Rask Madsen 2007, 155.

39 Krisch 2008, 206. See also Helfer & Slaughter 1997, 307-328.

40 Janis et al. 2008, 88, quoting Beddard 1980, 4; Rask Madsen 2007, 139, 148. The same is true regarding the Commission. 'In the early years, this involved strong elements of diplomacy: the EComHR often assumed a mediatory rather than adjudicatory role, much to the dismay of many legal scholars, but with the result of allaying member states' fears of an overly aggressive enforcement of human rights.' Krisch 2008, 206. Issues are dismissed by the Commission during the application phase, and political sensitivity is sometimes proffered as the rationale for dismissal. Janis et al. 2008.

41 Rask Madsen 2007, 148-149.

> confronted with high-political questions related to decolonization or high national politics.[42]

'In its early decisions, the Court seemed anxious to reassure its member states that it would be sensitive to their concerns and traditions'. It was not until 1968 that the Court rendered a judgement against a member state (the *Neumeister* case).[43] The Court needed to gradually convince 'the member states that it should be taken seriously'.[44] However, from the end of the 1970s onwards a new set of Strasbourg judges were 'increasingly ready to upset member states with decisions that stretch the language of the Convention'[45]:

> However, this readiness to upset states was a risky business. States did not need to accept either the jurisdiction of the Court or the right of individual petition. Both were optional clauses, part of the compromise reached in the process of drafting the Convention. If the Court was perceived by a state as going 'too far', then the state could decide not to renew its acceptance of the optional clauses.[46]

Therefore, if we consider the Court in its early existence to be 'a sleeping beauty, frequently referred to but without much impact'[47], once private parties are allowed the right to petition the Court it awakes from its dreamlike state.[48] One can question, however, whether the Court feels assured by the new group whose legitimacy it enjoys and who it feels it represents.[49] '[T]he Court increasingly represented an important legal forum for contesting claims of a broader group of applications, including the media, trade unions and many others.'[50] At this time human rights centres, such as the Danish Institute for

---

42 Rask Madsen 2007, 138.

43 Janis et al. 2008, 75-76. See also Rask Madsen 2007, 150-151.

44 Rask Madsen 2007, 151. The Court portrays itself as 'reliable, respectable, and legally conservative'. 'In other words, the ECHR system appeared to pose no significant threat to the specificities of the national ways of securing human rights and justice-as long as they were *justified*.' Rask Madsen 2007, 151.

45 Janis et al. 2008, 76; Rask Madsen 2007, 152-154. See also Morrisson 1981, 19. Voeten describes this trend in terms of an increased activism on the part of the Court. Voeten 2008, 422. See also Mowbray 2005, 57-79. However, a unanimous Court is not in the making: instead both progressive and conservative forces are at work, seen primarily in the many dissenting opinions of Judge Sir Gerald Fitzmaurice. Rask Madsen 2007, 153.

46 Janis et al. 2008, 76.

47 Frohwein 1984, 8.

48 Janis et al. 2008, 74-75.

49 A recently interviewed judge has concluded that: 'The way of thinking is different to all other multicultural institutions that I worked in: we all share a common approach and a mutual understanding for the differences on the surface level, and we share the same fundamental approach. (…) There are differences of style which could be described by national differences, but those are at the surface. And in the deeper sense, what I understand as legal culture, the deeper values, there I don't see any real difference (…) The ideal has always been to enhance the rule of law and to help individuals against the state…'. Anonymous judge, interview quoted in Arold 2007a, 320.

50 Rask Madsen 2007, 154.

Human Rights and the Raoul Wallenberg Institute of Human Rights and Humanitarian Law in Sweden, are established throughout Europe.[51]

As mentioned previously the member states of the Council of Europe met the establishment of the Court with scepticism, and the main cause of this scepticism pertained to the role of the Court. Member states exhibited wariness in allowing the international legal examination of 'national' affairs, expressed as an initial caution in agreeing to the optional clauses (the right to individual petition and the jurisdiction of the Court) to the ECHR. Legitimacy here is in some manner connected to representation. It is not self-evident who is representing whom. The optional clauses allow the Court, in relation to member states, to act as a representative for those individual citizens who claim that their human rights are being violated in a specific state. This then begs the question: what of state sovereignty? Again, the establishment of the European human rights system seemingly challenges modern conceptions of state sovereignty.

The Court (and the Commission) initially lacked institutional autonomy and institutional legitimacy.[52] However, over time, the Court appeared to enjoy legitimacy in and of itself and not merely as an extension of governmental (state) action. This is discernable in the change in perception regarding individual petition that states had. When first established, individuals could not at address the Court directly; instead the Commission referred a case to the Court and acted on behalf of the applicant initiating the proceedings. This was first changed in 1994 when the circle of who could refer a case to the Court (through the Commission) was expanded and last changed in 1998 when the Commission and Court were merged and individuals (including groups of individuals and non-governmental organisations) were given the right to bring cases against state parties in relation to the ECHR.[53] The optional clauses that had, until then, been *de facto* accepted by member states were now legally mandated.[54] Again, as mentioned previously, one should remember that these clauses had for some time already been considered *politically* obligatory.

Thus the Court is today seemingly more established. Member states are not hesitant in signing up to the ECHR, even if the possibility exists that a specific judgement could go against them. Member states not directly affected by a judgement are expected to take due note of Court 'precedents'. The legitimacy of the Court is thus in this manner manifested in member states' *acceptance* of the judgements of the Court. In this volume, the legitimacy of an institution and the legitimacy of a specific action, judgement or law are differentiated between. Thus the legitimacy of the Court is not dependent on whether or not a specific judgement or rule is deemed legitimate. Even if it runs contrary to its wishes and

---

51 Rask Madsen 2007, 154.
52 Rask Madsen 2007, 137-138, 148-159.
53 Janis et al. 2008, 72-73.
54 Janis et al. 2008, 88; Voeten 2008, 418.

interests, a state may still abide by a judgement because the judgement has been issued by a body which that state regards as authoritative. Nevertheless, even if other aspects related to a ruling are also important, the legitimacy of a judgement is not independent of the legitimacy of the Court:

> The legitimacy of a given judicial decision thus stands and falls in large measure on the logic and argumentation of the signed judgement, not the structural legitimacy of the entire judicial apparatus from which it hails.[55]

Mark Janis also connects the legitimacy of specific judgements to the legitimacy of an institution itself when discussing the European human rights system:

> [T]he actors within the [Strasbourg legal] system, both governments and individual litigants, as well as their lawyers, recognize the Strasbourg rules *and* the Strasbourg institutions as legitimate.[56]

As previously mentioned, the efficacy of the Court can be linked to the question of its legitimacy. Janis, too, emphasises this link by stating that 'there is little doubt that the efficacy of the European Court of Human Rights depends in good measure on its perception as a 'legitimate' institution, accepted as a rule enforcer across Europe'.[57] The Committee of Ministers oversees compliance with Court judgements. The ultimate sanction available in cases of non-compliance is the expulsion of a state from 'the club'. The only country to have ever withdrawn from the Council of Europe, by denouncing the ECHR and disavowing itself from the supervision of the European Commission, is Greece. Greece withdrew from the Council in 1969 to prevent the Council from ejecting the country in 1970 due to its significant human rights violations. On the whole, however, states have voluntarily 'complied' with the decisions of the Commission and the judgements of the Court and have overseen administrative and legislative remedies such as amendments of national legislation and the provision of monetary compensation to victims[58], despite some variation in attitudes. Janis explains that in practice 'perceptions of the legitimacy of the Court vary'.[59]

55 Lasser 2004, 338.

56 Janis et al. 2008, 107.

57 Janis et al. 2008, 109.

58 Janis et al. 2008, 64-66, 74; Voeten 2008, 419. Yet some caution is needed when asserting that states comply with Court judgements. There has been no general pan-European study of the issue. This is also true for the substantive legal framework. 'What is missing are general studies about how Strasbourg legal rules, whether in the form of the Convention's substantive provisions or in the precedent-like norms created by the Strasbourg institutions, have or have not influenced the actual practice of states or governments.' Janis et al. 2008, 104-106.

59 Janis et al. 2008, 109. See also Voeten 2008, 319, for examples of recent public criticism of Court judgements. Hertzberg makes a similar observation regarding the concept legitimacy

For Janis the question of legitimacy becomes 'the most crucial 'practical' test' of the efficacy of the legal system. Janis nonetheless notes that testing the 'recognition of the legitimacy' is difficult and that it has generally not been attempted, only asserted. In trying to focus on legitimacy, Janis highlights factors mentioned previously in this section: the vast caseload of the Court, the acceptance that prior to 1998 the optional clauses were in essence politically mandated, the fact that states accede to the Council of Europe and ratify the ECHR. These factors, Janus argues, 'point to individuals, governments, and lawyers in Europe taking the system more seriously and perhaps to the conclusion that the players increasingly recognize the system's legitimacy'.[60] Janis nevertheless does recognise that legitimacy is *relative* and that while an 'increase' can be discerned it is difficult to come to any definite conclusion other than this. Moreover, every relationship between a state and the legal system is unique:

> [T]ests of recognition of legitimacy do not easily form part of either legal or, even, political analysis. Gauging recognition of legitimacy of legal systems may be more a psychological, rather than a legal or political, exercise and in any case difficult to ascertain in any sort of definite way. This may well be true for most any legal system, domestic or international. [61]

It is conceivable then that to a certain degree an institution implicitly acquires legitimacy by forming part of the life of a community over time, for example the community made up of the Council of Europe and its member states. The evolution of the Court indicates a trend that the legitimacy of the Court as an institution is increasing. At the very least it is possible to maintain that the Court today enjoys a different kind of legitimacy than previously.

We understand that legitimacy is not something that is settled definitely but is rather something that may or may not be a feature in a relationship and is, as Janis points out, relative. Legitimacy can be gained and it can be forfeited. The Court accordingly continuously struggles with the question of how sensitivity is shown to a member state, that is to say how member states are 'represented' or taken into consideration, while through its judgements the Court simultaneously takes a stand in internal conflicts in relation to the acceptability of the actions of public authorities.

A judgement can challenge previously accepted views on to what extent states may emphasise national interests, needs and assumptions when they interpret the rights delineated in the ECHR. Some member states have lamented the increased activism of the Court, a result of the more 'legalistic and dynamic

---

in another contribution to this volume. A certain political entity can enjoy 'varying degrees of legitimacy'.

60 Janis et al. 2008, 107-108.

61 Janis et al. 2008, 108.

understanding'[62] of the ECHR that the Court has developed, arguing that they did not 'sign up' for such intrusions into their domestic sphere[63].

We consider that what is being questioned here is the limits of legitimate rule. Certain subject matters, which may vary from state to state, are essentially considered a matter of national concern. We maintain that the Court in its explicit argumentation does demonstrate sensibility towards political and societal realities. As will be demonstrated in a later section in this article, it would appear that the Court is not beyond the influence of such realities when determining whether a human right has been violated in a specific situation. This appears to be the case even if the judges of the Court sit in their so-named individual capacity and not as representatives of specific states. Whether (and to what degree) this is conscious or unconscious, sporadic or systematic, is another matter.[64]

We do not seek to question the impartiality of the Court as such by highlighting 'judicial discretion' but instead seek to understand which elements influence international human rights adjudication. As will be demonstrated later in this article, sensitivity has found its way into the legal discourse through the development of explicit legal doctrines that tend to the need of contextual interpretations of rights:

> Later, as the judicial function became increasingly settled, Strasbourg developed doctrinal tools to navigate the thorny issues: the evolutive approach and the margin of appreciation. Both of these tools are well known; together, they allowed for an incremental expansion of the reach of the Convention, responsive to the pace of progress in member states, but in a doctrinal, not openly political framework.[65]

Thus, as Hertzberg asserts elsewhere in this volume, an issue does not necessarily need to be framed explicitly in terms of legitimacy for one to consider certain actions and attitudes as being indicative of legitimacy or illegitimacy. Yet, as we will demonstrate in section 4, such sensitivity does permeate the proceedings of the Human Rights Committee (the Committee) in the form of explicit 'legitimacy arguments' from time to time. Committee experts interpret their own role in relation to state parties of the International Covenant on Civil and Political Rights differently.[66] Such consciousness also shines through in interviews with the judges of the Court:

---

62 Rask Madsen 2007, 138.

63 Voeten 2008, 422.

64 Voeten argues that no systematic biases can be found as regards 'legal cultural or geopolitical affinities between the judge's home governments and the government under review'. However, personal preferences do shape the decisions that international judges reach 'in significant ways'. Voeten 2008, 430.

65 Krisch 2008, 206.

66 For studies of the judges of the Court and their possible national, cultural, vocational and legal biases, see e.g. Arold 2007a; Arold 2007b; Bruinsma 2006; Bruinsma & de Blois

> I am convinced that too much activism detracts from the credibility of the Court and a lack of activism undermines its legitimacy. We have to steer a middle course between judicial activism and supervision versus judicial self-restraint and subsidiarity.[67]
>
> One can speak of judges who are concerned about problems of the *raison d' état* and others who sympathize with the applicants. The *raison d' état* is more present here than I would have thought possible, I may add.[68]

When attempting to formulate an understanding of legitimacy in the context of an international human rights body, it is important to highlight an 'internal' perspective on the issue. How does the issue of legitimacy affect the work of the experts working for such a body? How does the issue of legitimacy affect the self-image of said experts? What is the role of the Court and what is the role of each individual within the Court? Such queries can be contrasted against an 'external' perspective on the issue, including how legitimacy constitutes an element in the relationship between a human rights organ and contracting states. One should not forget, however, that the internal perspective, presented here in section 4, is connected to the external (institutional) perspective, presented in section 3.

An internal perspective on legitimacy

The UN Human Rights Committee (the Committee) and the Court operate within different human rights systems and are endowed with different competences. In contrast to the fully judicial Court, with its legally binding decision-making powers, the Committee is a quasi-legal body composed of competent independent experts who practise an adversarial procedure but do not render judgements with formal binding force. This fundamental difference between the two should be kept in mind when reading this article. It may be more important for the Committee to be perceived as legitimate than the Court, which presumably can be discerned in the trends seen in the respective treaty interpretations by the Committee and the Court. However, both bodies comprise a 'last resort' in relation to issues arising under the International Covenant on Civil and Political Rights (ICCPR) and the ECHR respectively, and they are

---

1997; Eudes 2000; Kuijer 1997; Voeten 2007; Voeten 2008, who notes 'we know remarkably little about international judicial behaviour'. Concerning the Court, Voeten goes on to conclude that 'ECtHR judges are politically motivated actors in the sense that they have policy preferences on how to best apply abstract human rights in concrete cases, not in the sense that they are using their judicial powers to settle geopolitical scores.' Voeten 2008, 417.

67 Judge Costa in Bruinsma 2008a, 41.

68 Judge Tulkens in Bruinsma 2008a, 41.

ascribed a key normative role when it comes to interpreting the meaning of the norms expressed in human rights treaties. Given their key role in treaty interpretation, it is of interest to examine both bodies in relation to the overall aim of this article. Despite potential differences in the presentation of facts, the manner in which the Committee and the Court present different positions may, in abstraction, allow us to discern something more general about what acting as an independent expert (at times specifically in the form of a judge) in an international organ entails.

Given that one of the authors of this article served from 1997-2004 as a member of the Committee, we are able to present a personal, 'insider' perspective on how issues of legitimacy function during the deliberations of the Committee when an individual case is brought against a state (in those instances where the state has accepted the competence of the Committee to consider such a complaint and, through its reasoned expert opinion, judge whether a violation of the ICCPR has occurred and, if so, what an effective remedy should entail.) Respecting the rule that the Committee deals with individual cases behind closed doors, the insider perspective is presented in the form of metaphors that seek to capture general observations of how issues of legitimacy figure in such debates conducted between 18 individual experts hailing from different parts of the world.

Our first observation concerns the question to whom an aspiration towards legitimacy is owed. Our article primarily addresses the legitimacy of the interpretive activity of a human rights court or other expert body in relation to states or governments which, as primary subjects of international law, are perceived to simultaneously constitute the critical audience of any interpretive performance and the constituency who determines the 'rules of the game', either through the adoption of treaties or through consistent state practice that constitutes the agreement of the parties. However, this view of legitimacy is too one-dimensional for an internal perspective. Legitimacy in relation to applicants, the individual victims of human rights violations and their legal representatives, is also of importance. The same can be said about legitimacy in relation to a broader human rights discourse, where non-governmental organisations and academic scholars constitute another exacting audience eager to critique the performance of the judges of the Court or expert body members.

As a second general observation we note that an insider perspective confirms a healthy 'cross pollination' between various human rights courts and treaty bodies: a line of interpretation convincingly adopted under one treaty is easily transferred to another treaty interpretation scheme as the correct, or in essence legitimate, interpretation. While historically the importation of interpretations has mainly occurred from the ECHR system to other human rights treaties,[69] examples also exist where the Court follows the interpretive lead of the Committee.[70]

The metaphor of a path helps us sum up our initial presentation of the insider perspective. A large portion of the legitimate interpretive activity of a human rights body consists of discerning 'what is already there', that is to say determining what the correct interpretation of a human rights treaty provision that is open to textual interpretation is so that, as soon as it has been articulated, the outcome is recognised as the legitimate, legally correct interpretation. The concept of a 'foreordained' path comprises the common denominator between the positions taken by the different members of a human rights expert body and also represents the idea of legitimacy being built through consistency and continuity. An important source of legitimacy in any interpretive activity is the demonstration that one's position has followed the path of an earlier line of interpretation. Conversely, a person wishing to challenge an established line of interpretation must 'raze' the path of the previous interpretation. Such an individual faces an uphill battle in trying to make his or her position legitimate, both internally and externally.[71] While perceiving a human rights treaty as a 'living instrument' open to 'dynamic interpretation' certainly has its place in human rights discourse, those resorting to such a perception usually attempt to demonstrate that the dynamic adaptation they advocate in actuality emanates

69 *Vuolanne v. Finland* (1989), stating that any form of deprivation of liberty must be subject to court review over its lawfulness, follows *Engel and Others v, the Netherlands* (1976); *Toonen v. Australia* (1994), stating that the criminalisation of homosexual conduct between consenting adults constitutes a human rights violation, follows in *Dudgeon v. the United Kingdom* (1981); and *Ng v. Canada* (1993) follows *Soering v. the United Kingdom* (1989) in affirming that extraditing a person to face capital punishment in another country may, in certain circumstances, constitute a form of inhuman treatment analogous to torture.

70 In *Mamatkulov and Askarov v. Turkey* (2005) the Court follows the Committee in *Piandiong et al. v. the Philippines* (2000), that non-observance by a state of a request of interim measures of protection constitutes a breach of a treaty obligation concerning the right of individual complaint; in *Folgerø and Others v. Norway* (2007) the Court follows the Committee in *Leirvåg et al. v. Norway* (2004), that the Norwegian model of compulsory education in Christianity and other religions was in breach of what human rights law requires for freedom of thought, conscience and religion.

71 The consideration by the Committee of the periodic reports by certain African countries illustrates this point. Because *Toonen v. Australia* (see footnote 69* above) represents the established position of the Committee (that criminalising homosexual conduct between consenting adults is a human rights violation) no Committee member would contest this position or interpretation. However, while some of the (typically) Western members of the Committee would use *Toonen* to 'grill' the government delegates appearing before the Committee to defend a report by, for example, Uganda or Zimbabwe, some (typically) African members of the Committee choose to remain quiet on the issue in the public meeting where the government report is considered but then afterwards offer their expertise in private (during a closed meeting where the Committee is to adopt its Concluding Observations). The expertise these members offer pertains to their views on the 'sensitivities' in the region, that is to say the particular context of the countries in question. Without contesting the interpretation adopted in *Toonen*, they propose to not raise the matter in the Concluding Observations as it would weaken the legitimacy of the Committee in the region.

from earlier jurisprudence, that is to say follows the path laid down by a series of earlier cases. The continuum of cases related to the rights of transsexuals decided by the Court is an illustrative example of the presence of legitimacy considerations acting as a constraint to any sudden changes in jurisprudence; seldom do judgements stray from the path. While change is possible and legitimate, in order for it to be possible and legitimate one must first prepare the foundation so that it becomes foreseeable.

At this point we leave the metaphor of a path in search of new horizons. We will now present three alternative metaphors that provide further understanding of the insider perspective on the different mindsets that the individual members of an independent expert body may have: the Captain, the Fire Brigade and the Icebreaker. These metaphors emanate from an insider perspective on the 18-member Human Rights Committee, which is mainly composed of law professors and pensioned judges hailing from six continents. These members are elected on the basis of their individual expertise and by the very same states that will be subject to their review and it is these same members who determine whether a state complies or fails to comply with the ICCPR.

The Captain. Some members of the Committee possess the mentality of the captain of a large passenger ship, such as those ships that sail between Stockholm and Turku. The Captain knows where Turku and Stockholm are and knows that an invisible yet identifiable and correct course exists between the two cities which allows him[72] or her to skirt islands and rocks and navigate some rather narrow passages. What makes our Captain a professional is a sense of responsibility over the ship and its passengers, crew and cargo – an understanding that these 'actors' are vital to the overall legitimacy of his or her performance. What distinguishes the Captain from any recreational sailor is the capacity to avoid situations of risk or trouble, such as being slightly off course or needing to change course unexpectedly because of another ship appearing. The Captain knows how slowly a big ship turns or slows down, and therefore he or she does not even try to force things. The Captain is patient, observative and behaves in a foreseeable manner.

This metaphor is particularly well suited to describe the mentality of those Committee members who have previously served as judges of a regional human rights court or a national Supreme or Constitutional Court. For some others, these members may appear 'conservative', but not because of being guided by state interests. Rather, these members are 'conservative' because of the way they see the legitimate role of a universal human rights body.

---

72 Here we are reminded of the story about the son of a world-famous neurosurgeon. The boy is brought in to hospital with a severe head injury following a car accident that has killed his father and is lying unconscious on an operating table awaiting surgery. The surgeon who enters the operating theatre to perform the surgery looks down at the patient and exclaims, 'I cannot perform this procedure, this is my son!' Question: How is this possible? Answer: Because the world-famous neurosurgeon is the mother of the boy.

The Fire Brigade. The opposite of our patient and conservative Captain would be the Fire Brigade. Also for the Fire Brigade, knowledge of the correct route is imperative in order to reach the destination as quickly as possible without getting lost, and therefore a map or GPS device is invaluable in the completion of the primary task, extinguishing a fire. This Committee member however is driven by a passion for human rights, and he or she perceives human rights violations anywhere in the world as life-threatening fires that must be extinguished as quickly and efficiently as humanely possible. The Fire Brigade is willing to cut corners and break speed limits in order to achieve this goal. For him or her human rights do not necessarily pertain to how people should live their lives as good human beings but rather to the necessary preconditions for people choosing their own way of life. As such the Fire Brigade perceives his or her legitimate duty to solely include extinguishing a fire; the mess left behind is not his or her concern. It is up to ordinary people to clean up afterwards, and it would not even be legitimate for the Fire Brigade to start to reorder the bookshelf.[73] The Fire Brigade associates legitimacy with the end result, in performing a task dictated by the human rights treaty upon receiving an emergency call from an affected individual. This metaphor is particularly well suited to describe the mentality of those Committee members with a background as academics and who share close contact with the world of NGOs.

The Icebreaker. Our third metaphor provides the middle ground between the 'conservative' Captain and the 'swift' Fire Brigade. The Icebreaker is a special-purpose ship designed to break through ice-covered waters and thereby open a passage for other ships to follow. As Icebreakers are perhaps not so common in most parts of the world, the word may require some explanation. Many bodies of water and waterways in the Nordic countries, including the Baltic Sea, tend to freeze during the winter, with ice forming a relatively thin layer on top of the water. Icebreakers, with their strong hulls and powerful engines, are capable of breaking through this ice and open and maintain the sole navigable passages for civilian passenger or cargo ships. The dimension of 'leading' or 'showing the way' is predominant in the Icebreaker mindset of this Committee member. He or she understands that other ships (state parties) cannot arrive at their destinations unless the Icebreaker (the treaty body) first opens a passage. To safely reach their destinations, other ships must follow the Icebreaker precisely and at a close distance. Some Committee members strive to become an Icebreaker and see the

73 Here we are reminded of the story of a Fire Brigade Chief who lived in a small village and was always on duty, despite there never being a fire. He left for a weekend holiday, the first in his career, during which (of course) a fire broke out. The Fire Brigade extinguished the fire by themselves successfully. However, when the chief returned from his holiday the following morning and visited the site, he exclaimed: 'Erroneously extinguished!' Such a perspective is also evident in the field of human rights adjudication, seen for instance when members of the Committee discuss how another human rights body (a regional human rights court for example) has decided a case.

task of the Committee as opening a navigable legal course that states must follow in order to comply with the provisions of the human rights treaty. In theory, states can decide whether or not to follow the Icebreaker, but in practice they all queue up and follow at a close distance. Should a ship decide not to follow the passage opened by an Icebreaker, that ship will quickly become locked into the ice and, in the worst-case scenario, be destroyed through the crushing of its hull. The Icebreaker mindset of this Committee member focuses on opening a specific route (the human rights treaty) and is greatly assisted by the forces of nature, which provide states no other viable option than to 'voluntarily' comply.

Affirming shared practices and transcending the given

There are several dimensions to the questions of how and why those serving as independent experts on human rights bodies reach a decision. For instance, we can suppose that underlying assumptions regarding gender and sexuality implicitly guide the thinking of these experts when they determine what is 'normal' and so forth. In this article, however, the focus does not primarily lie on such 'knowledge formations' nor on the creation of 'truth' and 'fact' in legal arenas. While these perspectives are not entirely separate from the issue at hand we instead focus on how the issue of political legitimacy influences human rights adjudication.

Human rights bodies cater to an ideal of justice. They are extremely consumed with delicately tending to the consent of member states when fleshing out the facts of a case and deciding on the truth, that is to say whether or not a human rights violation has taken place. This is seen during their discussion of the 'practice' of a state. As previously mentioned, experts in international organs, such as the judges of the Court or members of the Committee, are aware that their ability to influence how contracting states act depends on their ability to be receptive to the sentiments and practices of member states. When successful in this undertaking the Court not only ensures that its judgements are viewed as legally correct but also that the Court itself is considered legitimate. The authority of the Court as the ultimate interpreter of the ECHR is acknowledged and member states yield to the power that the Court exercises through its adjudication.

The acknowledgment of the authority of the Court is also expressed when member states, even having been found to have violated certain rights in a previous case, appear anew as defendants in cases before the Court. States instruct agents to argue their case before the Court, agents who present 'evidence' during Court proceedings and formulate arguments in a manner likely to resonate with the Court: for example, by presenting state actions as being consistent with the aims and goals of the ECHR. Agents may also reference earlier Court judgements when defending the state's position in an attempt to explain why the current case is dissimilar to previous cases or to support their argument that the current case falls within the margin of appreciation of an individual state. However, indifference to the Court and its decisions is also seen. Russia for example has been content to pay damages to victims as ordered by the Court in successive judgements yet refuses to undertake any legislative or other changes in regard to its involvement in Chechnya. When states act in such a manner the Court lacks legitimacy, at least in some respect in the eyes of those states. The alternative interpretation of such examples would be that the state in question has prioritised its competing national concerns over the judgement of the Court.[74]

Let us move on then to the substantive issue of gender/sex, family and marriage in relation to human rights law. Human rights law is primarily concerned with discerning the outermost acceptable limits for how states may treat its citizens and other individuals living under its jurisdiction.[75] For instance, what influence may states exercise in relation to an issue such as marriage? How should states legislate this matter?[76]

Article 12 of the ECHR stipulates that states must respect the right of individuals to marry, but states are not required to promote the decision to marry and may even restrict the right to marry. But when states do restrict the right to marry they must abide by the following rules:

> [I]f States establish restrictions, they should be based only on rational, reasonable, and non-arbitrary grounds, and the restrictions should not be applied in a discriminatory manner. Marriage impediments that are absolute and permanent could be considered violations of the right to marry.[77]

If we study the different clauses that delineate the grounds for when states may restrict a specific right, or otherwise specify rights in the ECHR, a comparable line of reasoning is seen. In the ECHR, states cannot alone wholly interpret what a right entails: instead the scope of state freedom in this respect is *qualified*. If we look at what ECHR has to say on the issue of marriage:

---

74 During work on this volume, fellow researcher Tom Kettunen observed that political communities may compete with each other, from which follows split legitimacy.

75 The provision by states of more extensive rights protection is of course welcome by the ECHR. Article 53 of the ECHR asserts that 'a higher level of protection' of fundamental rights may be afforded at the national level.

76 States can restrict the right to marriage by for example setting age limits or prohibiting marriage between blood relatives. Some restrictions are not allowed, however, such as prohibiting interracial or inter-religious marriages or marriages between individuals from different nationalities.

77 Kirilova Eriksson 2002, 125.

> Men and women of marriageable age have the right to marry and to found a family, according to the national laws governing the exercise of this right.[78]

Commentators have however noted that what this specification actually means in regards to the liberty that a national legislator is provided is not entirely clear:

> The scope of this qualification is not clear. It is evident that the exercise of the rights guaranteed cannot be wholly governed by national law. (...) The correct view, therefore, seems to be that Article 12 imposes an obligation to recognize, both in principle and in practice, the right to marry and to found a family. This obligation implies that the restrictions placed on these rights by national law must be imposed for a legitimate purpose, for example, to prevent polygamy or incest, and must not go beyond a reasonable limit to attain that purpose. On the other hand, the precise scope of the restrictions may vary among Contracting States, as does, for example, the marriageable age.[79]

Bearing in mind our introductory remarks on human rights language, we can assume that in cases of adjudication the factual will most likely take precedence over a progressive articulation of 'the ideal' as asserted by applicants. Conservatism did for a long time influence the interpretation of both Article 8 (the right to privacy) and Article 12 (the right to marry) of the ECHR. In the case law related to these articles, the epitome of a family consisting of a mother, a father and one or more children is evident. In case law the protection of marriage is connected to the idea of marriage as the basis of family life and therefore the right to marry is interpreted in relation to the right to start a family[80]. Thus a 'traditional' view of marriage, between persons of the opposite biological sex, is reinforced. *Rees v. UK* (1986) and *Cossey v. UK* (1990), which relative to the right of transsexual persons to marry, provide examples of this perception[81]:

> In the Court's opinion, the right to marry guaranteed by Article 12 refers to the traditional marriage between persons of opposite biological sex. This appears also from the wording of the Article which makes it clear that Article 12 is mainly concerned to protect marriage as the basis of the family.[82]

---

78 'The phrase under Article 12 'according to the national law governing the exercise of this right' suggests that national authorities are entrusted to the task of delineating the ambit of protection of the right to marry based on their law, and providing both 'institutional guarantees' and conditions for the exercise of the rights under this provision.' Arai 2006, 342-343.

79 Ovey & White 2006, 251.

80 van Dijk 2006, 856.

81 *Rees v. United Kingdom*, ECHR Series A (1987) No. 106, 9 EHRR 56, para. 49; *Cossey v. United Kingdom*, ECHR Series A (1991) No. 184, 13 EHRR 622, para. 46.

82 *Rees v. United Kingdom*, ECHR Series A (1987) No. 106, 9 EHRR 56, para. 49.

These cases also demonstrate how the Court in its judgements notes what it sees as 'certain developments' in the legislation of certain member states, and as 'evidence of significant societal change' in the respondent state and elsewhere, yet still concludes that little common ground exists whereby a departure from its earlier interpretations of Articles 8 and 12 would be warranted:

> There have been certain developments since 1986 in the law of some of the member States of the Council of Europe. (…) [T]his is still, having regard to the existence of little common ground between the Contracting States, an area in which they enjoy a wide margin of appreciation (…). In particular, it cannot at present be said that a departure from the Court's earlier decision is warranted in order to ensure that the interpretation of Article 8 (art. 8) on the point at issue remains in line with present-day conditions. (…)
>
> Although some Contracting States would now regard as valid a marriage between a person in Miss Cossey's situation and a man, the developments which have occurred to date (…) cannot be said to evidence any general abandonment of the traditional concept of marriage. In these circumstances, the Court does not consider that it is open to it to take a new approach to the interpretation of Article 12 (art. 12) on the point at issue.[83]

The cautious approach of the Court is often supported by its argument that it does not wish to become a 'social harbinger' that dictates how 'marriage' ought to be understood. The Court supports its view by maintaining that a traditional understanding of marriage has not yet been abandoned by member states.[84] A state, therefore, is considered to have acted within its mandate when insisting on its own view of marriage: as such no violation has occurred. This is an example of how the Court considers itself unable to 'legitimately' expand the interpretation of a human right, at least for the present, by maintaining that it is not authorised by member states to do so. The perception of the Court is that it would not be widely supported if it were to expand the interpretation of, for example, marriage in that the prevalent, general opinions and legal framework of member states do not support such an expansion.

This approach is not only specific to the issue of marriage[85] or the practise of European human rights bodies. International institutions usually settle for a conservative or *status quo* interpretation when faced with a choice between different alternatives.[86]

During the late 1970s other sexual orientations do to some extent begin to garner the attention, with case law being introduced concerning individuals who have undergone gender reassignment surgery. National laws prohibited

83 *Cossey v. United Kingdom*, ECHR Series A (1991) No. 184, 13 EHRR 622, paras. 40, 46.
84 van Dijk 2006, 848.
85 Recent judgements pertaining to Islam display the wariness of the Court to explore new grounds.
86 Koskenniemi, 2005, 601.

individuals who had undergone gender reassignment surgery from subsequently marrying another individual of the – now – opposite biological sex. The emergence of this issue brought attention to the situation of gender reassigned (transsexual) individuals and the extent to which their new, post-operative sex is acknowledged or ought to be acknowledged in law so as not to equate to a human rights violation. As the cases of *Rees*, *Cossey*, *B. v. France* and *Sheffield & Horsham v. UK* show, for a long time national legislation that only allows individuals of the opposite biological sex to marry is not perceived as violating the 'essence' or 'core'[87] of the right articulated in Article 12 of the ECHR. That is to say states are allowed to choose whether laws allowing transsexuals to marry a partner, independent of biological sex, should be enacted.[88] To quote the telegraph-style summary of the Grand Chamber judgement in the case of *Sheffield & Horsham v. UK*:

> In Court's view, no scientific or legal developments in area of transsexualism since Cossey judgement which would persuade it to depart from its decisions in above cases — respondent State still entitled to rely on a margin of appreciation to defend its refusal to recognise in law post-operative transsexual's sexual identity — for Court, it continues to be case that transsexualism raises complex, scientific, legal, moral and social issues in respect of which there is no generally shared approach among Contracting States. (---)
>
> Having regard to those principles [laid down in Court's Rees judgement on scope and interpretation of Article 12], inability of either applicant to contract lawful marriage under domestic law of respondent State on account of authorities' insistence on biological criteria for determining gender for purposes of marriage cannot give rise to breach of that Article (...).[89]

Thus, while the Court in the cases listed above does note 'certain developments' among member states (the contracting parties to the ECHR), it does not consider this consensus sufficient to introduce a reinterpretation. Yet the opinions of the judges themselves differ. In a dissenting opinion in *Sheffield & Horsham v. UK* and in an attempt to shift focus away from domestic law, Judge van Dijk maintains that 'sex', precisely like 'family', 'home', 'person' and so forth, could be considered an autonomous concept:

---

87 The 'core' refers to the idea that while most legal human rights can be limited and derogated from, they simultaneously possess an absolute essence that states may not infringe upon through their actions.

88 van Dijk 2006, 846-850. The first transsexualism case before the Court, which was dismissed on procedural grounds, is *van Oosterwijck v. Belgium*, ECHR Series A (1991) No. 40, 3 EHRR 557. The European Commission for Human Rights had previously also addressed this same case but had not found any violation of human rights as delineated under Articles 8-12. Scheinin 1998, 28-29.

89 *Sheffield and Horsham v. United Kingdom*, Judgement of 30 July 1998, European Court of Human Rights, Appl. No. 31-32/1997/815-816/1018-1019, www.pfc.org.uk/node/343.

> I cannot see any reason why legal recognition of reassignment of sex requires that biologically there has also been a (complete) reassignment; the law can give an autonomous meaning to the concept of "sex".[90]

The notion of autonomous concepts implies that understanding of a legal concept within the ambit of the ECHR is not exhaustively understood by merely recapitulating the legislation and jurisprudence of (certain) member states but that, instead, looking 'behind appearances'[91] is required. Nonetheless, while to a certain extent a shift away from domestic law occurs, the interpretation of the Court it still based on the factual and consensual (in other words what the majority of member states agree upon):

> [In *Engel v. the Netherlands*], the Court ruled that autonomous concepts should be interpreted according to the 'common denominator of the respective legislation of the various contracting parties'. The introduction of this standard echoes a requirement of consensus: in constructing the meaning of the ECHR concepts, the ECtHR must seek to respect and accommodate a certain convergence on meaning among the various contracting states.[92]

Given this, it appears that in his dissenting opinion, van Dijk does not distance himself from prevalent Court argumentation in a 'technical' sense. Instead he disagrees in substance; his opinion expresses/articulates that justice is not being done. However, cases also exist where the Court hesitates to outright affirm the given. In such cases the Court can be inclined to refer to 'the emergence of a common standard'. This is seen for example in *Dudgeon v. UK*, when the Court states:

> [D]espite the width of the margin of appreciation, the criminalization of homosexual conduct between consenting adults over the age of twenty-one was not necessary in a democratic society. (…) [T]he emergence of a more tolerant attitude elsewhere in Europe (…) was said to reflect a European standard which ought to be taken into account when determining the necessity of the provision.[93]

This indicates that the judges of the Court, at least the majority of them, felt that affirming actual shared practice would subvert justice in this case. However, by invoking an emerging common standard, they simultaneously preserved shared practice as a cornerstone of human rights adjudication.

As regards the right to marry, a similar argument is seen the case of *Christine Goodwin v. United Kingdom*, where the judgement of the Court

---

90 Letsas 2004, 291; Judge van Dijk, Dissenting Opinion, *Sheffield & Horsham v. UK* (1998), Reports 1998-V.

91 Letsas 2004, 298.

92 Letsas 2004, 295.

93 Evans 1997, 323; *Dudgeon v. UK*, Ser. A. no. 59 (1983), para. 60.

appears to express a reinterpretation of Article 12. Goodwin, having undergone gender re-assignment surgery, wished to be formally recognised as a female so that she could marry her male partner. In its judgement the Court noted that 'significant social changes' had taken place since the adoption of the ECHR in 1950 regarding the perspective of member states on the institution of marriage. The Court therefore concluded that the right of transsexuals to marry belongs to the core of the right delineated in Article 12 and that, accordingly, states are not allowed to completely prohibit such marriages.[94]

What the Court actually primarily acknowledges in the *Christine Goodwin v. United Kingdom* case is that transsexual individuals who have undergone gender re-assignment have in fact changed sex. However, the Court is cautious in its formulation and it is improbable that the Court, emanating from *Christine Goodwin v. United Kingdom*, will in the near future conclude that the right of same-sex persons to marry is part of the core of the right to marry as formulated in Article 12. The reason why this is improbable is once again factual; few member states of the Council of Europe endorse such a right in their legislation.[95]

The position of the Court to date on the issue of same-sex marriage in relation to Article 12 is that Article 12 does not encompass a right to same-sex marriage.[96] Still, a trend towards viewing gender as something other than a strictly biologically defined category can be inferred from the increased protection of the rights of transsexual persons. As the Court states in *Christine Goodwin v. United Kingdom*:

> It is true that the first sentence refers in express terms to the right of a man and woman to marry. The Court is not persuaded that at the date of this case it can still be

94 van Dijk 2006, 850–851; *Christine Goodwin v. United Kingdom* (App. 28957/95), Judgement of 11 July 2002; (2002) 35 EHRR 447, paras. 84, 100. See also Ovey & White 2006, 277; *I v. United Kingdom* (App. 25680/94), Judgement of 11 July 2002; (2003) 36 EHRR 557.

95 van Dijk 2006, 851.

96 In *Schalk and Kopf v. Austria* (App. 30141/04), Judgement of 24 June 2010, the applicants, both Austrian nationals and a same-sex couple, alleged that the legal impossibility for them to marry in Austria violated their right to marry as protected under Article 12. They also invoked Article 14 (prohibition of discrimination) in conjunction with Article 8 (the right to respect for private and family life.) The Court, observing that at present no consensus among Council of Europe member states exists in regard to same-sex marriage, held that Article 12 does not impose an obligation on governments to grant same-sex partners access to marriage. Moreover, while granting that the relationship of the applicants complied with the Article 8 meaning of 'private and family life', the Court stated that the Convention is 'to be read as a whole' and that, as such, the Court disagreed that the anti-discrimination requirements of Article 14 and Article 8 would impose the obligation under Article 12 that a state grant a right to same-sex marriage. The ruling of the Court follows the Human Rights Committee case of *Joslin et al. v. New Zealand* (2002).

> assumed that these terms must refer to a determination of gender by purely biological criteria.[97]

Judge J. Hedigan has pointed out that the *Christine Goodwin v. United Kingdom* case is 'a classic example of the incremental way in which our case law can develop. The last was a big step but it was the last step on a long journey'.[98] There is certainly some truth to this statement. Nevertheless, it is not the case that the category of gender is being eradicated as a parameter or being interpreted strictly in social constructivist terms. Rather human rights protection is being extended to possible new partner and family constellations. Moreover, the institution of marriage is no longer automatically connected to the ability to procreate, even if a hierarchy of family constellations still exists. The heterosexual couple holds central position in this hierarchy:

> The political rationale of the ECHR is that it lends legitimacy to the member states in occasional landmark cases in which particular member States are found to violate codified human rights.
>
> The most daring landmark cases are violations of Article 8 (the right to respect for private and family life) where the stakes of a liberal State are low. The jewel in the crown (of the Council of Europe) as the epithet goes, is first and foremost an ideological beacon in the symbolic field of human rights lawyering.[99]

When it comes to an understanding of marriage and family, the ECHR has at times been interpreted as 'a living instrument'. This implies that the Court has taken prevailing circumstances into consideration when providing an interpretation of a situation[100]. In some cases this has been construed as support for the renewed interpretation the ECHR, while in other cases a reinterpretation has been rejected due to the ideas expressed in the preparatory work of the ECHR[101] or because the Court has taken prevailing circumstances into

97 *Christine Goodwin v. United Kingdom* (App. 28957/95), Judgement of 11 July 2002; (2002) 35 EHRR 447, para. 100.

98 Judge J. Hedigan as quoted in Bruinsma 2008a, 36.

99 Bruinsma 2008a, 43.

100 See e.g. *Marckx v. Belgium*, ECHR Series A (1979) No. 31, 2 EHRR 330, para. 58; *Cossey v. United Kingdom*, ECHR Series A (1991) No. 184, 13 EHRR 622, para. 42.

101 See e.g. *Johnston and Others v. Ireland*, ECHR Series A (1986) No. 112, 9 EHRR 203, para. 53. 'However, these tools have not always led to an extension of human rights protection; sometimes they have also allowed for retreat in reaction to national concerns.' 'Yet its general approach remained cautious until the early 2000s when the negotiations on Additional Protocol No 14 gave questions of execution greater political weight. Thus, in 2004, the Court returned to a more determined language, holding that states were obliged to modify their domestic law if this was necessary to end violations of the Convention and fully comply with ECtHR judgements. (...) shows the Court's particular sensitivity to the political process and its readiness to react to resistance as well as encouragement. After all, the process of accommodation in the ECHR framework is not a one-way street leading to ever greater authority of Strasbourg; instead, it is a mutual process in which signals from political actors, including courts, feed back into ECtHR jurisprudence.' Krisch 2008, 208.

consideration. Because of this varying practice, the Court has been accused of casuistry:

> This dynamism [evolution] in interpreting the Convention has often been criticised, and understandably so, as there are hardly any methodological guidelines for how it is to be applied – after all, it is a tool of judicial politics that grants the Court flexibility in responding to circumstances and opportunities.[102]

Thus, when rendering judgements, the Court is guided by its understanding of political preferences and the like. Yet, as seen in the case of Judge van Dijk in regard to *Sheffield & Horsham v. UK*, judges do not always concur in their verdicts and their understanding of what is just or, indeed, true. In his dissenting opinion on *Cossey*, Judge Martens places the term legal truth in quotation marks to indicate his view that the perceived 'untruthfulness' and injustice in the issue arises from national legal arrangements:

> That is to say nothing of the lifelong dread to which the BSD-system [the legal system in force in the United Kingdom] condemns them, by obliging them [transsexuals], every time that their sex is legally relevant, to make the painful choice between either hiding what legally is "the truth" - with all the legal consequences of such untruthfulness, such as making themselves liable to a criminal charge, dismissal or a demand for nullification of the legal act in question - or revealing that legal "truth" and facing at least the possibility of very humiliating or even hostile reactions.[103]

In case law related to marriage and family one sees that the judges of the Court can to a certain extent disagree with one another. Cases have been decided with a narrow margin. Dissenting opinions have been added to judgements, questioning the facts relied on by the Court and the mission of the Court given those facts:

> One cannot but conclude that the reasons given for the Court's refusal to accept the societal developments as material are based on a distortion of the real state of affairs and are therefore far from convincing.
>
> The explanation may be that behind these explicit arguments lie hidden policy arguments. From judgements such as those in the Marckx case, the Dudgeon case, the Rees case, the case of F. v. Switzerland and the Cossey case one gets the impression that the Court, at least as far as family law and sexuality are concerned, moves extremely cautiously when confronted with an evolution which has reached completion in some member States, is still in progress in others but has seemingly left yet others untouched. In such cases the Court's policy seems to be to adapt its interpre-

102 Krisch 2008, 207.

103 *Cossey v. United Kingdom*, ECHR Series A (1991) No. 184, 13 EHRR 622, Dissenting opinion of Judge Martens, para. 3.4.

> tation to the relevant societal change only if almost all member States have adopted the new ideas.
>
> In my opinion this caution is in principle not consistent with the Court's mission to protect the individual against the collectivity and to do so by elaborating common standards (…). Caution is indeed called for, but in another direction: if a collectivity oppresses an individual because it does not want to recognise societal changes, the Court should take great care not to yield too readily to arguments based on a country's cultural and historical particularities.[104]

Cases related to Article 8 of the ECHR generate the highest amount of dissenting opinions. This is attributed not only to the open texture of the ECHR article formulation but also the issues at stake.[105] The possibility to append separate opinions to a judgement, either dissenting or concurring, has at times been criticised with some maintaining that this possibility takes the edge of and undermines the authority of a verdict.[106] Still, the opposite has also been maintained:

> Our [Court] judges were overwhelmingly in favour of the use of concurring and dissenting opinions, because it demonstrated the nuances of human rights protection, promoted debate among Strasbourg judiciary, indicated the questions of interpretation and application were not always clear-cut, could provide consolation for the losing party who could know that some judges appreciated their position and arguments, and demonstrated openness and transparency. The motivation to write dissenting opinions was universally stated to be disagreement with the majority as to the outcome. Judge B expressed this sense of obligation very succinctly: … you believe strongly enough in your view that you feel you have to put it down on paper.[107]

Writing separate opinions, not least dissenting opinions, is (viewed as being) beneficial. It provides a manner whereby even the 'losing party' can be heard. The allowance of the inclusion of dissenting opinions as well as openness, transparency and engaging with the substance matter of human rights are connected to the issue of legitimacy, the role of the Court and the issue of representation as mentioned previously in this article.

This is where we presently stand. Given its role and position within the European human rights system and the Council of Europe, the Court is caught up in a delicate task when deciding whether a human rights violation has occurred or not. The Court examines the specific social situation of the state that has allegedly violated the treaty and investigates how the issue is understood by other member states. At times, the Court concludes that more political support is needed before it can expand the interpretation of a right in a direction not

---

104 *Cossey v. United Kingdom*, ECHR Series A (1991) No. 184, 13 EHRR 622, Dissenting opinion of Judge Martens, para. 5.6.3

105 White & Boussiakou 2009, 54.

106 White & Boussiakou 2009, 55; Bruinsma & de Blois 1997, 186.

107 White & Boussiakou 2009, 57.

previously seen or in a direction not (discernibly) supported in the preparatory work of the Court.

Quite understandably, criticism of how the Court addresses new situations or new claims is often directed towards the margin of appreciation doctrine[108] that the Court employs, which allows the Court to play a deferential or subsidiary role in relation to those national authorities more well acquainted (in the mind of the Court) with the facts of the case. The predicament such an attitude places the Court in is that, quite frequently, the issues such as those that the Court addresses, especially including those in which delicate lines exist between what is right and what is wrong, can only be truly perceived from a distance. Allowing those closest to the 'facts' to make the decisions may amount to being led by the blind.

Concluding remarks

State sovereignty is a basic principle of international law, albeit complicated by the attribution of the right of self-determination to peoples and not states or governments. As a rule, states are bound by that to which they have voluntarily submitted themselves. Moreover, the international community, among them various human rights organs, have few coercive means whereby to force states to comply with the international rules they have consented to. For this reason compliance largely relies on the will of individual states to live up to their international commitments. Such voluntary compliance is dependent on the trust a state has in an international institution; if voluntary compliance is to prevail, the state must deem the institution a legitimate representative of the international community and also sensitive towards the individual state and its interests and needs. Thus when interpreting the legally binding obligations of a state, it is imperative that human rights bodies be convincing in their reasoning.

'Independence' and 'impartiality' are important institutional features that contribute to human rights organs being perceived as legitimate. Certain procedural features are important as well. Nevertheless, the experts and judges who serve on international human rights organs are equally cognisant of the fact

108 Krisch 2008, 207. See also Yourow 1996, 193-196; Arai-Takahashi 2002, 203-204. Nonetheless, Krisch has also noted (in line with the observations made in this article) that in regards to a tool such as the margin of appreciation: 'the value of the resulting flexibility for a court that is in the process of establishing its authority can hardly be overestimated. It helps to avoid clashes with member states and their courts while keeping alive the promise of a more effective human rights protection in the future, thereby also alerting national authorities to the risk that particular policies might one day be regarded as violations'. Krisch concludes that the 'story of the treatment of transsexuals in Britain is a good illustration of this point'. The cases of Rees, Cossey and others show how the Court 'rather than merely stating the law, was administering change in a dialogue with national institutions that benefited much from the flexibility of its doctrinal tools'. Krisch 2008, 207.

that their authority and legitimacy is contingent upon them not voicing their opinions too antagonistically in relation to states. These experts and judges understand that voluntary compliance is connected to the quality and persuasiveness of their judgements or other findings and that they must steer carefully between 'providing too little protection to individual rights' and 'pronouncing judgements that are not compatible with fundamental views and legal or institutional constructs existing in a certain state'.[109]

This aspect of legitimacy, related to the need to be simultaneously persuasive before quite different audiences, has been the focus of our contribution to this volume. This article has looked at human rights issues related to gender, sex, family and marriage in order to illustrate how issues of legitimacy play out in practice. Analysis of the argumentation of the Court in judgements related to the aforementioned human rights issues, often described as sensitive issues, effectively shows how legitimacy forms an undercurrent in international human rights adjudication.

The Court determines whether member states of the Council of Europe act in accordance with the ECHR. The political legitimacy of the Court is contingent on states confirming it and its specific judgements. Hence, the perceived prevalent opinion of member states plays a role when the Court decides what the core of a right is comprised of and to what extent state parties are allowed the freedom to independently interpret rights. Such assessment likewise plays a role when reference is or is not made to prevalent state practice. The Court, and the Committee likewise, should attest to what 'everybody knows' to be true: to paraphrase Mariana Valverde, human rights law is built on an idea of 'common knowledge'[110]. This is implicit when talking about human rights. In practice, common knowledge is dependent on what states actually do and how they actually behave, not least in regards to human rights adjudication. When human rights are concerned, we move in our talk about them between consensus and non-consensus both as regards legal human rights and the broader concept of human rights. Human rights as legal rights receive meaning through a previously existing institutional and political culture.

Yet the decision-making of the Court concurrently upholds and tests its legitimacy. Human rights imply the promise of justice to-be-realised. The manner in which the decision-making of the Court is administered allows the Court to cater to the ideal of justice while also acknowledging political realities and ensuring the continual cooperation of states.

This dual aspiration forms a backdrop for adjudication in human rights bodies. In dissenting opinions, justice is sometimes explicitly mentioned. Additionally, in public discourse the status held by international law differs

109 Gerards 2008.
110 Valverde 2003.

from 'ordinary' national legislation. In the eyes of the public, human rights law deals with the 'big ideas' that we all should share.

In this article our analysis of the concept of legitimacy strives to reveal an aspect of factual human rights, as these rights come into view in the adjudication of international human rights bodies. In this article, factual signifies what the Court, through a judgement, deems that an individual actually has a right to. The ultimate *justification* of human rights should not be confused with the problem of legitimacy dealt with in this article. Their justification is related to a moral stance *towards* human rights. An individual embracing human rights as a moral stance and human rights organs showing contextual sensitivity in their reading of various specific rights are not the same thing.

The judgements of the Court determine what is unacceptable, what is illegal. Claimants may additionally view a judgement as providing confirmation of what they in a moral sense have perceived as being unjust. The debate on what is legally and morally correct is often couched in legitimacy arguments. In this article, however, we do not equate talk of legitimacy with, for example, concluding that a judgement is 'legal'. Nor do we wish to claim that legitimacy is the same as what is just or right even if it, for example, does not coincide with what is legally correct in a strict sense. Legitimacy here resides in neither law nor morals. Through a discussion of (political) legitimacy, as has occurred in this article, it is possible to capture an aspect or dimension of how a court or (other) human rights organ works which cannot solely be described in legal or moral vocabulary. Then it is another thing that many of the scholars mentioned in this article have noted that this 'dimension' of legitimacy has become, or may become, 'internal to law'.

Legitimacy has thus primarily been used in this article in a descriptive, elucidatory manner. The term legitimacy has predominantly been introduced into human rights discourse from the outside. Therefore in this article we have not merely sought to address instances in which actors have chosen to formulate themselves in terms of legitimacy. However, an internal, explicit narrative on legitimacy also exists. Arguments couched in terms of legitimacy can be heard, for example when a human rights organ discusses to whom it should address a human rights claim.

Reference in this article has been made to instances when issues of legitimacy have been raised within the Committee. Through our internal perspective into the work of the Committee we see both the loyalty of an individual member to a Committee position (the determination that the criminalisation of homosexual conduct between consenting adults is a human rights violation) and the policy disadvantages that would follow if this position were to be imposed on certain states (the loss of legitimacy for Committee work as a whole). Here the narrative of legitimacy has been used to justify 'shying away' from publicly expressing and defending the legal position of the Committee while not contesting that position as such.

A diametrically opposite application of the narrative of legitimacy can be detected in situations where the facts are unclear or unverified but a clear position of principle nevertheless needs to be voiced. In such a situation a human rights body may choose to express its established position on the matter but express its position in relation to a specific state indirectly through a legitimacy argument. For instance, if a state maintains a regime of *incommunicado* detention, that is to say prevents contact between a detainee and his lawyer, family or doctor, that state opens itself up to allegations of torture. Without stating that torture actually *exists* in the state concerned, a human rights body attempts to convince said state that eradicating incommunicado detention is the only method whereby the state can avoid being suspected of torture and gain legitimacy.[111] This example actually reveals a double usage of the legitimacy argument: the human rights body protects its *own* legitimacy by not expressing a clear position on the facts (the presence or lack thereof of torture), and by resorting to more diplomatic language that is designed to appeal to the good intentions of the state, the human rights body points to a legitimacy deficit on the side of the *state*. Through such action the human rights body shifts the burden of legitimacy onto the state itself, demonstrating that all actors in human rights discourse must be concerned with legitimacy.

Bibliography

Council of Europe, *Collected edition of the "Travaux préparatoires" of the European Convention on Human Rights.* The Hague/Boston/London/-Dordrecht/Lancaster/ Martinus Nijhoff, 1975-1985. 8 volumes.

Arai-Takahashi, Y

2002 *The Margin of Appreciation Doctrine and the Principle of Proportionality in the Jurisprudence of the ECHR*. Antwerpen / Oxford / New York: Intersentia.

2006 Chapter 5, The System of Restrictions. In van Dijk, P et al. (eds.), *Theory and Practice of the European Convention on Human Rights*. 4th revised ed. Antwerpen/Oxford: Intersentia, 333–350.

111 The example comes from the report by the UN Special Rapporteur on the promotion and protection of human rights and fundamental freedoms while countering terrorism (Martin Scheinin) of a 2008 mission to Spain: 'The Special Rapporteur recommends the complete eradication of the institution of incommunicado detention as this exceptional regime not only entails a risk of prohibited treatment against the detainee, but also makes Spain vulnerable to allegations of torture and as a result weakens the legitimacy of its counter-terrorism measures.' (A/HRC/10/3/Add.2, para. 62)

Arold, N-L

2007a The European Court of Human Rights as an Example of Convergence. *Nordic Journal of International Law* 2-3 (Vol. 76), 305–322.

2007b *Legal Culture of the European Court of Human Rights*. Brill Academic Publishers.

Bauman, Z

1999 *Vi vantrivs i det postmoderna* (övers. Sven-Erik Torhell). Göteborg: Daidalos.

Beddard, R

1980 *Human rights and Europe: A study of the machinery of human rights protection of the Council of Europe*. 2nd ed. London: Sweet & Maxwell.

Bruinsma, F J

2006 Judicial Identities in the European Court of Human Rights. In van Hoek, A et al. (eds.), *Multilevel Governance in Enforcement and Adjudication.* Antwerp: Intersentia, 203–240.

2008a The Room at the Top: Separate Opinions in the Grand Chambers of the ECHR (1998-2006). *Ancilla Iuris* 2008 (Vol. 3) 32–43.

2008b A Socio-Legal Analysis of the Legitimacy of Highest Courts. Found at: folk.uio.no/andreasf/Projects/2009-CAS/TXT/Bruinsma.doc (28.12.2009)

Bruinsma, F J & de Blois, M

1997 Rules of Law from Westpoint to Wladiwostok: Separate Opinions in the European Court of Human Rights. *Netherlands Quarterly of Human Rights* 2/1997 (Vol. 15), 175–186.

Dijk, P van

2006 Chapter 16, The Right to Marry and to Found a Family (Article 12). In van Dijk, P et al. (eds.), *Theory and Practice of the European Convention on Human Rights.* 4th revised ed., Antwerpen/Oxford: Intersentia, 841–862.

Douzinas, C

2007 *Human Rights and Empire: The political philosophy of cosmopolitanism.* Abingdon/New York: Routledge-Cavendish.

Eudes, M

2000 La légitimité du juge de la Cour européenne des droits de l'homme: Observations sur la représentativité et l'indépendance du juge de Strasbourg. *Revue québéquoise de droit international* 1/2000 (vol. 13), 131–166.

Evans, M D
1997 *Religious Liberty and International Law in Europe*. Cambridge/New York: Cambridge University Press.

Freeman, M
2002 *Human Rights. An interdisciplinary approach*. Cambridge/Malden, MA: Polity Press.

Frohwein, J
1984 European Integration Through Fundamental Rights. *Journal of Law Reform* 1984 (Vol. 18).

Gerards, J H
2008 Judicial Deliberations in the European Court of Human Rights. folk.uio.no/andreasf/Projects/2009-CAS/TXT/Gerards.doc (28.12.2009)

Hastrup, K
2003 Representing the common good: the limits of legal language. In Wilson, R A & Mitchell, J P (eds.), *Human Rights in Global Perspective: Anthropological studies of rights, claims and entitlements*. London/New York: Routledge, 16–32.

Helfer, L R & Slaughter, A-M
1997 Toward a Theory of Effective Supranational Adjudication. *Yale Law Journal* 2/1997 (Vol. 107), 273–391.

Janis, M et al.
2008 *European Human Rights Law: Text and Materials*. 3rd edition, Oxford/New York: Oxford University Press.

Kirilova Eriksson, M
2002 Family Rights and the United Nations Covenant on Economic, Social and Cultural Rights: Article 10(1). In Chapman, A & Russell, S (eds.), *Core Obligations: Building a Framework for Economic, Social and Cultural Rights*. Antwerp/Oxford/New York: Intersentia, 115–146.

Koskenniemi, M
2005 *From Apology to Utopia: The Structure of International Legal Argument*. Reissue with new Epilogue. Cambridge/New York/Melbourne/Madrid/Cape Town/Singapore/São Paolo: Cambridge University Press.

Krisch, N
2008 The Open Architecture of European Human Rights Law. *The Modern Law Review* 2/2008 (Vol. 71), 183–216.

Kuijer, M
1997 Voting Behaviour and National Bias in the European Court of Human Rights and the International Court of Justice. *Leiden Journal of International Law* 1/1997 (Vol. 10), 49–67.

Kurtén, T
1998 *Teologi i nutida sammanhang. Studier i kontextuell teologi, dess begreppslighet, metodologi och genomförande*. Åbo: Åbo Akademi.

Lasser, M
2004 *Judicial Deliberations: A Comparative Analysis of Judicial Transparency and Legitimacy*. Oxford: Oxford University Press.

Letsas, G
2004 The Truth in Autonomous Concepts: How to Interpret the ECHR, *European Journal of International Law* 2/2004 (vol. 15), 279–305.

Mahoney, P
1990 Judicial Activism and Judicial Self-Restraint in the European Court of Human Rights: Two Sides of the Same Coin. *Human Rights Law Journal* 1-2/1990 (Vol. 11), 57–88.

Merrills, J G & Robertson, A H
2001 *Human rights in Europe: A study of the European Convention on Human Rights*. 4th ed. Manchester: Manchester University Press.

Morrisson, C C jr.
1981 *The Dynamics of Development in the European Human Rights Convention System*. The Hague/Boston/London: Martinus Nijhoff Publishers.

Mowbray, A
2005 The Creativity of the European Court of Human Rights. *Human Rights Law Review* 1/2005 (Vol. 5), 57–79.

Ovey, C & White, R
2006 *Jacobs & White, The European Convention on Human Rights*. 4th ed., Oxford/New York: Oxford University Press.

Scheinin, M
1998 Sexual Rights as Human Rights – Protected under Existing Human Rights Treaties? *Nordic Journal of International Law* 1/1998 (Vol. 67), 17–35.

Slotte, P
2005 *Mänskliga rättigheter, moral och religion: Om de mänskliga rättigheterna som moraliskt och juridiskt begrepp i en pluralistisk värld*. Åbo, Åbo Akademi förlag [Diss.].

2007a ”Med rätten att synas och bli sedd” – Mänskliga rättigheter som rättsfigur och moralisk tolkningsnyckel. In Lindfelt, M & Gustafsson Lundberg, J (red.), *Uppdrag Samliv – Om äktenskap och samlevnad.* Stockholm: Verbum, 423–452.

2007b That’s no Way to Treat a Human Being! – Semantics, Recognition and the Human Rights Debate. In Meireis, T (Hg.), *Lebendige Ethik – Beiträge aus dem Institut für Ethik und Angrenzende Sozialwissenschaften. Hans-Richard Reuter zum 60. Geburtstag.* Münster: LIT Verlag, 81–101.

Rask Madsen, M
2007 From Cold War Instrument to Supreme European Court: The European Court of Human Rights at the Crossroads of International and National Law and Politics. *Law & Society Inquiry* 1/2007 (Vol. 32), 137–159.

Valverde, M
2003 *Law’s Dream of a Common Knowledge.* Princeton/Oxford: Princeton University Press.

Voeten, E
2007 The Politics of International Judicial Appointments: Evidence from the European Court of Human Rights. *International Organizations* 4/2007 (Vol. 61), 669–701.

2008 The Impartiality of International Judges: Evidence from the European Court of Human Rights. *American Political Science Review* 4/2008 (Vol. 102), 417–433.

White, R C A & Boussiakou, I
2009 Separate Opinions in the European Court of Human Rights. *Human Rights Law Review* 1/2009 (Vol. 9), 37–60.

Yourow, H C
1996 *The Margin of Appreciation Doctrine in the Dynamics of European Human Rights Jurisprudence.* Dordrecht: Martinus Nijhoff Publishers.

LEGITIMACY, CONSTITUTIONALISM AND EUROPEAN INTEGRATION

Mats Lindfelt[1]

Legitimacy in a post-national setting

Legitimacy is often perceived as being directly related to certain agreed values such as democracy and the rule of law. However, not all states or international organisations are based on a democratic model yet are nonetheless still perceived as being run by a legitimate government or organisation, at least by the international community. Not all states are members of the United Nations, for instance, yet can nevertheless be considered legitimate states under public international law. Recent events in Egypt and Libya in the first months of 2011 provide examples where regimes, the holders of power, are loosing their legitimate mandate to stay in power: legitimacy in these countries is seriously being questioned both internally (by citizens) and externally (by the international community). International organisations, such as the European Union (EU) for example, are struggling with legitimacy issues to a greater extent than ever before, partly due to an increased transfer of power from the nation state level to a post-national level. A common feature of what has been labelled a legitimacy deficit in respect to the EU is that a component of evident mistrust exists regarding the EU moving towards the ever-increasing integration of its constituent elements, its member states. The debate relating to this integration process and the direction that it is taking reflects an examination of what can and should occur versus what should not occur in regards to the integration of member states. The Treaty establishing a Constitution for Europe (TCE), also known as the Constitutional Treaty, provides an example of this debate in that it was intended to unite the EU member states under one constitution but has never been realised in the form that the member states have agreed to and signed.[2]

---

1 This article is based on my PhD dissertation, "Fundamental Rights in the European Union – Towards higher law of the land?", presented at Åbo Akademi University in 2007.

2 The TCE was signed on 29 October 2004. O.J., C 310, 16 December 2004.

To a large extent European integration is and has been based on an integration through law, where the broadening and extension of integration has been codified through the mechanism of an international treaty. The legal interpretation and application of laws has occurred under the auspices of an active and integrationist court of law, the European Court of Justice (ECJ). European integration initially emanated from the founding countries' common constitutional traditions. The EU member states still maintain that the legitimacy of European integration must emanate from the EU member states. Yet as the EU has developed a distinct legal order of its own, distinct from its member states, the indirect manner whereby the Union is provided legitimacy has become somewhat inadequate. It is no longer possible for the EU to derive its legitimacy solely from its member states. Another aspect significantly affecting the EU's integration process has been the adjudication of some of its member states' individual national constitutional courts to set constitutional limits for EU integration and to legally challenge, in particular, the constitutional principles developed by the ECJ.

The EU has struggled with legitimacy issues for quite some time. Legitimacy was brought to the forefront in the early 1990s when the European Community started to move from primarily focusing on economic integration towards seeking new dimensions of integration, that is to say taking the first steps towards a political union through the Maastricht Treaty. When trying to understand the overall lack of interest in EU affairs that EU citizens (the general public) demonstrate, one must understand that a legitimacy debate in conjunction with what has been labelled a democratic deficit plays an instrumental role.[3] The EU is perceived as being undemocratic in that its *accountability* is not an inherent organisational component; instead its democratic accountability *emanates from* the individual member states. The governments of the EU member states act as agents in the European Council and as such the European Council derives its democratic mandate from the citizens of each member state, not through any democratic mechanism rooted in the EU itself.

The term legitimacy deficit is often used in such a way as to suggest that a correlation exists to an alleged lack of democracy. While a strong correlation

---

3 A prime example of this lack of interest is the low voting rate throughout Europe in the European Parliament (EP) elections. The voting rate in the first EP elections was significantly higher compared with the two latest elections in 2004 and 2009. The increased powers of the EP, garnered through treaty reforms, have hardly had any impact in this respect. Many examples also exist of the problems that some EU member states have had in ratifying treaties. For example in a 1992 referendum the Danes at first refused to ratify the Maastricht Treaty, Ireland faced problems with the ratification process of the Nice Treaty in 2001 and the Intergovernmental Conference (IGC) 2003-2004 negotiated and took into account the problems surrounding ratification of the Constitutional Treaty. Furthermore, two founding member states of the EEC – the 'wrong countries' in that they were expected to provide support – had extreme difficulty garnering popular support for the referenda.

between democracy and legitimacy no doubt exists, legitimacy is more complex in that it helps individuals better understand the reason why the majority of citizens, without any hesitation, accept that societies are governed by the rule of law or why for instance a certain specific piece of legislation passes a democracy test but fails to pass a legitimacy test. It is assumed that when decisions are made under constitutionally recognised procedures, authority and respect for the outcome will be increased: that is to say citizen compliance and consent will be assured. However, legislation can be enacted by a parliament, in accordance with a constitution's requirements, and as such pass the democracy test but still be openly challenged by those citizens 'affected' by the legislation and not accepted as an authoritative act.

Democracy pertains more to the overall justification of a power structure in a democratic society. The justification of a power structure occurs by popular control and/or through representative democracy. Collective decision-making is democratically legitimated as long as it can be controlled by all of those affected on equal terms.[4] Deliberative democracy, along with representative democracy, is an important element of legitimacy but is not in and of itself the sole foundation for legitimacy. For Habermas, human rights and the sovereignty of the people are essential to understanding the legitimacy of legal systems. Democratic processes must be based on the mutual recognition of citizens as rights holders embedded with private autonomy. This private autonomy is then complemented with public autonomy and the right to participate in public discourse (the right to participation) on equal terms. The participants taking part in a deliberative democracy should be allowed to express their free will and the end result of such deliberation should be binding.[5] Legitimacy in accordance with a deliberative democracy model is based on providing the means for a free, rational and open debate.

In order for a legislative act to be considered legitimate, rights-bearing citizens should have the opportunity to participate in the collective formation of the will, that is to say the subjects of a law should also be the ultimate authors of the law. The precondition for this deliberative democracy model is that the subject of a law must accordingly be provided some basic concept of (fundamental) rights so that he/she may become capable of participating in the public debate: the freedom or the autonomy of the individual is presupposed. Habermas writes that, 'The law receives its full normative sense neither through its legal form per se, nor through an a priori moral *content*, but through a procedure of lawmaking that begets legitimacy.'[6] Habermas argues for a legitimate force of fundamental rights and an understanding of the process or conditions under which these are 'collectively defined' within a political

4 On deliberate democracy, see Habermas, 1998.
5 Maurer 2004, 326-328.
6 Habermas 1998, 135.

context. Such a proceduralistic conception of law, a belief in the discursive and procedural basis of the democratic will of the people, is for Habermas the central source for legitimacy. Collective decision-making can only be legitimated if it has occurred in a deliberative way. The deliberative model is thus reduced and justified through the concept of human rights and the principle of the sovereignty of the people. The deliberative democracy model secures the right to equitable participation in formulating the will of the people. Legitimacy can thus be reduced to what is right, to what is good (reflecting public interest) and to what extent a decision is the result of a fair procedure. Accordingly, issues of legitimacy are highly complex and require more than a mere correlation to legality.

Formal correctness in accordance with a predetermined set of accepted rules regarding how decisions are to be made (the outcome) is a precondition for legitimacy, that is to say it fulfils the criterion of legal validity. Weiler maintains that, 'Formal legitimacy is legality understood in the sense that democratic institutions and processes created by law on which it is based.'[7] Legality cannot be considered the sole manner whereby legitimacy is achieved. The rules of power must also by justified through reference to acceptance by both a governor and the governed, that is to say the rules of power must achieve a certain level of moral justifiability in the decision-making structure. Consequently, if legitimacy is to be realised, a need exists for the governed to consent to the power relationship between their governor and themselves (acceptability).[8] In other words 'social legitimacy' is needed.[9] Social legitimacy reflects a broad societal acceptance of the founding structure of a given legal system that is committed to values such as sovereignty of the people and human/fundamental rights considerations.[10] To gain social legitimacy, governments, states and international organisations must first enjoy formal legitimacy; to gain formal legitimacy, a state's legal system must be built on the rule of law. Formal legitimacy or correctness, however, does not necessarily entail that social legitimacy is secured; civil disobedience, for example, can lead to a change in the law. Consequently, formal legitimacy does not imply that a state/legal system would automatically enjoy social legitimacy. Social legitimacy reflects a broad social acceptance of a system or state committed to values such as justice, freedom and welfare. What is interesting in terms of legitimacy is not formal legitimacy but rather to what degree a people or states *de facto* assume that a system or state that produces legally binding norms are legitimate.[11] In such cases, those individuals and states subject to binding decisions base social legitimacy on consent and conferral.

7 Weiler 1999, 80.
8 Beetham 1991, 15.
9 On social legitimacy, see for instance Karlsson 2001, 107-109; Weiler 1999, 80-81.
10 Habermas 1998,135.
11 Karlsson 2001,107-109.

Generally speaking, legitimacy has a tendency to become apparent when acceptance and/or authority are being questioned. The EU provides an example of such. In the EU a lack of interest in public affairs exists at the European level and a form of civil disobedience in relation to certain specific legislation is seen not only at the individual level but also at the state level. In this article I seek to address the concept of legitimacy in relation to the EU as an international entity and the justification the EU presents in regards to its authority in relation to its constituent member states. I furthermore investigate whether legitimacy in the EU is connected to the justification of authority in the EU: not only in association with the EU member states but also through the ultimate holders of power within the nation states, namely the European people.

The authority and nature of EU Constitutional law

In a nation state the question of legitimacy primarily pertains to the relationship between the state and its constituent 'demos' – the people. Understanding the relationship that provides the justification for the authority of a power in a post-national setting is made more complicated by the fact that it is difficult to identify the 'demos' from which the legitimation for power could be derived. Such a scenario is perhaps most recognisable in the post-national discourse related to the EU, where a European people with a shared cultural conception and identity do not exist. A significant part of the legislation passed though national parliaments now emanates in one form or the other from the EU. Consequently, the transfer of powers from a nation state to an international entity such as the EU has increasingly raised legitimacy issues. If a legal system, rule or entire organisation is to be characterised as being legitimate, it must be endorsed with a degree of acceptance and conferred with authority. Legitimacy concerns arise when binding legal norms are external and democratic control is not particularly evident. Legitimacy concerns additionally arise when the powers of international organisations increase: not only as a result of the transfer of power from the nation state level to the supranational level but also through the mechanism of increased powers at the supranational level. The EU provides a textbook example of such. Also, the move away from unanimous decision-making to majority decision-making can cause the issue of legitimacy to arise. In the past decades the structure of the legislation process in the EU has through treaty revisions moved from having been mainly based on unanimous decision-making towards majority decision-making in ever-larger areas of competence within the EU.[12] Such specifically agreed settings naturally lead to a situation where the will of the majority prevails.

12 Due to the size of the expanded EU, a gradual transformation has occurred from unanimous decision-making towards qualified majority with the Nice Treaty and, with the Lisbon

International treaty obligations become binding for a nation state when domestically implemented by way of ratification through the state's democratically elected parliament– for example the wording/formulation of a finalised text that a parliament can no longer change. The fundamental problem is not the lack of democracy at the national level. The issue instead is how (and whether) a state can legitimise external, binding international treaties and norms. This problem can be illustrated in a discussion on the legitimacy of international norms such as the United Nations Charter obligations and/or international treaty obligations and through a discussion on the legitimacy of case law as defined in the European court of human rights.[13] In regards to EU case law[14], the constitutionalisation of the EU legal order has been occurring for several decades. One dimension of this constitutionalisation process is the manner in which the relationship between the EU legal order and the EU member states' national legal orders has developed, including how such development should be perceived.

The original treaty establishing a European Economic Community (the EEC, renamed the European Community (EC) in 1993) did not include any specific provision on the relationship between EU and national law, that is to say no reference to the principle of the primacy of EU law was included. Instead a simple reference to a principle of co-operation was included, a principle that could be interpreted as indicating that member states were not allowed to enact legislation that would conflict with member states' treaty obligations as defined in EU law. As such the specific provision of the primacy of EU law was not specifically delineated.[15] The doctrine of primacy of EU law proclaims that, 'In accordance with well settled case law of the EU Court of Justice, the Treaties and the law adopted by the Union on the basis of the Treaties have primacy over the law of Member States, under the conditions laid down by the said case

---

Treaty, the introduction of double majority decision-making in the European Council with 55% of member states representing 65% of the population, thus raising the issue of public justification. The double majority decision will enter into force in 2014 and will replace unanimity in several new areas. Taxation, social security, foreign policy and common defence issues are excluded and decided on through unanimity. The Lisbon Treaty entered into force on 1 December 2009.

13 For a discussion of the legitimacy of ECHR case law, see the text by Scheinin & Slotte in this volume.

14 The term and concept EU law is used throughout this article for the sake of clarity, even though EC law is more appropriate when referring to the law of the European Union and case law thereof.

15 The supremacy doctrine was introduced in the draft of the Treaty Establishing a Constitution for Europe, part I-6, para. 1 which prescribes that, 'The Constitution, and the law adopted by the Union's Institutions in exercising competences on it, shall have primacy over the laws of the Member States.' O.J., C 310/1, 16 December 2004. However, the Treaty of Lisbon, which amends the Treaty on European Union, does not include this principle. The Lisbon Treaty, a constitutional treaty, would have given EU primacy an explicit legal and constitutional status. Instead it includes a declaration on primacy (No. 17).

law.'[16] Defined so, EU law overrules inconsistent norms of national law regardless of the nature of the law in question: where EU law is applicable, it has precedence over national legislation.

The doctrine of primacy is a conflict-resolving rule used in relation to EU law *vis-à-vis* national law and applied to all of EU law. The groundbreaking principles of primacy seen in EU law constitute a legal quality of all norms under EU law.[17] Certain conditions must however be fulfilled in order for the primacy rule to be applied in the resolution of a norm conflict in a given case at the level of adjudication or implementation of EU law. Firstly, according to EU law norm conflicts should always, if possible, be solved by way of harmonious interpretation so that a conflict of norms can be avoided. Secondly, the relevant national norm should fall within the scope of application of EU law.[18] Thirdly, invalid acts of EU law adopted beyond the scope of attributed powers cannot prevail over national law, that is to say the criteria of formal legitimacy must be fulfilled. Consequently, if clear and unconditional EU law is applicable, conflicting national legislation is to be set aside irrespective of the hierarchical or chronological status of said national law. Thus primacy in and of itself does not invalidate conflicting national law but instead requires that a conflicting national law is simply set aside. As such primacy *per se* does not invalidate conflicting national provisions.[19] Primacy instead in this manner operates as a *lex superior* rule. This subsequent primacy of EU law implies that national legislators cannot adopt laws that conflict with EU law. Uniformity and efficiency are therefore seen by the ECJ as essential. The effectiveness of these EU measures would be compromised if they were to be reviewed in the light of national legal standards.[20] The creation of an EU that garners its powers from its member states' sovereign powers has resulted in a body of law that binds both the member states and the citizens of the member states. According to the ECJ, the nature of EU law makes it impossible for member states to not accept the primacy of EU law in that EU law is based on the need for unilateral implementation and acceptance by EU member states on the basis of conferral. The constitutional principles developed by the ECJ are highly authoritative and member states obey these constitutional principles because it is believed that the ECJ and its institutional setting hold a high degree of legitimacy. It has been perceived as a fundamental principle that limits be set for national discrepancy. Primacy creates a hierarchy of norms that legislators, all levels of national courts and civil servants must take into account. That the primacy doctrine was

16 Declaration on primacy (No. 17).

17 De Witte 2000, 148.

18 According to Weiler, 'The principle of supremacy can be expressed, not as an absolute rule whereby Community or federal law trumps Member State law, but instead as a principle whereby each law is supreme within its sphere of competence'. Weiler 1999, 21.

19 De Witte 1999, 190.

20 De Witte 1999, 191; Craig & de Burca 1998, 259.

developed outside the EU political realm and not originally recognised as a constitutional principle in treaty context has, for the most part, been accepted by the EU members states as necessary for the development of a unifying post-national legal order. The ECJ has played a central role in defining the constitutional character of this supranational legal order, which has in turn profoundly impacted member state sovereignty. As the final interpreter of EU law, it is the ECJ that determines the validity of EU law.

The authority of EU law under scrutiny - the case of fundamental rights

That EU law should take precedence is accepted, though not unconditionally, as one of the foundational principles of EU law. The precedence of EU law over member state law is not fully and completely accepted as a means whereby the uniformity and efficiency of EU law can be secured so that the aims set out in EU treaties can be achieved. Some member states' national constitutional courts have questioned the validity of the doctrine of primacy in cases dealing with constitutional values and principles. Over the years a series of cases dealing with this issue have been seen in national constitutional courts. In particular the German Federal Constitutional Court (GFCC) has addressed cases concerning the relationship between EU law and German national (constitutional) law. Such cases have primarily focused on questioning the absoluteness of the primacy of EU law by arguing that the foundation for the validity of EU law lies in the national constitutional setting rather than in validity external to the scope of common constitutional traditions. The complete denial of the primacy doctrine has not been the goal of such cases but instead what is reflected is an attempt to set 'the limits of penetration of EC law into domestic constitutional order'.[21] Such national constitutional resistance is exemplified in a line of case law that perceives EU law as compromising national constitutionally protected fundamental rights. The GFCC has maintained a position whereby the ultimate power in determining the limits of EU competence is interpreted as lying in the hands of the EU member states.[22]

The key issue in this constitutional resistance is the lack of adequate safeguards whereby fundamental rights are protected in the EU legal order: the GFCC has determined that an EU legal act should be considered invalid if fundamental rights are compromised.[23] Interpreted so, in the case of a norm

---

21 De Witte 1999, 201.

22 For a discussion on the recent years' increased readiness to question the absoluteness of EU primacy and related case law, see Lindfelt 2007, 57-64.

23 The GFCC proclaimed that the transfer of powers to international organisations did not include the power to open or amend the basic structure nor amend the inalienable essential feature of the German constitution, namely the protection of fundamental rights. Case 2 BvL 52/71, *Internationale Handelsgesellschaft mbH v Einfuhr- und Vorratstelle für Getreide und*

conflict the domestic protection of fundamental rights would overrule EU law. The GFCC later softened its position on the safeguarding of fundamental rights when the protection of fundamental rights was strengthened in the EU legal order. Nonetheless, the GFCC still maintains that the ultimate power in the determination of the limits of EU competence lies in the hands of the EU member states. This line of reasoning has gained support from those who emphasise that the domestic implementation of EU law should not be allowed to weaken the national protection of constitutional rights. Obviously such a perspective possesses the potential to induce tension between EU and national constitutional law; the ECJ continues to maintain that national law should be interpreted in conformity with EU law and not the other way around. However, offering more extensive fundamental rights protection on a national level than that which is protected in EU law neither violates nor contradicts EU law. The margin of discretion left to member states when implementing directives and framework decisions has made it easier to take into account national constitutional rights and other international human rights obligations.

The discussion of the relationship between EU and national law and how the issue should be resolved does not necessarily revolve around the issue of who is the final arbiter of constitutionality in Europe. Proponents of legal pluralism and the abandonment of a hierarchical legal structure, such as McCormick[24] and Maduro[25], argue that European law should not to be perceived in terms of a hierarchical understanding of the law. Legal pluralism is based on the theory that EU constitutional law emanates from a legal dialogue between the ECJ and EU member states' national courts. The legitimacy of European constitutionalism, according to Maduro, is based on the belief in a 'bottom-up' effect on the nature of the European legal order. Imposing a hierarchical conception of law in the context of understanding the relationship between EU and national law therefore leads nowhere. Dialogue and perspectives should instead stem from the level of legal interactions between different legal orders in a pluralistic setting, that is to say an interaction between international, EU and national law: norm conflicts between EU and national constitutional law cannot be solved by adhering to a hierarchical conception of law. Both the ECJ and member states' national courts assume themselves to be the final arbiter of European constitutionality. According to Maduro, 'It has now become usual to highlight how different national and European perspectives on the notion of ultimate authority in Europe require a constitutional pluralist conception of the

Futtermittel, judgement of 29 May 1974 in 2 CMLR (1974), 549. This judgement was handed down at a time when the EU lacked a codified fundamental rights catalogue.

24 McCormick 1998,1-18.

25 Maduro 2003, 501-537 (a); Maduro, 2003 (b), 95-100 emphasise the mutual engagement of national and European legal orders; Weiler 2003, 7-23 emphasises constitutional tolerance. See also Kumm 2005, 262-307.

relationship between European and national constitutionalism.'[26] Judicial bodies would have to strive for solutions that would ultimately circumvent direct conflict, that is to say strive towards constructive cooperation where both EU and national courts take into account the constitutional boundaries of the other and share as the ultimate guiding principle the principle of coherence. An example of such is a case that was related to the EU framework decisions on combating terrorism that proved to be problematic in terms of respecting national fundamental rights. The national implementation of the Council Framework Decision on the European arrest warrant in Finland (Act No. 1290/2003) was deemed to be in conflict with section 9 (3) of the Finnish Constitution, which absolutely prohibits extraditing Finnish citizens to another country against their will. The Finnish Constitutional Law Committee issued a general statement stating that the domestic implementation of EU measures could not diminish the level of national protection guaranteed under the Finnish Constitution.[27] Thus, in this interpretation, constitutional rights and international human rights together compromised to a certain extent a straightforward definition of the policy on extradition. The implementation of Act No. 1290/2003 in Finland would have made the prerequisites for extradition stricter than those delineated under the Framework Decision on the European arrest warrant.

Member State or EU citizen legitimacy?

The constitutional doctrines developed by the ECJ at an early stage of EU integration have had a profound effect of the nature of the European legal order. Another central constitutional principle is that EU citizens can demand that provisions of EU law be directly enforced by national courts under certain preconditions: the obligation imposed on member states must be clear, unambiguous, unconditional and not dependent on further action in creating rights for the individual. National courts should recognise EU law as valid and binding, that is to say as a source of law.[28] Thus the individual citizen, and not merely member states, becomes a subject of EU law, which consequently alters the very foundation of EU law. As such EU citizens are the subject and effect of EU law but are not, however, the *authors of the law*. EU law is still very much a creation of the European Council.[29] The Lisbon Treaty did not change this state of affairs. The EU legal order and the structure of decision-making in the EU still rest upon the principle of integration through law. Nevertheless, the

26 Maduro 2003 (a), 501.
27 Opinion of the Finnish Constitutional Law Committee 18/2003 vp.
28 On the doctrine of direct effect, see for example de Witte 1999, 177- 213.
29 Weiler 1997, 113.

outcome of implementation continues to be founded on national implementation and the means thereof.

The GFCC extensively addressed the nature of EU constitutional law with regard to the conformity of the Lisbon Treaty[30] with the German constitution. One central question related to the transferral of powers, specifically the legislative powers of the German Bundestag and Bundesrat in European law-making and treaty amendment procedures.[31] This case revealed brought to the surface a few points on legitimacy and how the relation between domestic legal systems and the relation to the EU legal system should be understood. The point of departure for the GFCC was that the Lisbon Treaty, while providing major changes to the pre-existing treaty system, does not alter the very nature of integration between sovereign states. The treaty does not transform the EU into a federal state. In its analysis the GFCC concluded that with regard to the issue of European competence, EU integration is still based on the conferral of powers (Article 5, TEU), which forms the basis for constitutional acceptability. The GFCC upheld, in short, that the citizens of the EU, represented by their member states, are the decisive holders of public authority at the national and EU levels and therefore constitute and provide the ultimate authority on which the EU rests. Yet current European integration is still based on the integration of sovereign states where the structure of integration emanates from the principle of the equality of states, a rule recognisable from public international law. The GFCC clearly maintains that European integration should emanate from the *people* of Europe and that Europe must therefore construct its legitimation accordingly. As for the democratic legitimacy of the European Parliament (EP), the GFCC dismissed the idea that the EP could provide EU decisions democratic legitimacy through the development of increased competence. The argument that the GFCC presents is based *inter alia* on the fact that the composition and election of the EP does not emanate from the principle of equality, that is to say the EP cannot be democratically legitimised as long as it is not composed in accordance with the principle of democratic equality as realised in a nation state. Even after the ratification of the Lisbon Treaty, the EU still does not possess a political deci-

30 The Lisbon Treaty is the latest treaty revision, marking a new phase in the EU integration process and increasing the transfer of powers from EU member states to the EU.

31 The Lisbon Treaty and related legislative acts were challenged before the GFCC. The act extending and strengthening the rights of the German Bundestag was challenged on the grounds that the Bundestag and the Bundesrat had not been equipped with sufficient rights concerning participation in matters of European law-making procedures and Lisbon Treaty amendment procedures. The GFCC held that the proposed act infringed on Article 38 in conjunction with Article 23.1 of the German *Basic law* stating that German citizens possess the right to vote and thereby determine the public authority effective upon them through the means of elections. The challenge on constitutionality was, in brief, based on the argument that the Lisbon Treaty was too far-reaching in transferring sovereign powers from EU member states to the EU and as such posed a threat to the constitutional principle of democracy by undermining the competences of the German Bundestag and thereby, through lack of democratic legitimisation, the EU. 2 BvE 2/08 of 30.6.2009.

sion-making body born out of equal elections by all EU citizens. The GFCC concluded that the EP cannot constitute a body of representation for the sovereign people of Europe because the composition of the body of the EP is not representative of EU citizens under the principle of electoral equality but is rather instead an electoral body and a representation of the citizens of the EU member states. The EP accordingly violates the principle of electoral equality when choosing nationality instead of the equality of citizens as its point of departure. One can thus speak of a structural democratic deficit when referring to the European public authority. The EP still represents the citizens of the EU member states but is not representative for a sovereign European people.[32] What the GFCC emphasised was that the legitimacy of the EU is derived from its constituent member states and that the competence of the EU is based on the principle of conferral. The position of the GFCC is that the EU draws its legitimacy from the representative democratic systems of its member states. The GFCC advocates that democracy first and foremost must be connected to the concept of a European people and the nation state. The EU, lacking a European people and as such falling short of being a nation state, cannot base its legitimacy directly on its member states' citizens. At best the democratic element of the EU is what has been termed a delegated democracy, with a foundation in the nation state setting. The interpretation of the status of the EP by the GFCC, even following ratification of the Lisbon Treaty, is as follows:

> Measured against requirements in a constitutional state, even after the entry into force of the Treaty of Lisbon, the European Union lacks a political decision-making body created in equal elections by all citizens of the Union and with the ability to uniformly represent the will of the people. In addition, connected with this is the lack of a system of organisation of political rule in which a European majority will carries the formation of the government sustained by free and equal electoral decisions and thus genuine competition, transparent for citizens, between government and opposition can come about. Even in the new wording of Article 14.2 Lisbon TEU, and contrary to the claim that Article 10.1 Lisbon TEU seems to make according to its wording, the European Parliament is not a representative body of a sovereign European people. This is reflected in the fact that it is designed as a representation of peoples in the respective national contingents of Members, not as a representation of Union citizens in unity without differentiation, according to the principle of electoral equality.[33]

The GFCC recognises the EP as a significant law-making body but nevertheless finds it unable to fulfil the same democratic criteria as defined in a nation state. The GFCC continues by stating:

---

32 For a critical review of the conception of democracy as related to the EU according to the GFCC, see Eriksen & Fossum, 2010.

33 2 BvE 2/08 of 30.6.2009, para. 280.

> As long as European competences are ordered according to the principle of conferral in cooperatively shaped decision-making procedures, and taking into account state responsibility for integration, and as long as an equal balance between the competences of the Union and the competences of the states is retained, the democracy of the European Union cannot, and need not, be shaped in analogy to that of a state. Instead, the European Union is free to look for its own ways of reducing the democratic deficit by means of additional, novel forms of transparent or participative political decision-making procedures. It is true that the *merely deliberative participation of the citizens and of their societal organisations in the political rule - their direct involvement in the deliberations of the institutions with the power to take binding political decisions - cannot replace the legitimising connection based on elections and other votes. Such elements of participative democracy can, however, complement the legitimation of European public authority.*[34] This encompasses in particular forms of legitimation to which civic commitment can contribute in a more direct, more specialised and more profoundly issue-related manner, for example by providing the citizens of the Union and the societally relevant associations (Article 11.2 Lisbon TEU: "representative associations") with the possibility of expressing their views in an appropriate manner. Such forms of decentralised participation based on the division of labour and has a potential to increasing legitimacy for their part contribute to making the primary representative and democratic connection of legitimation more effective.[35]

Here the GFCC makes an important point when denoting that this is an issue that is evolving: namely that European level civil society participation, which has already played a slight role during, for instance, the process of negotiating the EU Charter of Fundamental Rights (the Charter) at the turn of the 21st century, still exists in an embryonic stage.[36] The European Council called for a more profound and broader debate that included the EU Commission, the EP and representatives of national parliaments and civil society. The Charter Convention was composed of one representative of head of state or government from each EU member state, sixteen members of the EP, thirty members of national parliaments (two representatives each) and one representative of the President of the European Commission.[37] It has been said that, 'The process of drafting the Charter was always going to be at least as important -if indeed not more so- than the substantive document which eventually emerged.'[38] The acknowledgement of the GFCC in deeming the evolving deliberative democracy model as being *embryonic* gives rise to that hope that European citizens can eventually in a participatory way and as form of democracy enhance post-national legitimacy.

34 Italics author's own.
35 Ibid, para. 272.
36 Lindfelt 2007 on the Convention method, 109-111.
37 See the Cologne European Council decision of 3-4 June 1999, Annex IV, 76.
38 De Burca 2001,130.

Concluding observations

The legitimacy of the EU is to a large extent still significantly linked to that of its member states. The EU itself gains its ultimate power from its member states through conferral and this state of affairs is acknowledged in the Lisbon Treaty. The European Commission, constituting the executive, is the *primus motor* in issuing new legislative acts, but the European Council retains a strong position in acting as a legislature even though the EP has gained a stronger position as co-legislator. The European Council however is still not accountable to the EP but instead derives its legitimacy and accountability from the citizens of the EU member states. The EP is not a representative political body that represents the will of the people through equal elections amongst all EU citizens but is nevertheless an established co-legislator with budgetary powers that exercises democratic control over the European Commission. As an international organisation the EU is not particularly democratic, and it lacks direct democratic accountability. This democratic deficit has partly been addressed through the treaty revisions that began in the early 1990s with the increase of EP powers. Nonetheless, despite its over 700 members the EP cannot represent the interests and views of more than 400 million Europeans and cannot express the will of the *people.* The EP is nothing like a national parliament. Yet despite these limitations the EU is gradually taking the notion of representative democracy to a supranational level.

The legitimacy of the EU is very much state centred and forms the foundation for post-national European legitimacy. A feature of European integration is that it is very much a result of the constitutionalisation of the EU legal order, with its basis in the rule of law. The work of the ECJ in constituting a sort of EU constitutional court has played a central role in the construction of a post-national legal order. ECJ judgements possess a high degree of authority *vis-à-vis* EU member states, despite a certain evolving opposition that maintains that the ECJ does not possess an 'open mandate' to develop the EU legal order. EU law has evolved through treaties that created a new type of international organisation with specific characteristics and a new legal order under international law. The EU legal order is a self-contained regime that is distinct (though not wholly) from international law and the law of the EU member states. As previously mentioned, while the transfer of powers from a nation state to an international organisation limits the nation state's sovereign powers this does not imply that competence should be allowed to *carte blanche* override the basic principles of said nation state's constitution. The EU extensively derives its legitimacy from member state legitimacy. There is a long road ahead before EU legitimacy can emanate from the European people. Nevertheless, the Lisbon Treaty has strengthened the element of democracy in the EU by, for example, creating a role for national parliaments in European matters and introducing a European Citizens' Initiative.[39] These are small steps towards anchoring in an embryonic manner legitimacy in the European people. It is the EU member states themselves that set the boundaries for European integration as delineated in treaty context and they who emphasise that it is the member states and not EU citizens who provide the foundation for legitimacy for the EU.[40] European citizens play a small but direct role in the overall creation of EU legitimacy. The new openings adopted in the Lisbon Treaty can potentially increase and anchor EU legitimacy in the European people. EU citizens still express a significant amount of support for European integration even though their trust in the EU and the benefits of EU membership has suffered as a result of the recent global economic crisis, which has profoundly affected the European economy.[41]

Bibliography

Beetham, D
1991 *The Legitimation of Power*. Basingstoke: Macmillan Education.

De Burca, G
2001 The drafting of the European Union Charter of Fundamental Rights. In *European Law Review*, Vol. 26, 126-138. London: Sweet & Maxwell.

Craig, P & De Burca, G
1998 *EU Law, Text, Cases and Materials*. Oxford: Oxford University Press.

39 National parliaments act as 'watchdogs' in regards to the principle of subsidiarity. A new participatory democracy provision was introduced where one million citizens may take the initiative to invite the European Commission to submit any appropriate proposal on matters where citizens consider that a legal act of the EU is required for the purpose of implementing the Treaty of Lisbon.

40 Eriksen & Fossum 2010, 7.

41 Following the debt crisis in Greece and fears regarding the potential risk of contagion to other EU economies, European citizens' support for their country's membership in the EU and belief in the associated perceived benefits of EU membership has fallen according to the latest Eurobarometer poll from May 2010. The poll results show that support for EU membership has fallen to 49% (versus 53% in autumn 2009). Trust in the EU has also fallen from 48% in autumn 2009 to 42% in spring 2010. Eurobarometer 73. Public opinion in the European Union, August 2010.

Eriksen, E & Fossum, J
2010 *Bringing European Democracy Back in or how to read the German Constitutional Court's Lisbon Treaty ruling.* Oslo: Arena Working Paper No. 9. Available at: http://www.sv.uio.no/arena/english/research/publications/arena-publications/workingpapers/working-papers2010/

Habermas, J
1998 *Between facts and norms contributions to a discourse theory of law and democracy*; transl. by William Rehg. Cambridge: MIT Press.

Karlsson, C
2001 *Democracy, Legitimacy and the European Union.* Uppsala: Skrifter utgivna av Statsvetenskapliga föreningen i Uppsala.

Kumm, M
2005 The Jurisprudence of Constitutional Conflict: Constitutional Supremacy, Europe before and after the Constitutional Treaty. *European Law Journal*, Vol. 11/3, 262-307, Blackwell Publishing.

Maurer, A
2004 The Convention Method for Enhancing EU Democracy. *Deliberative Constitutional Politics in the EU*, Closa & Fossum (Eds.), 357-362. Oslo: Arena Centre for European Studies.

MacCormick, N
1998 Risking Constitutional Collision in Europe. *Oxford Journal of legal Studies*, Vol. 18, 517-532. Oxford: Oxford University Press.

Maduro, M
2003a Contrapunctual Law: Europe's Constitutional Pluralism in Action. *Sovereignty in Transition* Walker, N (ed.), 501-537, Oxford: Hart Publishing.
2003b *Europe and the Constitution: what if this is a good as it gets?* European Constitutionalism Beyond the State (Eds.) Weiler & Wind, 74-102. Cambridge University Press.

Lindfelt, M
2007 *Fundamental Rights in the European Union. Towards Higher Law of the Land. A study of the status of fundamental rights in a broader constitutional setting.* Åbo: Åbo Akademi University Press.

Weiler, J
1997 The Reform of European Constitutionalism. *Journal of Common Market Studies*, Vol. 35, No. 1, 97-131.

1999 Transformation of Europe, *The constitution of Europe "do the new clothes have an emperor" and other essays on European integration.* 10-101, Cambridge: Cambridge University Press.

2003 In defence of the status quo; Europ's constitutional Sonderweg. In *European Constitutionalism Beyond the State*, (Eds.) Weiler & Wind, 7-23. Cambridge: Cambridge University Press.

Witte B

1999 Direct effect, Supremacy and the nature of legal order in *The Evolution of EU Law*. (Eds.) Craig & de Búrca, 177-213. Oxford: Oxford University Press.

2000 Institutional Principles: A Special Category of General Principles of EC law. *General Principles of European Union law*, Bernitz & Nergelius (eds.),143-159. Hague: Kluwer Law.

RECONCILIATION, TRANSITIONAL JUSTICE AND THE LEGITIMACY OF THE STATE

Joakim Molander

Reconciliation is a concept frequently used to describe the process of building peace in societies torn apart by conflict. The manner in which the concept is used, however, has given rise to debate among researchers and also caused controversy in post-conflict societies. Such debate and controversy concerns issues such as whether reconciliation relates to changing interpersonal relationships or general societal attitudes. Another topic for debate has been the relationship between forgiveness and reconciliation, with some individuals arguing that it is morally incorrect to ask victims of conflict to forgive and reconcile. At the same time that some victims of conflicts have been disturbed by such requests, other victims have claimed that justice is sacrificed on the altar of reconciliation.

Many of these controversies derive from the fact that the concept reconciliation has a long history rooted in Judeo-Christian tradition where reconciliation is framed by its interlinkage to other moral concepts such as atonement, penance, punishment and forgiveness. Yet such interlinkage is not commonly acknowledged by peace researchers and 'peace practitioners'[1], who often try to define reconciliation as if the concept were devoid of a history or religious and moral connotations and as if it did not already hold a position in everyday vocabulary. Thus, as it currently stands the manner in which the term reconciliation is commonly used by peace researchers and peace practitioners often results in more ambiguity than clarity.

Some of the conceptual ambiguity arising when the concept reconciliation is used in post conflict contexts will be investigated in this article. I will also

---

1 This term refers to individuals involved in humanitarian assistance, post conflict management and development cooperation in conflict and post conflict societies. These practitioners typically work for multilateral organisations (such as the UNDP, UNHCR or OSCE), bilateral organisations (such as the USAID, the DFID or Sida) and large international NGOs (such as the Lutheran World Federation, the Red Cross or Caritas).

present the argument that the full richness of language is needed to describe the process that is often labelled 'post conflict reconciliation'.

'Reconciliation' in peace research

Maria Ericson argues that she is following the recent tendency of peace researchers and theologians when she defines reconciliation as 'the establishment of a positive and sustainable peace between individuals involved in armed conflict.'[2] According to Ericson, the concept has been identified with two particular processes in recent research and debate:

1. 'Bridging the divide' of negative attitudes, stereotypes and images held by individuals in conflict in order to build mutual trust and new relationships across divisions.
2. 'Dealing with the past' by healing the damage caused in the course of past conflict. Here the needs of victimised individuals or groups as well as the perpetrators of violence are looked at with the aim of building, restoring or transforming interpersonal relationships.[3]

Defined as such, reconciliation processes address two of the three pillars in the so-named conflict triangle[4], namely conflict attitudes[5] and conflict behaviour[6]. Ericson writes:

> Initiatives for reconciliation may address the *conflict behavior*, for instance by seeking to bring an end to armed conflict, or by establishing measures to redress the trauma and broken relationships caused by certain forms of conflict behavior. Reconciliation may also be interpreted as the alteration of negative *conflict attitudes* through the enhancing of mutual understanding and challenging of misperceptions and distrust.[7]

Even if Ericson does underscore some of the most important features of how the term reconciliation is used in peace research, various influential researchers in the field define the concept quite differently. Many, like Johan Galtung, emphasise that reconciliation is 'a process of healing the traumas of both victims

---

2 Ericson 2001, p. 86.
3 Ericson 2001, p. 21.
4 The conflict triangle was originally proposed by Johan Galtung in 1969 and is nowadays a widely accepted definition of conflict among peace researchers. See Galtung 1978, pp. 484-507.
5 This includes emotional orientations such as feelings of anger, distrust, resentment, fear, and envy and cognitive processes such as misperceptions and stereotyping. See Ericson 2001, p. 81.
6 Armed force used by one or many parties in a conflict.
7 Ericson 2001, p. 85.

and perpetrators after the violence, providing a closure of the bad relation.'[8] Priscilla Hayner similarly writes that 'reconciliation implies building or rebuilding relationships today that are not haunted by the conflicts and hatreds of yesterday.'[9] Thus Galtung and Hayner regard the essence of reconciliation as being the process of restoring relationships between individuals. Galtung, however, emphasises the psychological aspects of the reconciliation process while Hayner highlights the social dimensions. Other researchers are more concerned with the moral aspects of the reconciliation process. Hizkias Assefa, for example, writes that 'the essence of reconciliation is the voluntary initiative of the conflict parties to acknowledge their responsibility and guilt.'[10]

Still others define reconciliation as a concept that encapsulates all sorts of societal relationships. John Paul Lederach argues that 'reconciliation represents a space, a place or location of encounter, where parties to a conflict meet'[11] and states that 'the key lies in transforming the *relationship* of the conflicting parties, with all that the term encompasses at the spiritual, psychological, social, economic, political and military levels.'[12] Hugo van der Merwe shares a similarly broad understanding of the concept. According to him, reconciliation includes 'all initiatives which bring together, or engage, both sides in a pursuit of changing identity, values regarding interaction, attitudes, and patterns of interaction that move them to a more cooperative relationship.'[13]

In an attempt to bring some order to these rather different yet nonetheless similar perceptions, Karin Brounéus has argued that reconciliation 'is not exact and constant but quite vague and elusive processes that we need to box into definitions that hold for scientific investigation.'[14] Emanating from the common features of the various definitions of reconciliation seen in literature, she suggests that 'reconciliation is a societal process that involves mutual acknowledgement of past suffering and the changing of destructive attitudes and behaviour into constructive relationships toward sustainable peace.' She furthermore states that 'reconciliation mainly focuses on remembering, changing, and continuing with life in peace' and that it 'does not require forgetting, forgiving, or loving one another.'[15]

Brounéus, however, only presents views and quotations that correspond with her own definition of the concept, whereas in fact the term reconciliation is used in post conflict discussions in a tremendous number of ways. In such

8 Brounéus 2003, p. 17 who quoted from Ericson 2001, p. 85.
9 Brounéus 2003, p. 15. Originally in Hayner 2001, p. 161.
10 Brounéus 2003, p. 17. Originally in Assefa 1999.
11 Brounéus 2003, p. 15. Originally in John Paul Lederach, *Building Peace: Sustainable Reconciliation in Divided Societies* (Washington D.C.: United States Institute of Peace Press 1997), p. 30.
12 Ericson 2001, p. 109. Originally in Lederach 1997, p. 40.
13 Brounéus 2003, p. 16. Originally in van der Merwe 1999.
14 Brounéus 2003, pp. 19-20.
15 Brounéus 2003, p. 20.

discourse some individuals for example define reconciliation very broadly: as a process of peace building that involves everything from reconciliation between individual perpetrators and victims; as reconciliation between groups that have been on opposing sides in a conflict; and as used to address inequalities in society. Inspired by the notion of 'structural violence', Robert J. Schreiter for example argues that reconciliation is 'not only a matter of healing memories and receiving forgiveness, it is also about changing the structures in society that provoked, promoted, and sustained violence.'[16] And South African Itumeleng J. Mosala stresses that 'black people insist that any talk of reconciliation between them and whites must begin with an appreciation of the history of their alienation. It is in this history that the roots of the black people's perspective on reconciliation lie.'[17] Interestingly, the Truth and Reconciliation Commission in South Africa subscribed to Mosala's point of view by pointing out that 'economic development and redistribution would be essential for reconciliation, underlining *the responsibility of the white population as a whole, as beneficiaries of apartheid.*'[18]

Viewed from Mosala's broad perspective, reconciliation mainly concerns reconciling groups of people, in this case blacks and whites in South Africa. Brounéus, like Ericson and most of the researchers she quotes, also focuses on reconciliation between groups in conflict. Yet in Ericson's and Brounéus' definitions, reconciliation refers to changing attitudes and behaviour rather than changing society. Perceived in this manner, the views promoted by Schreiter and Mosala do not fit into Ericson's and Brounéus' definitions.

Reconciliation and forgiveness

Nevertheless, both Brounéus and Ericson use the term 'reconciliation' in a much broader sense than is the case in everyday vocabulary, where reconciliation commonly refers to two individuals who settle a dispute. The Webster's Desk Dictionary (1990 edition) suggests that reconciliation is 'to make friendly again, as after a quarrel' and 'to harmonize or settle (a quarrel etc.).' And the Cambridge International Dictionary (1995) states that 'reconciliation is the process of making two people or groups of people friendly again after they have argued.' As these references demonstrate reconciliation as used in everyday vocabulary clearly differs quite substantially from the definitions attributed the term in peace research. For example, it would normally be quite strange in everyday vocabulary to use the term reconciliation to refer to two individuals who have not previously had a relationship prior to the wrongful act perpetrated

16 Schreiter 1992, p. 1. Quoted here from Ericson 2001, p. 109.
17 Mosala 1987. P. 21. Quoted here from Ericson, 2001 p. 429.
18 Ericson 2001, p. 370.

by one of the individuals. The reason for this is that reconciliation in everyday vocabulary is usually understood as the mutual undertaking of two individuals who *re-establish* a relationship that has been damaged by conflict (a quarrel for example).

But this is not the only way the word reconciliation can be used. In cases of wrongdoing by one party towards another, for example, reconciliation is not a mutual undertaking; the initiative instead rests with the victim. In such instances, reconciliation is pursuant to a victim being willing to forgive the perpetrator. Conceptual considerations of this nature '[raise] the question of whether forgiveness should include (or at least imply willingness to) *(re)-establish a relationship* with (i.e. to be reconciled with) the person whom one forgives.'[19] As Maria Ericson found during her interviews in South Africa and Northern Ireland, various individuals perceive issues of this kind the concept of forgiveness differently:

> Various interpretations of *forgiveness* could be noted, ranging from overcoming bitterness but focusing on one's own future rather than being concerned about the perpetrator, to forgiveness as sufficient trust to (re-)establish a (preferably long-lasting) relationship with the perpetrator. A middle way would be the view that forgiveness would entail releasing a grudge and replacing it with empathy for the perpetrator.[20]

As previously mentioned, Brounéus claims that reconciliation 'does not require forgetting, forgiving, or loving one another.' It is noteworthy that Ericson and others, nonetheless, do perceive clear associations between forgiveness and reconciliation. In some relationships, for example between family members[21], it would also appear as if true reconciliation implies that the parties involved must begin to love one another again: without such love, this is the settling of a conflict, not reconciliation.

One of the reasons why such conceptual confusion exists could emanate from peace researchers having borrowed the term reconciliation from the vocabulary of restorative justice, in which the encounter between a victim and perpetrator is fundamental to the reconciliation process. In peace building, however, researchers mostly tend to refer to more general, collective processes rather than interpersonal reconciliation between victims and perpetrators. For this and other reasons the relationship between reconciliation and forgiveness is much debated by both the researchers and practitioners involved with post conflict reconciliation. Hugo van der Merwe for example noted in his interviews

---

19 Ericson 2001, p. 131.

20 Ericson 2001, p. 431.

21 As, for example, following a conflict between husband and wife, parents and children, or when members of the same family have fought on opposite sides in an external conflict such as a civil war.

in South Africa that some victims find the idea of reconciliation, and especially forgiveness, offensive. And Amy Gutmann and Dennis Thompson have argued that many citizens (including the victims themselves) may reasonably believe that it is morally inappropriate to forgive individuals who are unwilling to be punished for their crimes or unwilling to offer their victims restitution. Even the South African Truth and Reconciliation Commission has been heavily criticised for expecting too much interpersonal forgiveness and reconciliation, with the point being made that forgiveness is a personal rather than public matter. This was also implied when a South African woman, commenting on the testimony given at the Truth and Reconciliation Commission by the killer of her husband, stated: 'No government can forgive.' Pause. 'No commission can forgive.' Pause. 'Only I can forgive.' Pause. 'And I am not ready to forgive.'[22]

Extrapolating from her interviews in Northern Ireland, Maria Ericson notes that, 'While forgiveness was regarded as one important part of the Christian message there was, however, *a wariness about putting too great emphasis on interpersonal forgiveness by the individual victims of violence.*'[23] Thus in Northern Ireland communal rather than individual forgiveness was seen as necessary for peace. As one of Ericson's informants stated, 'What *is required* is that the community at large – battered, hurt and damaged by what has happened over the last 25 years – be prepared to enter into a more general process of being able to set aside the past – with all its enmities and demands for revenge – and start anew.'[24]

Charles Villa-Vicencio has distinguished between the concepts of reconciliation as 'peaceful coexistence' and reconciliation as 'the restoration or establishment of personal relationships.' Villa-Vicencio's term 'peaceful coexistence' shares much in common with Brounéus' definition of reconciliation in that restoring or building personal relationships, in Villa-Vicencio's own words, would imply 'that we learn to love one another.'[25] Villa-Vicencio makes an important distinction here. In regards to peace building, reconciliation is in many ways a more perplexing than clarifying concept. It is, at best, odd to speak about reconciliation between victims of war crimes or apartheid and the architects and perpetrators of such acts.

To use the term reconciliation in such a way is odd for a number of reasons. One reason is that it is implied that victims and perpetrators cannot become involved in a mutual process of reconciliation unless the victim first forgives the perpetrator. While it is perhaps possible that a victim could forgive a perpetrator even if the perpetrator does not acknowledge that what he has done is wrong, reconciliation would appear to require that a perpetrator understand that he has

22 See Gutmann and Thompson, p. 31.
23 Ericson 2001, p. 323.
24 Ericson 2001, p. 323.
25 See Ericson 2001, pp. 427-428.

committed a wrong and accordingly feels or demonstrates remorse. As such reconciliation becomes a mutual undertaking where two parties must reach common understanding or agreement on an event; reconciliation without such common understanding is flawed. Perpetrators who have committed human rights violations very seldom admit that they have committed a wrong, which is a second reason why it is erroneous to speak about reconciliation about such perpetrators and their victims. A third reason is that victims and perpetrators in such circumstances are typically strangers to one another when the offences occur and as such have no relationship to restore. A fourth reason is that it is patronising to speak of reconciliation in such a manner: from a moral point of view reconciliation, precisely like forgiveness, can only be established in a relationship if it is introduced by those individuals involved in the conflict.

However, even if Villa-Vicencio makes an important point he is incorrect to assume that building a personal relationship implies that individuals learn to love one another. Only some personal relationships contain the element love, many others work just fine without it. Consequently, terms such as respect or trust would better apply to the actual nature of personal relationships.

Reconciliation and justice

Another much contested issue in the practice and literature of reconciliation in peace building concerns the relationship between reconciliation and justice. As a former program officer for the Swedish International Development Cooperation Agency (Sida) at the Embassy of Sweden to Bosnia and Herzegovina, I have first hand experience of the heated discussions that took place in an attempt to establish a truth commission in Bosnia and Herzegovina in 2005-2006. Representatives of the OSCE in particular claimed that a truth commission would undermine the pursuit of justice for the victims of the atrocities committed during the Bosnian civil war, which spanned from 1993-1996. From her interviews in Northern Ireland Ericson similarly finds that, 'While none of my sources [...] advocated unrestrained vengeance, it was nevertheless argued that there were a variety of needs among victims and that the stress on forgiveness and reconciliation silenced legitimate calls for retribution as an alternative form of closure.'[26] In South Africa the amnesty given to the perpetrators who testified before the South African Truth and Reconciliation Commission has caused anger. In response to such criticism Desmond Tutu spoke of accepting amnesty in terms of making a personal sacrifice for the sake of the nation. He has written 'that is indeed a high price to ask for the victims to

26 Ericson 2001, p. 431.

pay, but it is a price those who negotiated our relatively peaceful transition from repression to democracy believed the nation had to ask of victims.'[27]

Indeed, justice is a highly important concept in relation to reconciliation, but different views on what justice might entail exist. Martha Minow has highlighted that victims often have very different requirements for dealing with what happened to them:

> Survivors of violence often ache for retribution against identifiable perpetrators, and for public acknowledgement of what happened. Some want financial redress; psychological or spiritual healing seems crucial to others. Some survivors, and their fellow citizens, place higher priorities on moving ahead with life, building or rebuilding trust across previously divided groups, and establishing or strengthening democratic institutions. Many believe that the entire society needs to stand behind efforts to punish wrongdoers, and to deter any such conduct in the future. People understandably may have great trouble sorting out priorities among these possibilities.[28]

The range of attitudes observed by Minow helps us understand that justice and retribution are not the same concept. Yet neither are justice and reconciliation the same concept. Instead, justice should ideally encompass a number of processes that are in many ways interlinked and bound together by concepts such as guilt, truth, confession, remorse, penance, atonement and punishment. By acknowledging the interdependence that exists between these concepts, the notion that the essence of justice is constituted by either punishment or reconciliation can be dispelled.

It is therefore of outmost importance that the moral conceptual landscape where these concepts belong be more closely examined. To start it is worth noting the moral significance of truth and remorse. As both Hugo van der Merwe and Maria Ericson found while interviewing victims of apartheid in South Africa, many victims, in the words of Ericson, 'emphasised the importance of truth as a basis for reconciliation, i.e. that they first needed to know whom to forgive and exactly for what. Some underlined that it was only after they had heard the story of the perpetrator and had heard him express remorse that they could take forgiveness into consideration.'[29] What victims sought was in reality more than 'mere' truth. Instead one can speak of the demand for a confession, since a real confession is also an expression of remorse. This inference is illustrated in the following observation made by Ericson:

27 Ericson 2001, p. 420. Originally in Tutu 1999, p. 52.
28 Ericson 2001, p. 102. Originally in Minow 1998, p. 4.
29 Ericson 2001, p. 352. See also van der Merwe 1999.

> While some victimised people thus expressed forgiveness and empathy, other victims *expressed frustration and anger after their encounter with the perpetrators.* They felt angry with perpetrators who seemed to evade the questions, who did not express remorse, and who appeared to be more interested in amnesty than in repentance.[30]

True remorse is important for victims since it expresses a wrongdoer's realisation that he is, or rather has become, a wrongdoer. Such a realisation is morally and psychologically demanding. One could say that for you as an individual to realise that you are a wrongdoer is a matter of realising that you have betrayed what you regard as being holy in life; you must realise that you have betrayed yourself and your fellow human beings, which in a manner means that you understand that you have distanced yourself from humanity. Raimond Gaita effectively summarises this insight when he states that 'those who, in remorse, suffer in guilty recognition of what they have become, are radically singular, and for that reason remorse is a kind of dying to the world.'[31]

Gitta Sereny describes how a wrongdoer can gain such insight in her book *Into the Darkness*. *Into the Darkness* is based on a number of interviews Sereny conducted with Franz Stangl, commandant for the Treblinka extermination camp during the Second World War. In her book Sereny attempts to understand Stangl's actions, and she maintains that an explanation is that Stangl did not truly understand what he did. She writes:

> As our talks progressed, it became clear that what he was most concerned about until the last two days were what one might call the lesser manifestations of moral corruption in himself; once again, what he *did* rather than what he *was*. It was his "deeds" – his relatively mild deeds – he was at great pains to deny or rationalize rather than his total personality change.[32]

However, during and through the interviews with Sereny, Stangl comes to understand what he had become. During the final hour of the last interview he attempts to maintain his perception that he never intentionally harmed anyone but is overtaken by remorse:

> He gripped the table with both hands as if holding on to it. "But I was there," he said then, in a curiously dry and tired voice of resignation. These few sentences had taken almost half an hour to pronounce. "So yes" he said finally, very quietly, "in reality I share the guilt. … Because my guilt… my guilt… only now in these talks… now that I have talked about it for the first time…" He stopped.
>
> He had pronounced the words "my guilt" – but more than the words, the finality of it was in the sagging of his body, and on his face.

30 Ericson 2001, p. 361.
31 Gaita 1991, p. 48.
32 Sereny 1995, p. 129.

> After more than a minute he started again, a half hearted attempt, in a dull voice. "My guilt," he said, "is that I am still here. That is my guilt."

Stangl died 19 hours after this confession. Everyone, including Gitta Sereny, thought he had committed suicide, but the post-mortem concluded that he died of heart failure. Sereny writes in the last words of *Into the Darkness* that she thinks Stangl died because of his realisation of who he had become and the guilt and remorse associated with this insight.

Reconciliation and atonement retributivism

A sincere confession, such as Stangl's, is a prerequisite for atonement but cannot be regarded a means to such an end in that a sincere confession cannot in any manner be regarded a means to an end. A confession is instead an individual's *expression* of the insight that he has done wrong and that he has thereby become a wrongdoer. It is an expression of guilt and remorse, particularly if the confession is public. The question of whether an individual has atoned or expiated by confessing arises from such reasoning. No doubt many would argue that the sincerity of an individual's remorse, and the suffering he subsequently brings upon himself by publicly declaring his guilt, is sufficient for atonement and that it would be pointless to punish him since he incurs that which a punishment ideally would have conferred. Accordingly, they would argue, a sincere confession and expression of remorse should be enough for forgiveness and even reconciliation.

Punishment, however, cannot be an instrument that the wrongdoer wields. A wrongdoer can come to the realisation that he is a wrongdoer and, as a consequence of this insight, confess and do penance. But if the wrongdoer uses his confession and penance as a means to atonement, reconciliation or even forgiveness, he has not actually understood the essence of his wrongdoing. The point here is, as Socrates writes in *Gorgias*, that an evildoer is 'pitiable as well as miserable.'[33] Gaita has, I think, fully grasped the content of Socrates' rather esoteric point in the following quotation:

> I think that Socrates says that if we do not pity an evil-doer then we do not know what evil is, that indignation in the face of evil is a failure to understand what we are confronted with. That means that we would misunderstand Socratic pity for the evil-doer if we asked: but what of the hard-hearted, those who acknowledge the harm evil-doers do themselves but who say that it is no more than they deserve.[34]

33 Plato 1960, p. 53.
34 Gaita 1991, p. 61.

An example of such understanding is seen in Sonya's pity for Raskolnikov in Dostoyevsky's *Crime and Punishment*. Sonya pities Raskolnikov because she realises what he has become, and this insight brings her to the realisation that he must be punished. Punishment in this example is not an act of vengeance or retribution but of grace. Or, in the words of Simone Weil:

> Just as the only way of showing respect for somebody suffering from hunger is to give him something to eat, so the only way of showing respect for somebody who has placed himself outside the law is to reinstate him inside the law by subjecting him to the punishment that is ordained by the law.[35]

Through punishment, society brings a wrongdoer back from solitude into the community of mankind. Thus, Weil argues, punishment is a vital need for the soul and it accordingly 'must be an honour.' Punishment in this sense strives not only for understanding but also for acceptance:

> Just as the musician awakens the sense of beauty in us by sounds, so the penal system should know how to awaken the sense of justice in the criminal by infliction of pain, or even, if need be, of death. And in the same way as we can say of the apprentice who injures himself at his trade, that is the trade which is getting into *him*, so punishment is a method for getting justice into the soul of the criminal by bodily suffering.[36]

If an evildoer comes to accept his punishment, the punishment can achieve its full potential as a form of atonement. The evildoer can then reconcile with other human beings. If an evildoer never fully accepts his punishment, reconciliation cannot occur; the evildoer continues to be an evildoer even after punishment. This is what happens to Raskolnikov. He finally gives himself up and, rather than confessing, reluctantly pleads guilty in the legal sense of that expression. As such he never really comes to terms with his guilt. He is tormented by his conscience but uses utilitarian argumentation to overcome remorse. Guilt is internally connected to remorse; an individual does not truly understand that he is guilty without becoming remorseful. Raskolnikov fails to listen to his conscience and ultimately fails to see that he has perpetrated wrongs.

I would like to label the perspective on punishment delineated above atonement retributivism. Atonement retributivism should not be regarded as a theory that allows for the justification of punishment. Instead it is a label that can be applied to a form of moral vocabulary that derives from a Judeo-Christian tradition and finds its strongest expression in the death of Christ. Central to the story of the death of Christ is that God is able to overcome his wrath by allowing the suffering of Christ to serve as penance for the sin of men. The severity of

35 Weil 2002, p. 21.
36 Ibid, p. 22.

Christ's penance illustrates the gravity of evil in men and is able to awake remorse in mankind. By the grace of God an act of evil was turned into an act of atonement, and mankind was thereby reconciled with God. [37]

Reconciliation, trust, tolerance, acceptance and legitimacy

The story of the death of Christ shows that the term reconciliation is interlinked with a moral vocabulary in which concepts such as evil, wrath, penance, remorse and atonement are fundamental. Consequently it is difficult to understand the meaning of reconciliation without comprehension of the conceptual landscape that it derives from. Peacc researchers and peace practitioners repeatedly miss this point. Still, Hugo van der Merwe has made an attempt to address some of the conceptual problems discussed here. Van der Merwe distinguishes between reconciliation defined as relationship building and reconciliation defined as a process aimed at addressing the structural causes of conflict and also argues that these two dimensions of reconciliation are interdependent as parts of a broader peace building process. He further develops a three-dimensional view of reconciliation concerning the different spheres of a relationship that need to be addressed (identity, values relating to interaction, conflict behaviour, conflict attitudes), the different substantive components of reconciliation (justice, truth, security, healing) and the different levels of reconciliation (national, community and interpersonal).[38]

In his analysis van der Merwe calls attention to many crucial aspects of peace building and proposes a broad yet simultaneously differentiated manner of using the concept of reconciliation in such contexts. Although it is clear that the term reconciliation can be used quite differently in various circumstances, thereby making a straightforward definition difficult, I cannot see why it would be necessary to attempt to label all the processes van der Merwe refers to as being processes of reconciliation or processes whose predominant aim is to bring about reconciliation. It would instead be advisable to employ a variety of different terms to describe these varying circumstances.

When referring to conflicting groups whose 'representatives' are entangled with each other in numerous different ways, for example, it is neither possible nor necessary to use the term reconciliation for all of the diverse changes that need to occur in their relationships before a state of peaceful coexistence can be realised. However, in those instances when a conflict has divided former friends or family members, for example, it is sometimes certainly appropriate to apply the term reconciliation. Nevertheless, even in such instances one concept alone cannot fully encapsulate the complicated, damaged nature of the interlinked

37 For reference see Molander 2009, pp. 178-196.
38 van der Merwe 1999. See Ericson 2001, p. 48.

interpersonal relationships in the situation. It takes nothing less than the full richness of language to describe such complex relationships. When it comes to describing the 'restoration' of damaged relationships between individuals who do not know each other and have perhaps never met, reconciliation seems to be a misguided concept altogether. In such circumstances it is more appropriate to speak in terms of *mutual trust*, *tolerance* or *acceptance*.

A further crucial aspect inherent to the restoration of the social fabric in a damaged society is the restoration of individuals' trust in government and state institutions. Peace researchers and peace practitioners often apply the term transitional justice to such a process[39]. Yet the term is often regarded as a means whereby to achieve reconciliation. The August 2004 report of the United Nations Secretary-General, for example, states that 'the notion of transitional justice comprises the full range of processes and mechanisms associated with a society's attempt to come to terms with a legacy of large-scale past abuses in order to ensure accountability, serve justice and achieve reconciliation.'[40] But the concept of reconciliation is not fitting here. Transitional justice should instead refer to a manner whereby the *legitimacy* of a state can be rebuilt, with the underlying assumption that a legitimate state provides the framework for peaceful coexistence between its citizens.

By widening our vocabulary through the inclusion of the concepts described here, we are able to fine-tune analysis of the different processes that must occur in post conflict settings if sustainable peace is to be achieved. For example it would be illuminating to speak of the current constitution of Bosnia and Herzegovina, which divides the country between ethnic groups and is based on the Dayton Peace Agreement, as an obstacle to building the legitimacy of the state rather than an obstacle to reconciliation. Doing so allows for the realisation that a constitution that rests on the fragile division of power between ethnic groups undermines the legitimacy of the state; one can clearly see that such a constitution nurtures a form of distrust that then shapes the political landscape. Political problems of this type are not necessarily linked to processes of forgiveness or reconciliation between former neighbours, colleges and friends; the introduction of moral and religious language in such a political discourse therefore causes both confusion and anger.

To conclude the current discussion surrounding the concepts of transitional justice, peace building and reconciliation would benefit greatly from a change in

39 On 24 September 2003 the United Nations Security Council met at the ministerial level todiscuss the role of the United Nations in establishing justice and the rule of law in post conflict societies. This started a process that was concluded with the presentation of a report from the UN Secretary-General in August 2004 entitled "The rule of law and transitional justice in conflict and post-conflict societies", through which the term 'transitional justice' was established. The notion of transitional justice as discussed in the UN report comprises individual prosecutions, reparations, truth-seeking, institutional reform, vetting and dismissals or a combination thereof.

40 UN Secretary-General 2004, §8.

vocabulary. Even if concrete examples of concepts that can help sharpen the thinking surrounding these issues have been presented in this essay – concepts such as acceptance, tolerance, trust and legitimacy – the discussion found here should nevertheless be interpreted as a preliminary conceptual view of the issue.

Bibliography

Assefa, H
1999 "The Meaning of Reconciliation" in ed. Paul van Tongeren, *People Building Peace: 35 Inspiring Stories from Around the World*. Utrecht: European Centre for Conflict Prevention.

Brounéus, K
2001 *Reconciliation – Theory and Practice for Development Cooperation.* Sida, 2003.

Ericson, M
2001 *Reconciliation and the Search for a Shared Moral Landscape – An Exploration Based upon a Study of Northern Ireland and South Africa*. Lang: Frankfurt am Main.

Gaita, R
1991 *Good and Evil. An Absolute Conception*. Houndmills: Macmillan 1991.

Galtung, J
1978 "Conflict as a Way of Life": Chapter 15, in Galtung J: *Peace and Social structure, Essays in Peace Research*, Vol. III. Copenhagen: Ejlers, 1978.

Hayner, P B
2001 *Unspeakable Truths: Confronting State Terror and Atrocity.* New York: Routledge.

Lederach, J P
1997 *Building Peace: Sustainable Reconciliation in Divided Societies.* Washington D.C.: United States Institute of Peace Press.

van der Merwe, H
1999 *The Truth and Reconciliation Commission and Community Reconciliation: An Analysis of Competing Strategies and Conceptualizations*. Fairfax: George Mason University.

Minow, M
1998 *Between Vengeance and Forgiveness – Facing History after Genocide and Mass Violence*. Boston: Beacon Press.

Molander, J

2009 "Atonement Retributivism" in *Studia Theologica – Nordic Journal of Theology* Vol. 63, No. 2, pp. 178-196.

Mosala, I J

1987 "The Meaning of Reconciliation –A Black Perspective", in *Journal of Theology for Southern Africa*, No. 59.

Plato

1960 *Gorgias*. London: Penguin books.

Schreiter, R J

1992 *Reconciliation – Mission and Ministry in a Changing Social Order.* New York: Orbis.

Sereny, G

1995 (1974) *Into the Darkness – from Mercy Killing to Mass Murder.* London: Pimlico.

Tutu, D

1999 *No Future Without Forgiveness.* London / Sydney / Auckland / Johannesburg: Ryder.

UN Secretary-General

2004 "The rule of law and transitional justice in conflict and post-conflict societies", §8.

Weil, S

2002 (1049) *The Need for Roots – Preludence to a Declaration of Duties towards Mankind*. London: Routledge classics.

THE QUEST FOR LEGITIMACY IN CONFLICT RESOLUTION THROUGH RESTORATIVE JUSTICE

Heidi Jokinen

The concept of legitimacy is multi-faceted, as the collection of articles in this volume demonstrates. Still, as a simplified primary definition, I wish to start by proposing that legitimacy is often associated with approval: approval of political entities, approval of the laws and procedures of a political entity or approval of individuals as representatives of such entities. An institution can be considered legitimate when it is perceived to possess the right to independently make decisions that affect citizens and when citizens perceive the decisions of that institution to be worthy of obedience.

Defined so, the Finnish justice system can be viewed as an example of a legitimate institution. It enjoys the right to make decisions that affect individuals and its decisions are complied with. However, on closer look the concept of legitimacy might not be quite so straightforward. The decisions of a justice system are ultimately secured through the use of coercive power and as such citizen compliance is not necessarily voluntary. Instead citizens are forced to abide by these decisions.

In my view this brings us directly to a fundamental problem in understanding legitimacy as defined above, as mere approval. As compliance with certain rules is not always derived from the will of the parties involved in the matter but instead from something external to them, such as coercion, it is not clear in what manner and to what degree one could claim that the parties involved actually approve of the process. I therefore maintain that external coercion affects the legitimacy of conflict resolution.

In their contribution to this volume Tage Kurtén and Ville Päivänsalo argue that the legitimacy of a rule of law should primarily be considered as being taken for granted by citizens until something occurs which disturbs that fundamental trust in the system or in the authority representing the system. It is only then that the question of legitimacy becomes of interest.[1] In my view this is exactly what happens in the context of conflict resolution. The legitimacy of a legal procedure is often assumed yet signs indicate that this process is not imperfect and that, in fact, the legitimacy of legal procedures as a method of conflict resolution can be called into question. The traditional method for conflict resolution, a court process, does not always fully address the legitimacy claims of the parties involved and, consequently, they can become profoundly disappointed in authorities.

The purpose of this particular article is to examine how victim-offender mediation, in the context of conflict resolution, contributes to the legitimacy claims of the parties involved in the mediation.[2] Restorative justice provides an alternative or complement to adversarial legal processes. The restorative approach responds to crime and wrongdoing in a non-coercive manner. The parties involved are provided the authority to, by themselves, jointly identify the harms and needs that, in their opinion, should be addressed when resolving the conflict. As such restorative justice presents an internal rather than an external approach to conflict resolution and emphasises the personal participation of the parties involved.

I demonstrate that the quest for restorative justice can be interpreted as an expression of lost trust in the retributive system. Restorative justice, an attempt to amend the failure of traditional adjudication, can therefore be interpreted as enhancing the legitimacy of the conflict resolution process. I will also illuminate some further aspects of legitimacy as well.

Legitimacy of the criminal justice system questioned

Throughout history societies have implemented rules that delineate which behaviour is accepted and which behaviour is prohibited in an attempt to ease interaction between individuals in a community and protect citizens from different types of injustice. Such rules nowadays predominately take the form of laws and regulations.

In that rules are perceived as protecting the wellbeing and cohesion of a society, behaviour that deviates from that which society deems acceptable must be addressed. Society therefore takes measures against individuals who engage in prohibited actions. One belief deeply rooted in human culture is the belief that an offence can be made right through punishment. It is a society itself that determines and institutes rules and any violation of a rule is understood as a

1 See the article by Tage Kurtén and Ville Päivänsalo in this volume.

2 I call this method victim-offender mediation in that it, in my view, is a well-established concept in the context of conflict resolution. However, in Finnish legislation this method is officially termed 'conciliation'. See for example the Act on Conciliation in Criminal and Certain Civil Cases 1015/2005, section 1; Zehr 2002, 8 – 9.

violation against the whole of society. Punishment in this manner is accordingly provided collective meaning.[3]

Consequently, when dealing with offences in western societies, the victims of an offence are often only allowed to play a subordinate role. An important source of the discontent directed towards the criminal justice system of today is that the system primarily focuses on the wrong done to society rather than the wrong done to victims.[4] Punishment is something externally imposed on the parties involved and, as such, is problematic in relation to conflict resolution for the legitimacy claims of the parties involved.

Of course a certain rationale exists behind why an external approach to punishment prevails. In modern adjudication the avoidance of arbitrariness is central. In *Discipline and Punish* (1995), Michel Foucault maintains that this belief has its roots in the Enlightenment, which fostered in western societies the strong ideal of equality between all citizens and which is consequently applied to the domain of punishment. In the name of equality the personal will of a legislator should neither determine nor influence an issue and, irrespective of social class or status, offenders must be punished equally for comparable offences. So that equal treatment might be guaranteed, the legal system in western societies has been made as foreseeable as possible. Authorities make known in advance what punishment is connected to what crime and, consequently, the criminal justice system claims universality.[5]

Universality here is often perceived as the compliance of the parties involved with the criminal justice system. In that the parties involved are cognisant of the fact that the system is constructed in accordance with certain pre-accepted rules, it is believed that the system affords all individuals equal treatment and is objective or that, at least, the system is not in any manner subjective.

Still, the idea of an objective legal system is not quite as unproblematic as it would appear. That which is paradoxical in regarding positive (written) law as being universal and objective has been pointed out by Kaarlo Tuori among others. Tuori demonstrates how the emergence of pluralist societies challenges the legitimacy of positive law. According to Tuori, when the good of each individual is no longer presumed but rather up to each individual to define, no specific value can claim universality. Thus positive law in essence employs a subjective choice of values.[6]

As such the pre-accepted rules inherent in positive law do not necessarily express the will of each and every individual but instead merely constitute one manner of determining relationships between individuals in a society. One

3 Leer-Salvesen 1999, 240; Frände 2003, 4.
4 Leer-Salvesen 1999, 240; Frände 2003, 4.
5 Foucault 1995, 104 – 105.
6 Tuori 1990, 7.

particular individual might wish to define the rules in a completely different manner and, consequently, is prepared to challenge the legitimacy of positive law.

Nonetheless, the criminal justice system does not necessarily require the approval of the individual in order to function. Those rules that determine what is right and what is wrong also define the limits that authorities might take in relation to offenders and allow for a certain degree of coercion. For example, as long as court proceedings adhere to a certain regulatory procedural framework, a court continues to enjoy the right to enforce judgement without the consent of the parties involved. In other words, the coercive power of the state is inherent in such a legal order and the enforcing power of the state affects the parties involved whether they consent to judgement or not. Hence an offender has very little choice but to submit to the judgement of the court and consequently the punishment that the court deems appropriate.[7] Thus one can say that it is not that the parties involved wish to comply with the criminal justice system but instead that they must.

It is such qualities of the criminal justice system that are in my view significant when considering the meaning of legitimacy in relation to this system. Firstly, the attempt to believe in one single set of rules is not always quite as legitimate as one would expect and, secondly, the coercive powers of authorities, which results in the compliance of individuals, does not always necessarily indicate that those individuals believe in the legitimacy of that authority.

Questioning the legitimacy of the criminal justice system in a western context, where the system is typically considered to be highly reliable and where citizens predominantly trust both the system and its representatives, is perhaps unexpected. One possible reason behind why this system can be questioned is the fact that in legal discourse legitimacy is often identified with legality. The legitimacy of a specific norm is considered sufficient if that norm conforms to and is recognised by the formal requirements and procedures of a particular legal system. Such legitimacy does not necessarily reflect the opinion of the individual but is instead connected to the institution and its rights. [8]

Legitimacy here is therefore considered to be connected to a formal validity and efficiency of law, and the risk exists for a vicious circle: a law is considered legitimate only when it satisfies the requirements of legitimacy as established by the law itself. Hence the definition of the concept of legitimacy must contain some other aspects as well.

The prevailing tendency of the criminal justice system to focus on a formal validity also leads to a particular source of criticism against the system,

7 See for example Tuori 1990, 1 – 3.

8 For a legal positivism that does not recognise any grounds for legitimacy outside the legal system, see Petev 1989, 202, 205; Tuori 1990, 1 – 3.

with the accusation being made that the legal system has become excessively structured. In the late 1970s Nils Christie, a Norwegian criminologist, published a famous article entitled *Conflicts as property* where he pointed out that the professionalisation of legal proceedings had gone too far. Christie maintains that professionals not only overly dominate the legal system but that they also appear to have stolen legal conflicts from their rightful owners, namely the parties actually involved in the matter.[9]

Individuals not normally involved with the legal system can find it difficult to understand proceedings and consequently need help navigating the legal 'jungle' of rules and regulations. This difficulty that outsiders have in navigating the legal system constitutes a problem and the central source of the discontentment felt towards the justice system and even hints at some important aspects of legitimacy.

Christie criticises the current legal system as being rigid and not taking the specific circumstances of the parties involved into consideration. Christie maintains that in this system equal treatment is preserved in regards to judgements and punishment but that no consideration is given to the concept of justice in broader terms. The offence itself is the decisive factor in the judgement: not the wishes and needs of the victim, not the individual qualities of the offender, not the specific circumstances of the surrounding society.[10]

Other studies have also indicated that the so-named courtroom model cannot always be considered very satisfactory when viewed from the point of view of the parties involved. The disappointment these parties express is very often connected to their lack of involvement in legal proceedings. In *Court Work in Transition* (2002), Vaula Haavisto studied the Finnish civil litigation system prior to its reform in the early 1990s. Haavisto found that criticism of the litigation system existed and that especially the parties involved directed criticism towards the manner in which interaction occurred and the lack of dialogue during the entire process.[11] Similar results were seen in Tuula-Riitta Välikoski's study, *The Criminal Trial as a Speech Communication Situation* (2004). Välikoski's study found that no genuine discussion occurred during legal proceedings and that those formal discussions taking place were difficult for the parties involved to follow.[12]

When dealing with an offence the parties involved could contribute numerous things to the litigation process. Yet the strict behavioural codes of the court are unable to accommodate all the wishes of the parties; it is the court that determines what is legally relevant and what is not. The most important perspective for the parties involved is not always the same perspective that the

9 Christie 1977, 4.
10 Christie 1977, 8.
11 Haavisto 2002, 13 – 14.
12 Välikoski 2004, 51, 104. For examples of the failures of the criminal justice system, see also Leer-Salvesen 1999, 83 – 100.

court deems important. For the parties involved a strong need exists to not only being heard but to also be understood. Each of the parties involved desires an understanding of his or her particular and specific perspective.[13]

The perspective that the parties involved wish to garner attention for often involves aspects related to moral questions. Joakim Molander discusses the inability of the criminal justice system to countenance the needs of the parties involved in *Straffets grammatik* (2002). Molander argues that the legal manner in which matters are dealt with objectively and technically leads a court to overlook the morally relevant aspects of a criminal offence. However, the conflicts between individuals that are addressed during a litigation process are very much moral events. Yet within the current system no room exists for existential guilt in courtrooms, and as a consequence an important aspect of conflict is ignored.[14] The criminal justice system does not take the needs of the parties involved into account but instead addresses the needs of the system itself.

Still, another problem exists that is connected to the submissive role that the parties involved in the litigation process play. Tage Kurtén maintains that the value of a non-professional is undermined when that individual is not provided the opportunity to take responsibility for his actions. When society relies on external rules to determine what is morally correct, in this case rules emanating from professional experts, society disregards the meaning of responsibility and the role that the conscience of each individual plays. In that laymen cannot always understand the information needed to make determinations, they are deprived of the right to their own morals.[15] Externally imposed rules can therefore be problematic, with the problem extending to the judgement handed down as well.

If the parties involved cannot discern the basis for and outcome of a litigation process, the judgement (and thus accordingly the punishment) subsequently handed down may also be bereft of significance. If the parties involved do not consider a judgement fair or reasonable, the consequences can be dire. In such a situation the inhibitory effect of punishment weakens, and an offender who does not perceive the harm his actions have caused is more likely to offend again. Thus the meaningfulness of punishment in such cases can be questioned.

In sum, the lack of connectedness to a litigation process that both victims and offenders alike can feel may be caused by several different factors. Not sufficiently understanding proceedings is one factor while a second factor is the need for the parties involved to have some particular aspect be taken into account during proceedings, such as an existential guilt or the need for

13 Christie 1977, 4.
14 Molander 2002, 136. See also Paul Leer-Salvesen (1999, 89), whose interviews with convicted murderers confirm that the manner in which facts are dealt with during courtroom proceedings do not always correspond to the manner desired by offenders.
15 Kurtén 1998, 14 – 15.

reconciliation on a personal level. Whatever the cause of the dissatisfaction that the parties involved feel in regards to the litigation process, their dissatisfaction profoundly effects their assessment of the legitimacy of the process and, thereby, the criminal justice system as a whole.

Here we arrive at a central point. In regards to an individual actor, formal criteria alone are not sufficient when determining the legitimacy of a legal system. Legitimacy depends upon something other than external factors such as written law and regulations. Despite the occurrence of formal, correct proceedings during a litigation process (which, as stated previously, ultimately only represent externally imposed standards), the parties involved may perceive the judgement handed down to be incomprehensible.

Such perceptions are connected to the personal assessment that the parties involved make of the initial offence. An offender may not perceive his actions to be incorrect, even following judgement, and as such the entire litigation process, and not least sentencing, may to him seem unfair. Hence, again, despite formal, correct proceedings the parties involved may challenge the legitimacy of both the litigation process and its outcome.

Therefore it would seem to be evident that there exists more to the concept of legitimacy than mere conformity to law. The legitimacy claims of the parties involved include aspects that a third party many not necessarily be able to comprehend. Thus I will more closely examine this issue by analysing a concrete example of an alternative method of conflict resolution, victim-offender mediation. Victim-offender mediation can be considered an expression of how the legitimacy of the mainstream criminal justice system is sometimes challenged. Such conflict resolution can, therefore, highlight important aspects of the concept of legitimacy.

Victim-offender mediation as an alternative

Criticism of the criminal justice system has led to the search for a more legitimate way of solving conflicts.[16] Restorative justice is commonly perceived to be a theory of criminal justice that considers crime to be an offence against another individual or community rather than the state. In such a definition, room exists for the personal involvement of the two parties involved and allows these individuals to express their opinions during conflict resolution. While a

16 See Zehr 1995, 158 – 159 and Iivari 1991, 137 for the origins of the so-named Kitchener project in Ontario, Canada in 1974. The Kitchener project is the result of a group of Mennonites who gathered to discuss a Christian response to thieving. This group proposed that victims and offenders be allowed to meet face to face, which also occurred. This project is often considered an important milestone in the creation of the victim-offender mediation movement seen today.

multitude of different practices fit under the umbrella concept of restorative justice, in this article I specifically focus on victim-offender mediation.[17]

Tracing the origins of victim-offender mediation is rather complicated in that the concept does not derive from one single theorist or idea. Instead victim-offender mediation has developed from a variety of concurrent movements that build upon an ancient idea. Mediation is not a new phenomenon invented in our times; similar practices have been used all around the world throughout the history of mankind. For example, the restorative practices of the aborigines in Australia and New Zealand are often mentioned as examples of how important it is that methods be suitable for a particular culture and society when seeking legitimate manners of conflict resolution.[18] Once again we understand that it is important to realise conflict resolution that is meaningful for the parties involved rather than a solution that merely guarantees legal rights. Again, at times the experience of justice is more connected to personal views and attitudes than laws and regulations.

Victim-offender mediation is practiced outside and away from courtrooms to allow the parties involved a chance to informally meet and discuss the mental and material harm caused to the victim by the offence. This meeting does not however address the judicial rights and wrongs of the situation. Victim-offender mediation highlights the importance of a human, inter-personnel perspective on the restorative process. The parties involved are provided the chance to settle the issue personally and express their accountability in the case. In victim-offender mediation the parties involved become subjects instead of mere objects.

In victim-offender mediation a meeting takes place in the presence of a neutral third party, the mediator. In contrast to the role of a judge in a courtroom, the role of the mediator is facilitative. In a balanced manner and without any determinative or advisory aspects, the mediator guides the parties involved in their dialogue so that they best can resolve their conflict. The mediator does not take sides in the case but is, rather, an active listener. The role the mediator plays is based on a fundamental idea in mediation: that the parties involved themselves know what is best for them.[19]

During this meeting the mediator does not propose the manner in which the conflict should be resolved; instead the parties involved themselves 'single-handedly' identify and agree on a suitable resolution. The outcome usually takes the form of a written agreement signed by the parties involved at the end of the meeting. It is imperative that the agreement reflects the opinions and needs of

---

17 Other restorative practices include, among others: Family Group Conferences, where not only victims and offenders but also their families are involved, and Circles, where participants arrange themselves in a circle and speak in the order they are seated in the circle. Zehr 2002, 47 – 52.

18 Braithwaite 2001, 26.

19 Pelikan & Trenczek 2008, 81 – 82. See also the Act on Conciliation in Criminal and Certain Civil Cases 1015/2005, section 17.

both the parties involved. Their desires and wishes play an important role when they discuss the consequences of the offence and restitution. While the nature of the offence should, of course, be taken into account the course of the discussion in a specific meeting and the other matters decided on emanate entirely from the parties involved in relation to that particular meeting and that particular offence: some cases are settled with an apology whereas others are settled with monetary restitution.[20]

Victim-offender mediation and its relationship to the criminal justice system are widely discussed. Although mediation is considered a supplementary judicial process in that it occurs external to courtrooms and professionals, the legal system nonetheless still exerts significant control over victim-offender mediation. In Finland victim-offender mediation can be realised during all stages of a criminal litigation process; it can thus be deceptive to speak of mediation as an alternative. In the Finnish model, victim-offender mediation can be initiated by either of the parties involved or the police or prosecuting authority. Victim-offender mediation in Finland, therefore, constitutes more than a mere alternative; it is in actuality a very important part of the official system of punishment. Moreover, the agreement brokered by the parties involved may lead to significant judicial consequences.[21]

Depending on the nature of an offence, a legal process can be avoided through the use of victim-offender mediation. Firstly, the parties involved broker an agreement, which both parties should find satisfactory and consider acceptable. Secondly, following mediation the police or prosecuting authority is informed of the outcome of the process and the prosecutor either confirms or throws out the agreement. In this process no guarantee exists that a formal litigation process will be avoided, even if the agreement expresses the wishes of the parties involved. The prosecutor holds the right to accept or dismiss the agreement. So while further legal action may be deemed necessary, the agreement can also constitute an adequate reason for non-prosecution.[22]

---

20 Braithwaite 2001, 12; Mielityinen 1999, 46. Even though formally it does not matter what the actual agreement consists of, and the autonomy of the parties involved is in this respect underlined, advocates of restorative justice emphasise that not every kind of resolution should be considered viable. The restorative justice process should be connected to restorative values such as apology, repairing of harm, forgiveness and reconciliation. Braithwaite 2001, 12.

21 The Act on Conciliation in Criminal and Certain Civil Cases 1015/2005 sections 3, 13; Pelican & Trenczek 2008, 82 – 83. The Finnish model of mediation does not fully correspond to Christie's model, in which mediation is delineated as being something external to and independent of the court system. Christie's model would entail a risk that many cases would never progress to mediation. In the Finnish model mediation can also exert a renewing effect on the official, 'formal' criminal justice system. Iivari 1991, 75.

22 The Act on Conciliation in Criminal and Certain Civil Cases 1015/2005 section 16; Frände 2003, 196 – 200.

The positive effects of victim-offender mediation are numerous. It humanises criminal justice processes through personal encounters and increases the personal accountability of an offender through direct contact between the parties involved. Mediation also provides satisfying roles for the parties involved through active participation, meaningful restitution for victims and the possibility for alternative consequences for offenders. These all contribute to the positive legitimacy claims of mediation. Restorative practices such as victim-offender mediation can be considered expedient, 'fruit-bearing' opportunities and legitimate experiences of justice. Justice through victim-offender mediation becomes tangible in the lived experience of citizens who desire a more meaningful experience of justice.[23]

The legitimacy of restorative justice

This article has already addressed the distinction between legality–legitimacy, which is aptly exemplified when reflecting upon the views of the parties involved in regards to the criminal justice system. Victim-offender mediation, which emanates from the personal attitudes and opinions of the parties involved, further underlines the distinction between legality and legitimacy, clearly accentuating the meaning of legitimacy.

In *Social Consent and the legitimacy of Law: Marginal remarks on the Murikka Symposium* (1989), Krzysztof Pałecki claims that the legal system is subordinate to the normative sphere and dependant on the inner criteria of the same system. Yet legitimacy concerns something moreover. Pałecki emphasises that acting in a legal manner is not always sufficient for legitimacy and vice versa. Legitimation does not automatically imply that a given act is legal.[24] The manner in which the parties involved question the legitimacy of a litigation process provides us with an example where acting in a legal manner does not always sufficiently equate to legitimacy.

Still, something that is legally 'incorrect' can be regarded as being legitimate and can at times comprise the objective of victim-offender mediation. An offender might believe that his action, though technically illegal, is ultimately perfectly legitimate. Accordingly, in victim-offender mediation, the offender can explain his actions and motivations to the victim and they then together can discuss the matter, during which different aspects of the issue emerge.

---

23 See for example Mielityinen 1999, 129 for concrete examples on how, in their own words, the parties involved compare court proceedings and victim-offender mediation.

24 Pałecki 1989, 184 – 185. See also Knuts 2006, 236 – 237, 249 for a situation where the legitimacy claims of the parties involved differ from the applicable criteria that determines the legality of a certain action.

Thus I would like to maintain that restorative justice is a particularly legitimate method of conflict resolution and clearly emphasises the concept of legitimacy. However, upon reflecting on restorative justice in relation to legitimacy, it soon becomes clear that the concept of legitimacy has at least two relevant aspects. Mediation in conflict resolution primarily concerns society handing over some of its rights to the parties involved. Hence, in regard to the legitimacy of victim-offender mediation, we can distinguish between the perspective of an agent and the perspective of a spectator.

The agent's perspective implies that legitimacy claims related to victim-offender mediation are made by the parties involved in the case. This perspective is something internal to the parties involved in that they are required to personally decide the manner of this particular type of conflict resolution. The spectator's perspective implies that legitimacy claims are made by an individual not personally involved in the process and are therefore external. It is the perspective of society as a whole, the perspective of a third party that assesses the legitimacy of victim-offender mediation.[25]

The agent's perspective is the main objective of victim-offender mediation. It is also the agent's perspective that is at times disregarded in the litigation process. As far as the parties involved are concerned, a conflict is not necessarily resolved before positive legitimacy claims about a particular outcome can be made. When legitimacy is challenged it has a negative effect on conflict resolution and the consequences of conflict resolution. It becomes a significant impediment to positive change in regards to the future behaviour of the parties involved and their attitude towards the offence. It is therefore the agent's perspective that brings added value to conflict resolution.

Nevertheless, the positive perspective that an agent might have in regards to legitimacy should not be confused with compliance with externally imposed rules; the concept of legality is not completely unrelated to the agent's perspective. For example, even if an offender complies with a specific judgement his perspective on the legitimacy of the particular legal process that that judgement stems from might be negative. Due to the coercive powers of the criminal justice system the offender has no other choice but to comply with the judgement handed down. If the offender does not comply, the coercive powers of the state are flexed. In such a situation conflict resolution is imposed on the offender externally and the offender may not necessarily perceive the resolution of the conflict as being legitimate. Legitimacy should therefore primarily be identified as an expression of an internal approach to conflict resolution.

I will now highlight the differences between the perspectives of the agent and spectator in legitimacy claims in the context of restorative justice through the work of Peter Winch, in which a distinction is made between these two

---

25 Another way of describing the perspectives of the agent and spectator would be to refer to first person and third person perspectives.

perspectives in regards to the concepts of reward and punishment. Winch draws on Wittgenstein's distinction between the two different senses of the term punishment, the usual sense and the ethical sense.

In the usual sense the term punishment is understood as merely being the consequence of an action. The role of punishment is to deter or induce certain future actions. Thus understanding of the term in this manner is connected to certain externally imposed standards.[26]

Examples of the usual sense of punishment are plenty when considering that conflict resolution traditionally takes place in a courtroom. In *Poetic Justice* (1995), Martha C. Nussbaum maintains that in a criminal justice system it is commonly accepted that during decision-making reason is maximised and emotional standpoints are irrelevant. It is believed that decisions must be based on facts and not the emotional state of a judge. Utilitarian and retributive perspectives primarily prevail in such a traditional criminal justice system, despite the eventual needs of the parties involved. The needs of the parties involved are often considered to be based on feelings and emotions and are, as such, characterised as being irrational or as needs that merely drive an individual helplessly back and forth.[27] Restorative justice challenges this situation by challenging thinking that idolises reason and denies the value of the personal opinions of the parties involved regardless of what those opinions are based on, be it feelings, emotions, reason or any other grounds.

Still, it is typical for our time that reason, and not a subjective matter such as emotions, reigns. Courts practice positive modern law, where reasonability is the guiding principle. Yet litigation processes do not always meet the expectations of the parties involved. Whether victim or offender, the parties involved are very much guided by their emotions when confronted with an offence. The incomprehensibility of the judicial language used and the ensuing need for highly specialised knowledge, which the parties involved do not posses, can lead the parties involved to feel as if they are mere bystanders during the litigation process. Such an off-putting experience negatively affects the legitimacy claims of the parties involved in relation to the proceedings as a whole.

Winch points to other effects that the usual sense of punishment can have. He maintains that when an individual has 'nothing against the sort of action he has committed' that individual is likely to draw two kinds of conclusions regarding the potential consequences of that action. In the first conclusion, punishment is considered to fulfil utilitarian aims and the offender draws the conclusion that he should not commit a further offence. This individual had

---

26 Winch 1972, 211 – 212.

27 Nussbaum 1995, 55, 57. For example, the need for revenge is a reality and must be respected. In a state governed by law this need, however, is typically 'channelled' through the court system where an attempt is made to 'cool down' strong feelings of revenge within a framework offered by the state. Christie 2005, 152.

learnt his lesson but in a rather superficial sense. In the second conclusion, an offender may be highly annoyed at having been apprehended. The conclusion this individual then extracts from punishment is that he must not be apprehended the next time he commits an offence.[28]

The first conclusion, not re-offending, satisfies everyone, especially society. Recidivism decreases because the offender does not wish to commit any further offences. Yet from a moral point of view the reasoning of the offender here is quite revealing. Winch maintains that conforming to demands as a result of inducements is not the same as acting morally. In the second conclusion, punishment resides in the action itself.[29]

If an individual considers the events following an offence in a manner that constitutes a difference to the understanding of that individual in regards to what the wrong actually was, punishment entails an ethical sense for that individual. In such a conclusion punishment and reward lie in the action itself. What is of special importance here is that the offender himself must come to this conclusion; a third party cannot impose such understanding.[30] I will now address these conclusions in regards to the effect such can have in relation to victim-offender mediation.

Again, the agent's perspective is key in this context. Victim-offender mediation does not seek justice through court verdicts, prior sentencing or any type of judicial decisions but instead seeks justice through the relationship between the parties involved. At its best, a face-to-face meeting in conflict resolution can entail a meaningful experience for the parties involved. Martin Buber is a philosopher whose idea of existence as an encounter can help illuminate the meaning inherent in meeting another individual, the other party, as a human being.

In *I and Thou* (2004), Buber describes his thesis of dialogical existence through the word pairs *I-Thou* and *I-It*. These word pairs exemplify an individual's manner of being conscious, of interaction and of being in the world. *I-Thou* is a relationship that stresses the mutual and holistic existence of two beings. It is a concrete encounter in that *I* meets *Thou* in an authentic existence without special aims or expectations of any sort. In an *I-Thou* encounter, infinity and universality are made actual in the present. Then again, in *I-It* the two beings do not actually meet. Instead, *I* treats *It* as an object.[31]

Restorative justice transcends mere restitution and reparation and brings a dynamic dimension to the determination of justice. Thus the consent of the parties involved comprises an important starting point in the search for justice and justice becomes implausible without the active participation of the parties

28 Winch 1972, 217.
29 Winch 1972, 211 – 212.
30 Winch 1972, 214.
31 Buber 2004, 15 – 18.

involved. In restorative justice, the parties involved hopefully gain an understanding of the other as *Thou*. Resolving a conflict with *Thou* becomes important and meaningful. The parties involved are given the possibility to exchange viewpoints and reflect on those moral standpoints and actions that they hold to be valid. When such occurs, the righting of a wrongful action makes a difference in the lives of the parties involved. Due to the participatory nature of the process, mediation is likely to produce a comprehensive solution to those problems arising from an offence or those problems that initially led to the offence.[32]

Seen from the agent's perspective, the legitimacy of the agreement that the parties involved reach derives from the fact that the parties involved have personally negotiated the agreement. Individuals wish to personally have a say in that this provides a manner whereby they can ensure that the resolution of a conflict is congruent to the resolution they desire. Mediation offers individuals the possibility to express their perception of an offence and influence the outcome. Again, it is personal determination that makes individuals more comfortable with abiding by those decisions that directly affect them. Involvement and sharing not only ensure that an outcome is perceived as being legitimate but also that the entire process is legitimate from the agent's perspective.

Mediation well suits the needs of the parties involved in their search for a legitimate outcome. I therefore want to highlight the importance of the agent's perspective in regards to legitimacy. The agent's perspective that Winch describes encourages the enthusiasm of the parties involved in relation to agreement and garnering meaning from the mediation process. This particular type of conflict resolution can truly resonate with the parties involved. Conflict resolution can also positively affect the spectator's perspective on the legitimacy of victim-offender mediation. Even from the perspective of society, it is extremely important that the parties involved garner a lesson from conflict resolution.

I will now address yet another aspect of the concept of legitimacy in relation to the particular context that is victim-offender mediation, namely that both an institutional and an individual aspect to legitimacy exist, separate from the perspectives of the agent and spectator. The institutional aspect is pertinent when reflecting on victim-offender mediation as a system, where a society governed by law has entrusted some of its powers in the area of conflict resolution to the individual parties involved. The individual aspect is relevant when reflecting on the actual meeting between the parties involved and their definition of an acceptable resolution to the conflict.

From the agent's perspective, the individual aspect of legitimacy is most meaningful. For the parties involved the opinion of the general public or

32 Pelikan & Trenczek 2008, 65 – 66.

authority might not matter after all. Here we see that the perspectives of the agent and spectator do not necessarily correspond in content. Where an agent makes positive legitimacy claims about a certain issue, a spectator might make negative legitimacy claims about the exact same issue and vice versa. Such situations are actually quite common in victim-offender mediation.[33]

We can envision a situation where the parties involved come to an agreement but that this agreement is found to be completely inadequate by authorities. According to the manner in which victim-offender mediation is organised in Finland today, it is a prosecutor who ultimately determines whether an agreement brokered during mediation complies with the formal criteria of law.[34] Thus given the role that the police or prosecuting authorities play when assessing an outcome, we understand that the legality of the final agreement is considered important. It is believed that such definitive control by an official authority ensures that no capricious decisions are made. However, in some cases such an approach has proven to be problematic.

If the parties involved have, on their own, reached an understanding and settled an issue it is extremely difficult for these individuals to comprehend why the state, through a prosecutor, feels it should have anything more to say on the matter. The parties involved are largely unable to consider the matter in a broader context external to their own personal sphere.[35] For these individuals, the institutional aspect of legitimacy is not associated with 'their' conflict resolution and the victim and offender take the agent's perspective, whereas the state feels that the institutional aspect must be taken into account and the state takes the spectator's perspective.

In this article I mostly concentrate on the aspect of legitimacy as linked to the individual, but institutional legitimacy is by no means irrelevant. Public opinion may not support victim-offender mediation in the sense of the parties involved independently resolving the conflict on their own. Victim-offender mediation would seem to contravene the retributive, punishing manner of solving conflicts typically used and accepted by the public at large. Thus I maintain and emphasise that the spectator's perspective on the institutional legitimacy of mediation must ultimately emanate from the agent's perspective on the individual legitimacy of a particular mediation. If such occurs, mediation can be understood as a legitimate method for conflict resolution in that it develops from the positive legitimacy claims of the parties involved.

---

33 Such situations are also rather common in the context of the criminal justice system, as I have demonstrated previously in this article. In that in a legitimate conflict resolution the spectator's perspective does not necessarily correspond to the agent's perspective, the parties involved may become dissatisfied with the conflict resolution even after the matter has judicially been resolved.

34 The Act on Conciliation in Criminal and Certain Civil Cases 1015/2005 sections 13, 16; Frände 2003, 187 – 193.

35 Mielityinen 1999, 130.

The need for a legitimate conflict resolution of our time

In this second to last section I will relate the emergence of restorative methods to some more general late-modern developments in society. I do this because I believe that these societal developments are also relevant to the call for legitimate conflict resolution that has resulted in the emergence of restorative justice practices. Furthermore, I believe that the general conditions seen in present day society help us better understand the perspectives of the agent and spectator.

Late-modernity places more emphasis on the singular context than the universal and generally valid context. This challenges most aspects of life. It challenges the legitimacy of the justice system and the rationale whereby the justice system bases its belief on a single entity that can accommodate all situations and all individuals. It also challenges any interaction between individuals in that a universal set of rules is lacking. An overarching system of ideas no longer conclusively defines what is right and what is wrong, in that these are felt to differ from one context to another. Individuals' understanding of what is right and what is wrong becomes diluted in that individuals create their own definitions of right and wrong.

Nevertheless, in a human community a common understanding of right and wrong is still of utmost importance in that it provides the foundation for any interpersonal interaction. The importance of a continuous moral discussion, of an exchange of ideas and opinions on moral issues, should therefore be emphasised. By defining what is right and wrong for each particular situation, human beings can achieve mutual understanding. Our time then is characterised by the need for moral communication yet very few instances allow for such communication. In my opinion victim-offender mediation accommodates this need for moral discourse. Victim-offender mediation also provides an example of an individual context that disregards predefined, generally valid rules. Victim-offender mediation thus challenges the traditional understanding of what a 'proper' and 'suitable' punishment for an offence should be.

This paradigmatic shift is typical for late modern times. In *La condition postmoderne* (1979), Jean-François Lyotard examines the postmodern challenge through different kinds of knowledge. Thus far in history scientific knowledge has constituted the primary and exclusive form of knowledge. Yet narrative knowledge has begun to gain more and more importance, which poses a problem in regards to the role that knowledge plays in late modern societies. Those who advocate and play the prevailing scientific language 'game' are incapable of approving of knowledge that stems from a source that, according to their rules of scientific knowledge, cannot be proven.[36]

Victim-offender mediation exemplifies this narrative shift. The meeting that occurs during victim-offender mediation consists of the parties involved recounting ideas and understandings related to the offence being discussed. In victim-offender mediation no formal need exists to establish a special kind of truth based on certain formal criteria. Instead the parties involved are allowed to determine which information they find important and relevant. In this manner their personal attitudes and opinions shape the outcome of the mediation, the resolution of the conflict in that particular case.

Lyotard's idea of the legitimacy of knowledge can also partly explain why victim-offender mediation and the legitimacy of victim-offender mediation can be called into question and can especially illuminate the spectator's point of view in regards to this issue. In times of firm modern conviction, where rationality is used as the solution to the problems of mankind, narrative knowledge is not highly valued. By definition, restorative justice is a unique exception in western societies that are otherwise profoundly rooted in the rule of law and the equality of all mankind. The legitimacy of restorative justice develops from the personal opinions of the parties involved as they are made in a particular context during mediation. Hence one cannot maintain that the outcome would necessarily reflect any rational reasoning.

The grounds for the legitimacy claims of the parties involved, which are based on a singular context, are therefore not always accessible when seen from the spectator's perspective, which emanates from general standpoints. Accordingly, from the spectator's perspective, victim-offender mediation can be considered wholly problematic, which therefore contributes to negative legitimacy claims from the spectator's perspective.

Conclusions

Victim-offender mediation provides a fruit-bearing opportunity in regards to the understanding of the concept of legitimacy as it has been developed in response to the questioned legitimacy of the criminal justice system. In that victim-offender mediation is entirely voluntary and either one of the parties involved can terminate the process at any time and continue the conflict resolution within the official litigation system, the legitimacy of mediation is highly important. If the two parties involved do not consider victim-offender mediation legitimate, they will not participate. Restorative justice seeks to satisfy both the parties involved by allowing them to resolve the conflict by themselves, which

36 Lyotard 1979, 48.

underlines the importance of personal determination when forming legitimacy claims.

Still, legitimacy is not a self-evident prerequisite in the restorative system itself. The restorative system is not an institutional system of victim-offender mediation, where each and every situation is legitimate, nor are individual mediations always legitimate. The legitimacy of the restorative system is confirmed every time a particular victim-offender mediation is realised. It is in such cases that the legitimacy claims of the parties involved play a central role in the context.

In this article I maintain that a difference exists between the concepts of legitimacy and legality. Legitimacy expresses something more than mere legality, even though (especially in judicial discourse) the two are often identified with one other. Legality primarily refers to the formal criteria of the litigation process, which is of utmost importance to the criminal justice system. Nevertheless, this kind of legitimacy is external to the parties involved in the process. Seen from the viewpoint of one of the individual parties involved, not all aspects of legitimacy depend on external factors such as written law and regulations.

Disparity often exists in regards to legitimacy as seen through the eyes of the parties involved and as exemplified in the criminal justice system. Victim-offender mediation emerged from this disparity. Even after perfectly legal proceedings and a formally valid judgement, the parties involved can still sincerely believe that their opinion was correct and that the formal judgement was incorrect. Moreover, the court process may be considered unfair even though it officially and formally was fair and just and, as such, cannot be contested. Thus from the perspective of the parties involved, legitimacy to a great extent is something that is internally related.

Accordingly, in the context of victim-offender mediation, the perspectives of the agent and spectator play an important role. In the Finnish model of victim-offender mediation the parties involved independently reach an agreement. This agreement takes the form of a legitimate resolution of the conflict when seen from the agent's perspective. The spectator's perspective is actualised thereafter when an official authority assesses and determines the legitimacy of the agreement in accordance with the formal criteria of the law.

The twofold aspect of the concept of legitimacy can help us understand that even when there is no legitimacy from the spectator's perspective there might well be legitimacy from the agent's perspective and vice versa. Restorative justice thus emphasises the connection between legitimacy and personal involvement. From the agent's perspective neither the mediator nor authorities guarantee the legitimacy of the victim-offender mediation. It is the parties involved themselves who constitute the legitimacy of victim-offender mediation through engaging in an activity that they feel comfortable with.

Again, what is perfectly legitimate in one context with certain parties might be considered wholly illegitimate in another context with other parties.

By acknowledging that some victim-offender mediations are legitimate and some are not, seen from either the agent's or spectator's perspectives, we discern yet another aspect of the concept of legitimacy, namely that both an institutional and an individual aspect of legitimacy exist. When talking about legitimacy in the context of victim-offender mediation one must distinguish between a meeting where the parties involved in a conflict meet to resolve said conflict and a societal institution where the two parties involved are provided the possibility to autonomously resolve their conflict. In this article I have primarily focused on the individual aspect of legitimacy: the agent's perspective in regards to the assessment of legitimacy by the parties involved in their own case and the spectator's perspective in regards to a particular victim-offender mediation.

Yet the institutional aspect of legitimacy in regards to victim-offender mediation indicates an important paradigmatic shift in society. Positive law no longer solely and always forms the definitive basis for conflict resolution in that society has delegated some of its powers in conflict resolution to an institution such as victim-offender mediation. Moreover, extra-judicial aspects can now be taken into account in conflict resolution. In my view, the introduction of restorative justice can be regarded as a late-modern contravention of modernity. The modern positivist legal system is giving way to a more late modern idea of restorative justice, where in victim-offender mediation the parties involved are allowed to agree upon a resolution suitable for them specifically, with their personal desires and wishes providing the sole guiding principles.

Victim-offender mediation maintains and enhances personal moral responsibility and the role of the conscience of the parties involved by allowing them a decisive role in the matter. The parties involved are invited to personally, in their own words, reflect on what has happened. They are stimulated to discern the meaning of the offence together with the concrete other sitting on the opposite side of the table. In victim-offender mediation the moral understanding and meaning of an offence becomes internal to the parties involved and is not allocated to outside experts, as is often the case in the criminal justice system. Restorative justice can be considered a new manner whereby the legitimacy of conflict resolution can be defined and the legitimacy of some more traditional methods can be questioned.

The purpose of this article was to illuminate some aspects of legitimacy that are pertinent to the context of restorative justice and more closely examine how victim-offender mediation contributes to the legitimacy claims of the parties involved. Victim-offender mediation not only highlights how an important aspect of the concept of legitimacy in actuality lies in the agent's perspective (built on the involvement of the parties involved) but also exemplifies a wider paradigmatic shift in society's claims of legitimacy in regards to conflict resolution.

Bibliography

Act on Conciliation in Criminal and Certain Civil Cases, 1015/2005. Entered into force 1.1.2006.

Braithwaite, J

2001 *Restorative Justice and Responsive Regulation*. Cary, NC, USA: Oxford University Press.

1989 *Crime, Shame and Reintegration*. Cambridge et al: Cambridge University Press.

Buber, M

2004 *I and Thou*. London: Continuum.

Christie, N

2005a *Lagom mycket kriminalitet*. Stockholm: Natur och Kultur.

1977 Conflicts as property. Pp. 1 – 15. *The British Journal of Criminology*. Vol 17.

Foucault, M

1995 *Discipline and Punish*. New York: Vintage Books.

Frände, D

2003 *Brott och rättegång*. Helsingfors: Publikationer utgivna av juridiska fakulteten vid Helsingfors universitet.

Haavisto, V

2002 *Court Work in Transition. An Activity-Theoretical Study of Changing Work Practices in a Finnish District Court*. Helsingfors: Helsinki University Press. Diss.

Iivari, J

1991 Rikosten ja riitojen vaihtoehtosovittelu refleksiivisen oikeuden konseptiossa. Sosiaali- ja terveyshallitus. *Tutkimuksia* 12/1991. Valtion painatuskeskus: Helsingfors. Diss.

Knuts, G

2005 *Förfarandegarantier vid domstolsanknuten medling*. Helsinki: Suomalainen lakimiesyhdistys. Diss.

Kurtén, T

1998 Det handlande subjektet och det moraliska kravet. Studier i etikens och trons roll i mänskligt handlande. Åbo: *Skrifter utgivna av institutet för ekumenik och socialetik.*

Leer-Salvesen, P
1999 *Menneske og straff: en refleksjon om skyld og straff som et bidrag til arbeidet med straffens etikk.* Oslo: Universitetsforlaget.

Lyotard, J-F
1979 *La condition postmoderne.* Paris: Les éditions de minuit.

Mielityinen, I
1999 Rikos ja sovittelu. Valikoituminen, merkitys ja uusintarikollisuus. Helsinki: Oikeuspoliittisen tutkimuslaitoksen julkaisuja 167.

Molander, J
2002 *Straffets grammatik.* Åbo: Åbo Akademi. Diss.

Nussbaum, M C
1995 *Poetic Justice. The Literary Imagination and Public Life.* Boston: Beacon Press.

Pałecki, K
1989 Social Consent and the Legitimacy of Law: Marginal Remarks on the Murikka Symposium. Pp 165 – 189. In Aarnio, Aulis and Kaarlo Tuori (eds): *Law, Morality, and Discursive Rationality.* Helsinki: Publications of the Department of Public law, University of Helsinki D:8.

Pelikan, C & Trenczek, T
2008 Victim offender mediation and restorative justice. The European landscape. Pp. 63 – 90. In Sullivan, Dennis & Larry Tifft (eds): *Handbook of restorative Justice.* London et al: Routledge.

Petev, V
1989 Socio-Ethical and Political Conceptions of Major Groups within the Society as Reasons for the Legitimacy of the Law. Pp. 199 – 213. In Aarnio, Aulis and Kaarlo Tuori (eds): *Law, Morality and Discursive Rationality.* Helsinki: Publications of the Department of Public Law, University of Helsinki. D:8.

Tuori, K
1990 Johdanto: Modernin oikeuden legitimitettiperiaatetta etsimässä. Pp. 1-27. In Tuori, Kaarlo and Jaana Matikainen (eds): *Yhteiskuntasopimuksesta yhteisöön.* Helsinki: Publications of the Department of Public Law, University of Helsinki. D:10.

Välikoski, T-R
2004 *The Criminal Trial as a Speech Communication Situation.* Tampere: Tampere University Press. Diss.

Winch, P
1972 *Ethics and Action*. London: Routledge & Kegan Paul.

Zehr, H
2002 *The Little Book of Restorative Justice*. Intercourse, PA: GoodBooks.
1995 *Changing Lenses. A New Focus for Crime and Justice*. Scottdale, Pennsylvania: Herald Press.

LEGITIMACY CHALLENGES IN GENDER POLITICS – CHALLENGES TO POLITICAL LEGITIMACY IN PARLIAMENTARY DEBATES CONCERNING LGBT RIGHTS, ASSISTED REPRODUCTION AND DOMESTIC VIOLENCE

Lise Kanckos & Malena Björkgren

In this article we examine the concept of political legitimacy in relation to issues concerning gender and sexuality. We focus on how the legitimacy of political authorities or particular laws is challenged in political discourse concerning sexuality, gender, violence and reproduction. For reasons of practicality and the purposes of this article the concept *gender politics* is used as an umbrella concept to encompass these types of political issues even though the concept gender politics is wider than the cases examined here. We examine a number of cases where the legitimacy of particular laws is questioned and where, consequently, the legitimacy of standing political authorities is also questioned. The material we analyse consists of government bills and minutes from commissions and sessions in the Finnish parliament. The laws we in particular focus on relate to various issues that have been on the political agenda in Finland during the last two decades: 1) registered partnership and other issues concerning LGBT rights, 2) domestic violence and 3) assisted reproduction.[1] The examples we present are relevant for many reasons, not least as regards the facilitation of a discussion on transitions between the private and the public spheres but also to demonstrate how the rise of human rights and feminist perspectives has changed political discourse in Finland.

This article specifically seeks to answer the following question: if a law is considered essential by the public, in the sense that something crucial would be

1 Lise Kanckos has authored those sections concerning the empirical examples of assisted reproduction and registered partnership and, to a large degree, the theoretical portions of this article while Malena Björkgren has authored the section concerning the examples of domestic violence.

missing if this law did not exist, what form might the challenge to the legitimacy of political authorities take? In the case studies presented here the questioning of legitimacy often originates in common arguments concerning issues such as discrimination, gender neutrality, equality and the transition of private concerns to public matters.

What happens, though, when a group in society views a particular law as illegitimate with reference to religious, ideological or identity-based reasons? Legitimacy may be challenged in gender politics through judgements rooted in either liberal ideas on how legislation should be developed so that discrimination is prevented or conservative claims regarding, for example, how the development of LGBT rights in society 'threatens' the basic values of society. At the same time that differences between the opinions of individual policy-makers and politicians may exist, a discrepancy between what policy-makers and politicians value and what the public or groups in society value may also exist. In the cases presented here legitimacy judgements mainly concern political authorities or specific laws rather than the state or entire political system.

The legitimacy concept

Political scientists and philosophers hold different views on how the concept of legitimacy should be defined and how it should be discussed in relation to the rule of law or particular laws. In this article we do not primarily consider legitimacy to be a moral evaluation of particular laws, which is a common interpretation of the concept, but rather view legitimacy judgements as an expression of the commitment of individuals to political authorities. It is also important to note that accepting a political system or a particular law as legitimate can be an expression of what an individual values in life. In this sense the acceptance of the individual is not free from moral dimensions. We consider legitimacy to possess a self-evident character until something happens that calls attention to the question of the legitimacy of political bodies. Interpreted so the concept is similar to the concept of trust.[2] In this article we primarily study legitimacy judgements that are made internally by those who live under the purview of a political system. In other words, we focus on legitimacy judgements that are expressions of the allegiance of citizens to political authorities, not an external justification of the authority of the state.[3]

We endeavour to include both the content of debates and performative or communicative aspects of the production of laws and their connection to legitimacy in this article, and as such the production of law is focused on in the

2 See the article by Tage Kurtén and Ville Päivänsalo in this volume.
3 See the article by Lars Hertzberg in this volume.

form of government bills and minutes of commissions and parliamentary debates. For Jürgen Habermas the connection between legitimacy and communication is essential. According to Habermas, the production of law is a matter of communication and communication produces legitimacy.[4] We use Habermas' discussion on legitimation crisis as a starting point for this article. Habermas combines theories concerning legitimacy with crisis theory when he talks about legitimation crisis and perceives legitimation crisis to be a failure of institutions in society to legitimate their position and maintain a requisite level of mass loyalty, thus leading to a general crisis in society.[5] Habermas explains that one can speak of crisis 'only when members of a society experience structural alterations as critical for continued existence and feel their social identity threatened.'[6] He also uses Durkheim's concept anomie to describe a crisis condition. Anomie refers to a state of normlessness and a social condition in which individuals have been disintegrated from society.[7] Habermas maintains that a legitimation crisis may, for example, appear as a consequence of an economic crisis if the crisis management of a government fails to repair the damage.[8] Nevertheless, Habermas does not discuss legitimation exclusively as an administrative activity by political authorities. He also uses the concept legitimacy to describe a combination of validity claims formulated in discourse between policy-makers and the public.

Habermas argues that in order to be considered legitimate a law must pass the discursive tests of different so-named validity claims. Habermas distinguishes between four validity claims: truth, related here to the likely consequences of different legal options; rightness, related here to the moral rightness or justness of different legal options; truthfulness, concerning the authenticity of different options in relation to shared values and history; and comprehensibility, pragmatic claims about which option would be feasible or more efficient.[9] Habermas maintains that if an ideal speech situation is to be realised all four validity claims should be tested. In this article we do not present a detailed discussion of what these validity claims would imply in practice. However, in practical situations relating to lawmaking processes, many conflicts of interest arise that cannot always be solved through rational political discourse. Many laws are the result of political compromises. Habermas' validity claims and his emphasis on communication illuminate what might

4 Guibentif 1996, 56–61; Habermas 1996, 103–104.
5 Barker 1990; Habermas 1989 [1973], 46–48.
6 Habermas 1989, 3.
7 Durkheim 1951 [1897].
8 Habermas 1989, 68–69.
9 Bohman & Rehg 2008; Habermas 1979. The terminology used varies somewhat in discussions on Habermas' validity claims. Cukier et al. 2004, 239. The terminology used in this article (truth, rightness, truthfulness and comprehensibility) follows *Communication and the Evolution of Society* (Habermas 1979).

happen when trust-based legitimacy is questioned and when attempts to regain that legitimacy are introduced.

According to Rodney Barker legitimation is a central characteristic of government, and a state of unstable legitimacy is a normal feature of transitions.[10] Habermas, who has a more crisis-theoretical approach to legitimacy, maintains that the politicisation of certain issues that used to belong to a private sphere may contest the legitimacy of political authorities. These issues used to be culturally presumed but have become the object of administrative planning: educational planning, regional and city planning, planning of the health system, family planning, marriage laws and child-rearing, for example. When such issues were culturally presumed they existed in a sphere of self-legitimation but are nowadays the object of public regulation and legitimation.[11] Habermas' argument is summed up in the following quotation:

> At every level, administrative planning produces unintended unsettling and publicizing effects. These effects weaken the justification potential of traditions that have been flushed out of their nature-like course of development. Once their unquestionable character has been destroyed, the stabilization of validity claims can succeed only through discourse. The stirring up of cultural affairs that are taken for granted thus furthers the politicization of areas of life previously assigned to the private sphere.[12]

Barker criticises Habermas for a lack of historical perspective because, according to Barker, issues such as marriage law or birth control have also in the past been politically contested. Barker's main point is that, if a line is drawn between normal times and occasions of legitimacy crisis, viewing something contemporary as being novel is problematic when discussing legitimacy.[13] We nonetheless agree with Habermas that the process of the politicisation of some previously 'private matters' is a transition that may challenge the legitimacy of government authorities, even though we believe that the descriptions of these transitions should be nuanced and described in a longer historical perspective. These transitions are often better described as an oscillation rather than a shift, and different social groups or political parties usually hold conflicting views on the private or public character of these matters. Still, our approach to legitimacy differs from Habermas' on some essential points. First, unlike Habermas we do not intend to develop the theoretical or moral grounds for legitimacy[14] but instead investigate selected empirical examples of how the legitimacy of authorities is challenged in gender politics. Second, we prefer not to use the term

---

10 Barker 1990, 40–41.
11 Habermas 1989, 71–73.
12 Habermas 1989, 72.
13 Barker 1990, 40–41.
14 Barker 1990, 88–89.

'crisis' but instead employ the terms 'challenge' or 'questioning'. We primarily examine the debates related to laws that rarely cause a general societal crisis. The legitimacy claims expressed by Members of Parliament (MPs) during such debates may, when seen from a historical perspective, remain quite marginal. Calling such examples instances of a legitimacy crisis might therefore be slightly excessive.[15]

It follows our understanding of legitimacy judgements as expressions of the commitment of individuals to political authorities that we have chosen to study claims in Finnish society relating to the legitimacy or illegitimacy of particular laws and, consequently, political authorities. One separate claim made by a single individual rarely entails a real challenge to the legitimacy of political bodies. Thus the arguments we distinguish between and the quotations we provide are considered examples that illustrate discourses rather than separate claims made by individual MPs.

When legitimacy is challenged

The legitimacy of political authorities may be challenged or questioned when a particular law or proposed law results in strong disagreement in a society, during which conflicting views appear to be impossible to overcome. Debate is nonetheless an essential part of a democratic and legitimate system. This is also emphasised by Habermas, who describes the discursive process of lawmaking as a democratic principle for legitimacy[16]. Our use of the term 'questioning' does not necessarily imply that the concept legitimacy occurs in the debate itself. Rather, legitimacy is often questioned indirectly, through the use of moral arguments for example, and in a subtler manner. We therefore seek to understand what form this questioning takes in political discourse and, more specifically, in political debates on sexuality, gender, violence and reproduction.

Legitimacy judgements may transpire either explicitly or implicitly in a debate on a proposed law and may also have various objects.[17] The object of the legitimacy judgement may be the government or other politicians but can also be comprised of other institutions that represent the authority of the state, for example the police. The object can moreover be somewhat diffuse.

In a plural society the legitimacy of political authorities is sometimes challenged when particular laws are perceived to lack the support or confidence of the citizens in that society. Legitimacy is especially sensitive to political issues that are in some manner connected to individuals' worldviews and issues

15 However, on one occasion Habermas mentions that 'legitimation needs *do not have to* culminate in a crisis.' Habermas 1989, 74; italics in original.

16 Habermas 1996, 110.

17 See the article by Lars Hertzberg in this volume.

that elicit moral reactions. The public can at times perceive that policy-makers and politicians place value on the wrong issues. Bureaucracy and instrumental approaches to issues that people encounter in their daily lives may alienate the public from political authorities whose legitimacy can thereby be challenged. The best solutions in a policy-making process are often created by the individuals closest either professionally or personally to these issues and not through external commentators.[18] This is especially true regarding issues where the line between the public and private is blurred.

In the cases discussed here, a renewed desire to regulate issues politically is seen. The rise of human rights and feminist perspectives have increased awareness that groups of people or specific issues have been excluded from or neglected in legislation. LGTB rights, violence against women and assisted reproduction comprise such political issues. The regulation process concerning these issues has also led to discussions in the media, the church and society in general.

LGTB rights and discrimination

A legitimacy problem is clearly evident if we look at the development of LGTB rights as a process in Finnish society. In 2001 Finland became the last Nordic country to pass a law on registered partnerships. In comparison to the other Nordic countries Finland was also late in instituting a law on assisted reproduction, with a central and contested issue in this particular discussion being whether lesbian couples and single women should be allowed access to assisted reproduction.

In society and public discourse in general, the view on homosexuality has gradually changed during the 20th century. Discourse changed from a description of homosexuality as a moral question, disease or crime to include the perspective of basic or human rights.[19] LGTB rights have during the last few decades been acknowledged in international law, and laws discriminating against homosexuals have in some countries been altered. A pattern in the order of the development of LGTB rights is discernable in various countries, beginning with decriminalisation and continuing on to registered partnership, gender-neutral marriage and adoption rights. Each step seems to induce the following step.[20] One change, in other words, tends to lead to the perception that other laws are discriminatory, thereby weakening the legitimacy of such laws.

In Finland homosexual relations were first decriminalised in 1971. That same year, however, the public encouragement of homosexual acts became a

18 Holden 2006, 29–30, 56.
19 Hiltunen 1996, 1.
20 Waaldijk 2001, 439–440.

criminal offence. A decade later in 1981 homosexuality was demedicalised and removed from the Finnish disease list. In 1995 the Criminal Code was renewed so that the discrimination of homosexuals became a criminal offense. It was first in 1999, through the renewal of chapter 20 of the Finnish Criminal Code, which legislates sex crimes, that the encouragement of homosexual acts was removed as a criminal offence. Yet the last ruling on this chapter and relevant specific paragraph occurred in the early 1990s when members of the Finnish LGTB rights organisation SETA (*Seksuaalinen Tasavertaisuus,* 'Sexual Equality') chose to ridicule this paragraph by encouraging individuals on a public square to engage in homosexual acts. SETA then duly reported these actions to the police.[21] This event was clearly meant to awaken public discussion regarding the (il)legitimacy of the paragraph. It also illustrates how the gradual development of LGTB rights could not continue by itself; changing the paragraph first required both grass root level political actions and then political will in the Finnish Parliament, with the latter obviously not being found before 1999.

Gradual improvements in LGTB rights continued with the renewal of Finnish constitutional law in 2000, including the prohibition of discrimination in 6 §, interpreted in the bill on registered partnership (HE 200/2000) as relevant to sexual orientation and accordingly used as an argument for passing the Act on Registered Partnership, also known as the Partnership act. However, as we will see later in this article, some conservative MPs perceived the Partnership act, which took effect in 2002, to be illegitimate. The Act on Assisted Reproduction followed in 2007 and has further improved the legal situation for those seeking reproductive help, especially lesbian couples. As a result of the Partnership act, official discussions on the blessing of same-sex unions were initiated in the Evangelical Lutheran Church of Finland. The next step in the development of LGTB rights in Finland was a bill that allowed same-sex couples living in registered partnerships to adopt each other's biological children (HE 198/2008), ratified by parliament on 15 May 2009. In Finland gay and lesbian individuals may petition to adopt a non-biological child but same-sex couples cannot jointly apply for non-biological adoption. As such the 2009 legislative change concerns only the rights of those living in a registered partnership to adopt the offspring of their registered partner. All of these examples can be viewed as the gradual development of change, where one change gave rise to the following change.

The development of LGTB rights in society exemplifies a process where matters formerly considered private gradually became public through a process of politicisation. When homosexuality was criminalised and medicalised, the hegemonic view on homosexuality in society was based on a perspective of discipline and punishment. More precisely, the criminalisation and medicalisation of homosexuality were processes through which homosexual actions were made a public concern; at the time it was felt that such 'deviant'

21 Hiltunen 1999, 45.

actions had to be disciplined. Yet in more recent legal changes sexuality has been emphasised as being a private matter while at the same time same-sex family relationships have increasingly become a public concern. As Habermas points out, such transitions between the private and public spheres may challenge the legitimacy of political authorities[22], and it is essential to discuss these transitions in a longer historical perspective. The social problem that is men's violence against women is another case where a distinction has occurred between private and public matters.

Demands for change - private becomes public

The development of laws concerning violence against women and other forms of domestic violence has been slow in Finland compared to many other Western European countries. It was not until 1994 in Finland that spousal or marital rape was criminalised.[23] Since 1995 assault in intimate relationships has been publicly prosecuted while laws pertaining to restraining orders came into effect in 1999. Researchers have attempted to discern the reasons underlying such slow development, both regarding legislation and other public measures relevant to the issue. Suvi Ronkainen maintains that there is a lack of responsibility in the actions of the state in regards to domestic violence in that a great deal of the service offered in Finland (for example shelters for abused women) is organised outside the public sector and must therefore often rely on insecure sources of funding. Ronkainen argues that this is not an issue of a lack of knowledge about the problem; surveys on domestic violence have been conducted in Finland since the 1970s.[24] Instead Ronkainen attempts to explain the distant interest of the government in dealing with and recognising victims of domestic violence as being the actions (or non-actions) taken by a traumatised nation. During the decades following the Second World War, Finnish society was characterised by a post war 'culture of silence' and the nearly insurmountable struggle to rebuild the nation. During this period neither the time nor the interest to acknowledge problems such as domestic violence existed.[25]

Even in the 1990s, when the issue finally came to the attention of the Finnish government, the attitude towards the matter was ambivalent despite the many changes taking place in legislation. The prevalent attitude of the time is best characterised as a lack of commitment to the problem of domestic violence and a lack of engagement for victims of domestic violence, but exceptions do exist. The Council for Gender Equality, Finland's Ministry of Social Affairs and

22 Habermas 1989, 71–73.
23 A similar law was legislated in Sweden in 1962 and in France in 1980, for example.
24 Ronkainen 2008, 391–392.
25 Ronkainen 2008, 393–394.

Health, undertook a massive project when it sought to criminalise spousal rape.[26] To a great extent UN treaties and declarations from the Council of Europe were used to motivate the demands for legislative change.[27] Through reference to the international treaties that Finland had signed, the government attempted to stress the seriousness of such crimes and the importance of realising the agreements that the Finnish state had entered into. As several MPs claimed during the parliamentary debates on the issue, Finland's international reputation was at stake.[28]

'Reputation discourse' can be interpreted as a manner whereby pressure to change a law can be exerted. In this respect signed treaties play an important and instrumental role. Treaties help indicate the types of arguments that can be effective when lobbying. Nevertheless, when the reputation of a state and treaties are wielded as tools in political discourse a risk exists that the focus of the discourse will be lost, resulting in a situation where the seriousness of the situation being discussed and the central meaning of the law being formulated are obscured. If the main focus merely lies on reputation and signed treaties, the real problem is not highlighted: that rape in marriage, for example, should and must be condemned. However, as Pamela Slotte demonstrates, invoking human rights discourse (which treaties can be said to represent) can highlight the occurrence or potential occurrence of something morally objectionable.[29] Still, even when supporting the same bill, MPs base their decisions on different grounds.

The situation becomes even more complex when we look at a statement made by a Finnish MP. The MP recounts how embarrassed she and other women have felt when, representing Finland at international conferences, attention has been called to the insufficiency of the country's laws on rape.[30] This recollection reveals the connection of these delegates to the nation and suggests that there could be more to reputation discourse than previously discussed in this article: this particular state and its legislation matter to these citizens. Olli Lagerspetz maintains that feelings of shame indicate a sense of allegiance and that loyalty towards a nation can be shown through the condemnation of a state or laws that a citizen perceives as being illegitimate.[31] Reputation discourse can consequently also be interpreted as an indication of a feeling of shame, which in turn demonstrates a connectedness to the state and the legitimacy that the state enjoys.

Human rights discourse opens up new perspectives in relation to legitimacy. In this article we study legitimacy judgements in the form of statements made by Finnish citizens in relation to the political authorities of the Finnish

26 Pehkonen 2003, 61–65; 89–90.
27 LA 25/1991, LA 28/1991, HE 365/1992.
28 PTK 16/1994: Hassi (The Greens); PTK 4/1993: Ojala (Left Alliance).
29 Slotte 2005, 114.
30 PTK 16/1994: Hassi (The Greens).
31 Lagerspetz 1998, 128.

state. In human rights discourse, global and international demands play an important role. Finland has entered into treaties and, as legislative bills and parliamentary discussions demonstrate, many MPs wish to realise these agreements: not only because it is important to 'follow the rule-book' but also because the agreements reflect their own views, for instance that violence against women should be prevented. It would, however, be an over-simplification to describe the development of such laws as a process whereby a clear 'no' to violence against women is always expressed and continuously supported by all members of the government. Domestic violence is still partially considered to be a private matter, and legislation in Finland has also reflected this sentiment. Between 1995 and 2004, for example, plaintiffs could request that a public prosecutor not prosecute an assault. The paragraph that apportioned plaintiffs this right was eventually removed as women experiencing violence in a partnership requested non-prosecution in almost all cases.[32] However, the paragraph allowing victims of sexual violence (rape) to request non-prosecution still exists as it is considered best to allow rape victims the right to avoid court proceedings given that these can be very trying for victims of sexual violence.[33] Yet even among the MPs themselves this argument in regards to legitimacy shows a lack of confidence in court procedure as an adequate and appropriate manner with which to express a governmental and legislatively based 'no' in relation to violence against women. Instead of focusing on victim support or how court procedure could be improved, the solution up until 2004 was (and still is in rape cases) to renounce some of the responsibility of the state for prosecution. This contributes to retaining the problem of violence in the private sphere, in other words as a private concern.[34] According to Johanna Niemi-Kiesiläinen, criminal policy in Finland has scarcely played any role in countering domestic violence, which makes the situation in Finland different from the other Nordic countries.[35] Furthermore, in Finland, mediation is still possible in cases of domestic violence, albeit with some special regulations.[36]

The examples discussed in this section demonstrate that the development of laws pertaining to violence against women in Finnish society has been an ambivalent process. Even though violence against women has to a greater extent become a public matter, the transition of the issue from the private to the public sphere is in reality an oscillation that reveals ambivalence. This ambivalence in turn affects the commitment of individuals to the state and, consequently, the

32 Valtakunnansyyttäjänvirasto 2000; HE 144/2003. As of 2011 the public prosecutor may also bring charges for petty assault if the victim is a partner or former partner of the perpetrator. HE 78/2010.

33 LaVM 3/1998.

34 For a discussion of responsibility and the right to institute criminal proceedings, see Niemi-Kiesiläinen 2004, 281–282.

35 Niemi-Kiesiläinen 2001, 297.

36 See the article by Heidi Jokinen in this volume.

legitimacy of government and political authorities. We understand that the demands for new laws indicate a challenge to the legitimacy of the state, but how wholly does Finnish society support this challenge and, moreover, what support is there for tackling violence against women among politicians or the public? In Finland only 12 percent of the women experiencing violence contact the police.[37] The reasons why this may be are numerous, but the low figure nevertheless clearly indicates that victims of domestic violence do not yet completely trust the police and thereby the state. This therefore constitutes a challenge for a state that wishes to take responsibility for the welfare of its citizens.

Gender neutrality

Political discussions on domestic violence in Finland have been characterised by gender neutrality—a fact that is seen in the widely used concept 'family violence'. Such a gender neutral approach is apparent for example in the late 1990s when restraining orders were discussed in the political realm and any reference to gender became an obstacle in parliamentary debate. The restraining order law (1999) in Finland was originally primarily intended to prevent violence in close relationships (HE 41/1998), yet it was first with the addition of a further paragraph in 2005 that individuals were given the right to obtain a restraining order against another individual living in the same household (HE 144/2003). In plenary sessions many MPs expressed their satisfaction with the law: finally an instrument existed to counteract violence against women. However, for each individual that emphasised the gender specific usefulness of the law and the gender specific character of violence against women, an equal number of individuals opposed and even questioned the inclusion of the aspect of gender:

> [To terrorize another person] has nothing to do with gender. Anyone can do it.[38]
> Violence and violent behaviour are not incarnate in men or women.[39]

It was not sufficient to merely present the restraining order law as an instrument with which to support abused women, it was also imperative to emphasise that the law did not solely apply to women. In a study of how male violence against women has been addressed in politics in Sweden, Maria Wendt Höjer finds gender neutrality to be an important legitimacy-supporting element:

---

37 Kääriäinen 2006, 112.
38 PTK 61/1998: Partanen (Social Democratic Party). Translation authors' own.
39 PTK 61/1998: Puisto (Social Democratic Party). Translation authors' own.

> In order to implement measures against violence, the problem had to be defined as general, as "universally human"; measures to protect only women lack legitimacy in the liberal schema.[40]

If gender neutrality characterised Swedish political discourse on domestic violence during the 1970s and 1980s in Finland a decade later it still played a strong role in discourse. In Finnish society, gender in relation to domestic violence became an issue of interest fairly late. Yet surveys show that in close relationships it is women who are the principal objects of violence and that it is men who are the main perpetrators.[41] This cannot have lain outside of MPs' field of knowledge; rather this demonstrates their disregard for the facts of the situation and also how difficult it is to address violence in connection to gender and power.[42]

New laws have emerged through a feminist and gender sensitive analysis of existing legislation, or as Wendt Höjer writes, 'Bit by bit the naturalness and banality of violence is eroded, and the question finds a place on the political agenda.'[43] Yet there concurrently seems to exist limitations to the capacity for a feminist perspective to gain consideration. Instead, arguments that embrace a gender neutral perspective are preferred. However, as many feminist scholars have observed, the abstract individual that a law presupposes is not (gender) neutral. Instead this abstract individual, that is to say the norm as presumed in legislation, closely mirrors a free, autonomous, heterosexual middle class male.[44] A strict gender neutral perspective does not discern a gendered subject but is instead sceptical to measures and laws that are supported by arguments couched in gender specific terms. Arguments based on gender specific terms are felt to threaten the objectivity and fairness required by the abstract individual and the legal system as a whole. So while arguments exist that political rhetoric should be gender neutral, Suvi Ronkainen reminds us that everyday social and cultural life is very much gendered, a fact she maintains is evident in working life, education, hobbies and in relation to parenthood.[45]

Gender neutral language relates to the issue of legitimacy by highlighting the following questions: 1) Whose problems are considered important enough for a society to address? 2) Are policy-makers willing to take action in regard to issues that might 'only' concern half of society, understanding here that 'concern' means 'suffer from' and that it is women who constitute the half of the population being affected? Legislative documents in Finland reveal an

40 Wendt Höjer 2002, 212.
41 Statistikcentralen 2005.
42 Marianne Notko understands this gender neutral stance as an example of an equality discourse that fears imposing guilt on men. Notko 2000, 21–22.
43 Wendt Höjer 2002, 214.
44 See Davies 1997.
45 Ronkainen 2008, 396.

attitude where violence against women in and of itself is not considered to sufficiently constitute an issue that should be addressed but that instead 'broader' argumentation is needed if the issue is to be considered important. Consequently, a danger exists that victims of violence (again, shown to be predominately female) will lose their trust in political bodies and the work of such bodies if meanings of gender and power are not taken seriously in work against violence.

Equality arguments

Reproductive technology can still be considered a new social phenomenon and before a law on assisted reproduction came into force on 1 September 2007 Finland lacked a uniform law on the issue. A need existed to regulate both the techniques used at fertility clinics and the availability of treatments. Both bioethical and family norms were first discussed and then created through laws. In Finland the discussion concerning assisted reproduction is, in a broad sense, an example of conflicting views on how or if social norms should be regulated through law. Some individuals maintain that assisted reproduction legislation should be as minimal as possible so that the autonomous procreative choices of citizens are protected and the legitimation of any specific moral or religious view does not occur.[46] It is maintained that such a perspective respects the plurality of family forms in society, including the families of lesbian couples and single parents. When preparing the law on assisted reproduction, the Finnish government obviously preferred this point of view, arguing that all women should have equal access to fertility treatments. However, it was emphasised that women's equal right to assisted reproduction was contingent on the condition that any children resulting from such treatment must be guaranteed a secure childhood. In other words, the principle of the best interests of the child was emphasised.[47]

In the political discourse a strong emphasis was placed on equality in the sense of equal rights for women regardless of marital status or sexual orientation. The Finnish government bills on assisted reproduction (HE 76/2002 and HE 3/2006) include a rhetorical argument of equality between women, including the right for lesbian couples and single women to seek treatment. Previously, lesbian couples and single women could seek reproductive treatments at private infertility clinics.[48] Earlier government proposals (1988, 1990 and 1997[49]) had denied lesbian couples and single women the possibility

46 Neri 1996, 154.
47 HE 3/2006.
48 Malin & Burrell 2004, 74.
49 Oikeusministeriön työryhmä 1988; Oikeusministeriön työryhmä 1990; Oikeusministeriön työryhmä 1997.

of receiving treatments in that it was felt that fertility care should be allocated on purely on medical grounds. The 1997 proposal gave rise to a public discussion of the issue, that is to say whether lesbian couples and single women should have the right to assisted reproduction. In 1998 another proposal[50] was put forth which included lesbian and single women in the category of women allowed to receive treatments with the stipulation that treatments could be provided only if the sperm donor had provided consent.[51]

Tangential to this discussion is the argument that each child has the right to a father, a view voiced frequently in Finland during parliamentary discussion of the two most recent government bills on assisted reproduction, HE 76/2002 and HE 3/2006. Upon revision of the first bill in 2002, the standing committee on laws suggested that access to fertility treatments should only be provided to heterosexual couples[52]. The committee explained its standpoint by saying that a child must always have the right to two parents, a mother and a father. The committee further supported its argument by stating that the other Nordic countries had not yet provided lesbian couples and single women access to assisted reproduction. After the committee's revision of the law proposal, the government decided to withdraw the bill. In February 2006 the government again presented a bill on assisted reproduction (HE 3/2006) that included the right to assisted reproduction for lesbian couples and single women. The standing committee on laws once more reached the same conclusion as in 2002, but this time the government did not withdraw the bill and the discourse continued in parliament. In 2006, during plenary voting, the government bill on assisted reproduction was passed despite the reservations of the standing committee on laws.

These examples demonstrate how equality arguments challenged the legitimacy of the government. In Finland it is unusual for a government to withdraw a bill following initial debate and the committee stage. The government appears to have been apprehensive that it would face a legitimacy problem unless the law on assisted reproduction provided all women an equal right to assisted reproduction. Such an interpretation is consistent with the manner in which legislation pertaining to LGBT rights in Finland has gradually been altered once earlier laws are perceived by citizens and/or policy-makers as being discriminatory.

50 Oikeusministeriön työryhmä 1998.
51 Malin & Burrell 2004.
52 LaVM 29/2002.

Conservative criticism as legitimacy claims

For those issues in political discourse that are considered to be moral issues, the various Finnish political parties do not demand party discipline from MPs. This allows MPs to individually decide how they wish to respond to political issues. Such issues often possess a symbolic character or are easily relatable to on a personal level. LGTB rights, for example, represents such an issue as does assisted reproduction. Such political issues in Finnish political discourse appear to be susceptible to conservative criticism, criticism that often is religiously legitimated.

Individual citizens may view a particular law as being illegitimate based on religious, ideological or identity-based reasons and legislation on the issue of LGBT rights is a good example of this. During preparation of the law on registered partnership in Finland, many MPs and citizens were of the opinion that the existing law was discriminatory against homosexuals. However, other conservative MPs and citizens were of the opinion that both general societal changes concerning attitudes towards homosexuality and changes in the legal situation of homosexuals were problematic. In the Finnish parliamentary debate on registered partnership, several opponents of the bill expressed dissatisfaction with the Partnership act and maintained that the purpose of the act was ambiguous. Conservative MPs described the bill as a seemingly superficial effort to improve the legal status of homosexuals that in actuality concealed a different, latent symbolic significance.[53] The conservative MPs consequently interpreted the legislation as an attempt to 'normalise homosexuality'.

Conservative critics argued that the Partnership act sought to deem same-sex relationships normative. During parliamentary debate many Partnership act opponents stated that instead of supporting registered partnership they would like to provide homosexuals certain rights so that the inequities existing in same-sex relationships and other shared household models might be eliminated. The critics often referred to the Evangelical Lutheran Church Council's statement on 5 October 1999, which emphasised the importance of marriage as the basic relationship model while maintaining that same-sex relationships should be considered comparable to other shared household models. In this statement the Church Council furthermore suggested that, rather than creating a new social institution (registered partnership), the legal conditions for shared households should instead be improved: for example for siblings sharing a household. During parliamentary debate, critics of the act suggested a change in the existing inheritance laws as an alternative manner whereby to address inequalities in relation to same-sex relationships.[54] A particularly illustrating

53 Kanckos 2003.

54 PTK 101/2001: This was, for example, suggested by Kari Kärkkäinen (Christian Democrats).

metaphor used during this discussion was when an MP stated that the Partnership act was a Trojan horse: the implication was that the elimination of inequalities for homosexuals concealed the so-named 'normalisation' of homosexuality in society.

> The gay law is a Trojan horse, by which Finland's traditional family and community values are being attacked. This battering ram must now be destroyed. If through the gay law this Trojan horse is now let into camp, there will be a continuation of this procedure every year.[55]

The MP here believes that, if the Partnership act is passed, other laws will be enacted in the same spirit (with the aim of improving LGBT rights in Finnish society). The MP mentions later in this same discourse that he believes that the real aim of the Partnership act is to equate registered partnership with marriage, and that, subsequently, the following step will be the right for same-sex couples to adopt children. This MP perceives these changes as an attack on traditional Christian values. This quote thus exemplifies a legitimacy claim: a particular law is presented as a challenge to the legitimacy of political authorities. The conservative MPs not only expressed their dissatisfaction with the Partnership act through their criticism, they also expressed their dissatisfaction with the state or legal system as a whole; for them the state lost its legitimacy and their confidence in those individuals holding power diminished. For conservative MPs, the perceived 'normalisation' of homosexuality in society through changes in attitudes and laws threatened values that conservative MPs and their constituents consider sacred. The Trojan horse metaphor can also be described as an example of one of Habermas' four validity claims; a rightness claim, related to the moral rightness or justness of legal options. We remember that Habermas maintains that if an ideal speech situation is to be realised, all four validity claims (truth, rightness, truthfulness and comprehensibility) should be tested. Yet unlike Habermas we do not argue for the necessity of consensus through rational political discourse. We do, nevertheless, believe that an isolated validity claim about moral rightness is usually not sufficient to constitute a judgement on the illegitimacy of political authorities.[56] Another relevant aspect is *how* arguments are represented. Legitimacy judgements can only be taken seriously if opponents to a proposed law express their reasoning in a thoughtful, open and sincere way and manage to communicate the reasons why a proposed law should not be implemented.

55 PTK 96/2001: Vistbacka (True Finns). Translation authors' own.
56 Habermas 1979; Cukier et al. 2004, 239.

Concluding remarks

In regards to gender politics, the human rights and feminist perspectives have to a large extent influenced the process whereby laws are re-evaluated. This article has sought to discuss those laws that certain groups in society have considered indispensible: for these groups if these laws did not exist something crucial would be missing from society. The contesting of rights in gender politics has largely meant the contesting of universalism, or as Kate Nash expresses it, 'challenging the exclusion of social groups who would not conform to the norm of white, heterosexual, male head of household.'[57] Many social movements have sought to challenge universalism during the last few decades and the women's movement and the LGBT rights movement have been the most prominent of these groups.[58] The application of human rights have also in many cases resulted in the re-evaluation of laws in regards to gender politics and, as such, a challenge to the legitimacy of laws that have been considered discriminatory. While Finnish MPs have customarily expressed their own human rights arguments in Finnish parliamentary debates on LGBT rights, domestic violence and assisted reproduction, these legitimacy claims are also relevant in an international context. By referring to the international treaties that Finland has entered into, Finnish MPs have called attention to the seriousness of crimes such as rape and the discriminatory element of existing laws while emphasising the importance of living up to human rights agreements. Yet the question remains: are political authorities in reality challenged from internal sources (citizens for example) or are they in some sense challenged externally? As seen here, the difference between internal and external legitimacy claims is not that distinct. In this article we have demonstrated that human rights discourse contributes a further dimension to the concept of political legitimacy. At the same time, however, we must still question the meanings of and reasons for the use of human rights arguments. Are human rights arguments used instrumentally, rhetorically or do they instead express a moral stance whereby a specific issue can be highlighted?

Through our discussion of LGBT rights, domestic violence and assisted reproduction we have distinguished between different claims regarding the political legitimacy or illegitimacy of political authorities. The arguments presented here concerning discrimination, gender neutrality, equality and the distinction between private and public issues overlap extensively. Legitimacy claims related to discriminatory laws and the need to develop laws on LGBT rights, domestic violence and assisted reproduction may also be described as claims that indicate that these issues should be moved from the private to the public sphere. Claims pertaining to equality and gender neutrality are often connected to the issue of discrimination. Still, equality and gender neutrality dis-

57 Nash 2000, 157.
58 Nash 2000, 156–157, 165.

course embodies two contradictory views on how gender politics should be developed, the so-named 'sameness-difference' dilemma. Should men and women have identical rights or should rights be gender-specific?[59] Gender neutrality also reveals its shortcomings in relation to gendered violence, seen in this article in the example of gender neutral discourse as related to domestic violence. How this will affect the legitimacy of the laws on and actions taken against violence against women still remains unknown, yet it is worth remembering the low number of women in Finland seeking help for such problems from public authorities.

Throughout history the political issues discussed in this article have many times oscillated between the private and public spheres. This oscillation can have an unsettling effect when traditions and social norms no longer are self-legitimating.[60] In a plural society different opinions tend to exist on whether laws concerning gender, sexuality, domestic violence and reproduction should be as minimal as possible or whether such legislation should be developed further so that the rights of the individuals and groups affected by this legislation are protected. It is obvious that certain laws affect some individuals more than others and, for those individuals, whether a law exists or not makes an immense difference. Extended rights for homosexuals, for example, do not affect opponents in the same way as those being given the extended rights. The dominating view in Finnish politics would appear to be that legislation should not legitimate a specific moral value or a religious community's values, particularly if the implementation of religious values results in the discrimination of minority groups, such as same-sex couples.

Bibliography

Legislative documents[61]

HE 365/1992 Hallituksen esitys Eduskunnalle laiksi rikoslain väkisinmakaamista ja vapautta loukkaavaa haureutta koskevien säännösten muuttamisesta. Laki rikoslain 20 luvun muuttamisesta. [The government proposal to Parliament with bill on sex offences, chapter 20 of the Criminal Code of Finland].

59 Nash 2000, 165–167.
60 Habermas 1989, 72.
61 The legislative documents we reference here are only available in either the Finnish language (predominantly) or, to a certain extent, the Swedish language. As such the translations of the document titles are the authors' own. We have referenced FINLEX, the database of Finnish acts and decrees, to aid us in the translation process. (Lainsäädäntösanasto 2010).

HE 41/1998 Hallituksen esitys Eduskunnalle laiksi lähestymiskiellosta ja eräiksi siihen liittyviksi laeiksi. [The government proposal to Parliament with bill on restraining order and other laws connected to this].

HE 200/2000 Hallituksen esitys Eduskunnalle laiksi virallistetusta parisuhteesta. [The government proposal to Parliament with bill on registered partnership].

HE 76/2002 Hallituksen esitys Eduskunnalle laeiksi sukusolujen ja alkioiden käytöstä hedelmöityshoidossa ja isyyslain muuttamisesta [The government proposal to Parliament with bill on the use of sex-cells and embryos in assisted reproductive treatments and the Act amending the Act on Paternity].

HE 144/2003 Hallituksen esitys Eduskunnalle laiksi lähestymiskiellosta annetun lain muuttamisesta ja laiksi rikoslain 21 luvun 17 §:n kumoamisesta. [The government proposal to Parliament with bill on amending the Act on the Restraining Order and repealing 17 § in chapter 21 of the Criminal Code of Finland].

HE 3/2006 Hallituksen esitys Eduskunnalle laeiksi hedelmöityshoidoista ja isyyslain muuttamisesta [The government proposal to Parliament with bill on assisted reproduction and the Act amending the Act on Paternity].

HE 198/2008 Hallituksen esitys Eduskunnalle laiksi rekisteröidystä parisuhteesta annetun lain 9 §:n muuttamisesta. [The government proposal to Parliament with bill amending the Act on Registered Partnership 9 §]

HE 78/2010 Hallituksen esitys Eduskunnalle laiksi rikoslain 21 luvun 16 §:n muuttamisesta. [The government proposal to Parliament with bill amending 16 § in chapter 21 of the Criminal Code of Finland].

LA 25/1991 Lakialoite O. Ojala ym.: Ehdotukset laeiksi rikoslain 20 ja 21 luvun sekä maksuttomasta oikeudenkäynnistä annetun lain 1 §:n muuttamisesta. [Members' initiative: Proposals with bill on chapter 20 and 21 of the Criminal Code of Finland and amending 1 § in the Act of cost-free legal proceedings].

LA 28/1991 Lakialoite Pykäläinen ym.: Ehdotus laiksi rikoslain 20 luvun muuttamisesta. [Members' initiative: Proposal with bill amending chapter 20 of the Criminal Code of Finland].

LaVM 3/1998 Lakivaliokunnan mietintö [The report of the standing committee on laws].

LaVM 29/2002 Lakivaliokunnan mietintö [The report of the standing committee on laws].

Oikeusministeriön työryhmä (1988) Ehdotus Hallituksen esitykseksi Eduskunnalle laeiksi ihmisen keinotekoisista lisääntymismenetelmistä sekä isyyslain muuttamisesta, Oikeusministeriön työryhmän mietintö, Lainvalmisteluosaston julkaisu 12/1988 [Ministry of Justice Working Group

(1988) Proposal for government proposal to Parliament with bill on human artificial reproductive methods, and amending the Act on Paternity, the Ministry of Justice Working Group Report, publication of the Law Drafting Division 12/1988].

Oikeusministeriön työryhmä (1990) Ehdotus Hallituksen esitykseksi Eduskunnalle laeiksi ihmisen keinoalkuisesta lisääntymisestä sekä isyyslain muuttamisesta, Oikeusministeriön työryhmän mietintö 18.12.1990 [Ministry of Justice Working Group (1990) Proposal for government proposal to Parliament with bill on human artificial reproduction, and amending the Act on Paternity, the Ministry of Justice Working Group Report 1990-12-18].

Oikeusministeriön työryhmä (1997) Sukusolujen ja alkioiden käyttö lääketieteellisessä hedelmöityshoidossa, Oikeusministeriön työryhmän mietintö 14.10.1997 [Ministry of Justice Working Group (1997) The use of sex-cells and embryos in medical fertility treatments, the Ministry of Justice Working Group Report 1997-10-14].

Oikeusministeriön työryhmä (1998) Ehdotus Hallituksen esitykseksi Eduskunnalle laeiksi sukusolujen ja alkioiden käytöstä hedelmöityshoidoissa ja isyyslain muuttamisesta [Ministry of Justice Working Group (1998) Proposal for government proposal to Parliament with bill on the use of sex-cells and embryos in fertility treatments, and amending the Act on Paternity].

PTK 4/1993 Report of the proceedings 1993-02-16.

PTK 16/1994 Report of the proceedings 1994-03-15.

PTK 61/1998 Report of the proceedings 1998-05-12.

PTK 143/1998 Report of the proceedings 1998-11-13.

PTK 96/2001 Report of the proceedings 2001-09-19.

PTK 101/2001 Report of the proceedings 2001-09-25.

Literature

Barker, R
1990 *Political Legitimacy and the State*. Oxford: Clarendon Press.

Bohman, J & Rehg, W
2009 "Jürgen Habermas". In Zalta, EN (ed.) *The Stanford Encyclopedia of Philosophy* (Fall Edition 2009). Available at: http://plato.stanford.edu/archives/fall2009/entries/habermas/ [Accessed 19 January 2011].

Cukier, W & Bauer, R & Middleton, C

2004 Applying Habermas' Validity Claims as a Standard for Critical Discourse Analysis. In Kaplan, B & Truex, DP & Wastell, D & Wood-Harper, AT & DeGross, JI (eds) *Information Systems Research. Relevant Theory and Informed Practice*. Boston: Kluwer Academic Publishers, 233–258.

Davies, M
1997 Taking the Inside Out: Sex and Gender in the Legal Subject. In Naffine, N & Owens, RJ (eds) *Sexing the Subject of Law*. Sydney: LBC Information Services.

Durkheim, É
1951 [1897] *Suicide: A Study in Sociology*. Glencoe: Free Press.

Guibentif, P
1996 Approaching the production of law through Habermas's concept of communicative action. In Deflem, M (ed.) *Habermas, Modernity, and Law*. London: Sage, 45–70.

Habermas, J
1996 *Between Facts and Norms. Contributions to a Discourse Theory of Law and Democracy*. Cambridge: Polity Press.
1979 *Communication and the Evolution of Society*. Boston: Beacon Press.
1989 [1973] *Legitimation Crisis*. Cambridge: Polity Press.

Hiltunen, R
1996 *Virallisesti ventovieraat. Samaa sukupuolta olevien parisuhteet lainsäädännössä*. Helsingfors: SETA-julkaisut.
1999 Rikoksesta kohti tasa-arvoa – homoseksuaalien oikeudellisen aseman kehitys. In Lehtonen, J (ed.) *Homo fennicus. Miesten homo- ja biseksuaalisuus muutoksessa*. Helsinki: Sosiaali- ja terveysministeriö, 41–53.

Holden, J
2006 *Cultural Value and the Crisis of Legitimacy. Why culture needs a democratic mandate*. Available at: http://www.demos.co.uk/files/Culturalvalueweb.pdf?1240939425 [Accessed 19 January 2011].

Kanckos, L
2003 *Normer och normalitet. Homosexualitet inom en politisk diskursordning*. Master's thesis. Åbo: Åbo Akademi University [unpublished].

Kääriäinen, J
2006 Väkivalta ja apuun turvautuminen. In Piispa, M et al. (eds) *Naisiin kohdistuva väkivalta 2005*. Oikeuspoliittisen tutkimuslaitoksen

julkaisuja 225. Yhdistyneiden Kansakuntien yhteydessä toimiva Euroopan Kriminaalipolitiikan Instituutti (HEUNI) Publication Series No. 51. Helsinki.

Lagerspetz, O
1998 *Trust. The tacit demand.* Library of ethics and applied philosophy; vol. 1. Dordrecht: Kluwer.

Lainsäädäntösanasto
2010 FINLEX. Available at: http://www.finlex.fi/data/muut/saadkaan/laki.pdf [Accessed 11 April 2011].

Malin, M & Burrell, R
2004 Unregulated Practices, Familiarity and Legality. In Blyth, E & Landau, R (eds) *Third Party Assisted Conception Across Cultures. Social, Legal and Ethical Perspectives*. London and New York: Jessica Kingsley Publishers, 73–93.

Nash, K
2000 *Contemporary Political Sociology. Globalization, Politics, and Power*. Oxford: Blackwell Publishers.

Niemi-Kiesiläinen, J
2001 Criminal Law or Social Policy as Protection Against Violence. In Nousiainen, K et al. (eds) *Responsible Selves. Women in the Nordic legal culture*. Aldershot: Ashgate.

Notko, M
2000 *Väkivalta parisuhteessa ja perheessä*. Jyväskylän yliopiston perhetutkimusyksikön julkaisuja 11. (Reports from the Family Research Centre, University of Jyväskylä.) Jyväskylä: Jyväskylän yliopiston perhetutkimusyksikkö.

Pehkonen, P
2003 *Naisen puolesta, ei miestä vastaan. Suomalainen naisliike väkivaltaa vastustamassa*. Sosiologian raportteja n:o 2. Joensuu: University of Joensuu, Department of Sociology.

Ronkainen, S
2008 Kenen ongelma väkivalta on? Suomalainen hyvinvointivaltio ja väkivallan toimijuus. *Yhteiskuntapolitiikka* 73 (4), 388–401.

Slotte, P
2005 *Mänskliga rättigheter, moral och religion. Om de mänskliga rättigheterna som moraliskt och juridiskt begrepp i en pluralistisk värld.* (Diss.) Åbo: Åbo Akademis förlag.

Statistikcentralen
2005 Familjevåld 1997–2005. Available at: http://www.tilastokeskus.fi.

Valtakunnansyyttäjänvirasto
2000 VKS:2000:4. Seuraamusluonteinen syyttämättä jättäminen pahoinpitelyrikoksissa.

Waaldijk, K
2001 Small Change. How the Road to Same-Sex Marriage Got Paved in the Netherlands. In Wintemute, R & Andenæs, M (eds) *Legal Recognition of Same-Sex Partnerships. A Study of National, European and International Law*. Oxford: Hart Publishing, 437–464.

Wendt Höjer, M
2002 *Rädslans politik. Våld och sexualitet i den svenska demokratin*. (Diss.) Malmö: Liber.

Šárka Waisová / Ladislav Cabada

Ethics in Foreign Policy

Postmodern States as the Entrepreneurs of Kantian Ethics

Frankfurt am Main, Berlin, Bern, Bruxelles, New York, Oxford, Wien, 2011.
195 pp.
ISBN 978-3-631-61255-2 · hardback € 39,– *

Two important positions might be observed in the discussion about the importance of ethics for international politics and the relevance of ethics for the theoretical analysis of international relations. Some deny any connection between ethics and international politics; others believe that moral values are an essential component of international relations. The contributors assume that in an epoch of military interventions waged in the name of humanity and just war it is impossible to deny moral and ethical demands in international politics. The main hypothesis of this book is that the post-modern states are playing the role of norm entrepreneurs and promote Kantian ethics in international relations. The articles analyse in five case studies the development in post-modern states towards a moral foreign policy. Canada, Germany, Norway, the Netherlands, and Slovenia are included in this analysis showing that Kantian ethics in international affairs is the ideal-typical position, and that some states have developed a foreign policy tending to this position.

Content: Postmodern States as the Entrepreneurs of Kantian Ethics in International Relations · Canada: A Humane Internationalist in the Shadow of a Large Neighbour · The Federal Republic of Germany: The Gentle Giant · Norway: A Humanitarian Superpower? · The Netherlands: Human Rights Above Own Interest? · Slovenia: Pioneer and Mentor of the Western Balkans?